Oral Medicine: A Handbook for Physicians

Editors

ERIC T. STOOPLER
THOMAS P. SOLLECITO

MEDICAL CLINICS OF NORTH AMERICA

www.medical.theclinics.com

Consulting Editors
DOUGLAS S. PAAUW
EDWARD R. BOLLARD

November 2014 • Volume 98 • Number 6

ELSEVIER

1600 John F. Kennedy Boulevard • Suite 1800 • Philadelphia, Pennsylvania, 19103-2899

http://www.theclinics.com

MEDICAL CLINICS OF NORTH AMERICA Volume 98, Number 6
November 2014 ISSN 0025-7125, ISBN-13: 978-0-323-32381-9

Editor: Jessica McCool
Developmental Editor: Yonah Korngold

Medical Clinics of North America (ISSN 0025-7125) is published bimonthly by Elsevier Inc., 360 Park Avenue South, New York, NY 10010-1710. Months of publication are January, March, May, July, September, and November. Business and editorial offices: 1600 John F. Kennedy Boulevard, Suite 1800, Philadelphia, PA 19103-2899. Periodicals postage paid at New York, NY, and additional mailing offices. Subscription prices are USD $255.00 per year (US individuals), $471.00 per year (US institutions), $125.00 per year (US Students), $320.00 per year (Canadian individuals), $612.00 per year (Canadian institutions), $200.00 per year (Canadian and foreign students), $390.00 per year (foreign individuals), and $612.00 per year (foreign institutions). To receive student/resident rate, orders must be accompanied by name of affiliated institution, date of term, and the signature of program/residency coordinator on institution letterhead. Orders will be billed at individual rate until proof of status is received. Foreign air speed delivery is included in all Clinics' subscription prices. All prices are subject to change without notice. **POSTMASTER:** Send address changes to *Medical Clinics of North America*, Elsevier Health Sciences Division, Subscription Customer Service, 3251 Riverport Lane, Maryland Heights, MO 63043. **Customer Service: Telephone: 1-800-654-2452** (U.S. and Canada); **1-314-447-8871** (outside U.S. and Canada). **Fax: 314-447-8029. E-mail: journalscustomerserviceusa@elsevier.com** (for print support); **journalsonlinesupport-usa@elsevier.com** (for online support).

Reprints. For copies of 100 or more of articles in this publication, please contact the Commercial Reprints Department, Elsevier Inc., 360 Park Avenue South, New York, NY 10010-1710. Tel.: 212-633-3874; Fax: 212-633-3820; E-mail: reprints@elsevier.com.

Medical Clinics of North America is also published in Spanish by McGraw-Hill Interamericana Editores S. A., P.O. Box 5-237, 06500 Mexico, D.F., Mexico.

Medical Clinics of North America is covered in *MEDLINE/PubMed (Index Medicus), Current Contents, ASCA, Excerpta Medica, Science Citation Index, and ISI/BIOMED.*

Printed in the United States of America.

MEDICAL CLINICS OF NORTH AMERICA

RELATED INTEREST

Otolaryngologic Clinics of North America, August 2013, (Vol. 46, No. 4)
Oral Cavity and Oropharyngeal Cancer
Jeffrey N. Myers and Erich M. Sturgis, *Editors*
http://www.oto.theclinics.com/

PROGRAM OBJECTIVE

The goal of the *Medical Clinics of North America* is to keep practicing physicians up to date with current clinical practice by providing timely articles reviewing the state of the art in patient care.

LEARNING OBJECTIVES

Upon completion of this activity, participants will be able to:

1. Discuss the evaluation and management of oral mucosal disorders, salivary gland disorders, and temporomandibular disorders.
2. Review the anatomical and examinations of the oral cavity.
3. Recognize common dental and orofacial trauma and periodontal disease.

ACCREDITATION

The Elsevier Office of Continuing Medical Education (EOCME) is accredited by the Accreditation Council for Continuing Medical Education (ACCME) to provide continuing medical education for physicians.

The EOCME designates this enduring material for a maximum of 15 *AMA PRA Category 1 Credit*(s)™. Physicians should claim only the credit commensurate with the extent of their participation in the activity.

All other health care professionals requesting continuing education credit for this enduring material will be issued a certificate of participation.

DISCLOSURE OF CONFLICTS OF INTEREST

The EOCME assesses conflict of interest with its instructors, faculty, planners, and other individuals who are in a position to control the content of CME activities. All relevant conflicts of interest that are identified are thoroughly vetted by EOCME for fair balance, scientific objectivity, and patient care recommendations. EOCME is committed to providing its learners with CME activities that promote improvements or quality in healthcare and not a specific proprietary business or a commercial interest.

The planning committee, staff, authors and editors listed below have identified no financial relationships or relationships to products or devices they or their spouse/life partner have with commercial interest related to the content of this CME activity:

Ramesh Balasubramaniam, BDSc, MS; Thomas Berardi, DMD; Edward R. Bollard, MD, DDS, FACP; Scott S. De Rossi, DMD; Martin S. Greenberg, DDS; Kristen Helm; Michaell A. Huber, DDS; Brynne Hunter; Gary D. Klasser, DMD; Arthur S. Kuperstein, DDS; Sandy Lavery; Frederick Liu, DDS, MD; Mansoor Madani, DMD, MD; Farideh M. Madani, DMD; Louis Mandel, DDS; Jessica McCool; Jill McNair; Lindsay Parnell; Prem B. Patel, DMD, MD; Santha Priya; Ziv Simon, DMD, MSc; David C. Stanton, DMD, MD; Andrew Steinkeler, DMD, MD; Megan Suermann; Bundhit Tantiwongkosi, MD.

The planning committee, staff, authors and editors listed below have identified financial relationships or relationships to products or devices they or their spouse/life partner have with commercial interest related to the content of this CME activity:

Eric J. Granquist, DMD, MD is on speakers bureau and has a research grant from Biomet, Inc.

Joel M. Laudenbach, DMD is on speakers bureau for Center for Oral Health & Kaiser Permanente and for InterDent, Inc.; is a consultant/advisor for Center for Oral Health & Colgate Oral Pharmaceuticals, Inc. and for DentalEZ, Inc.

Thomas P. Sollecito, DMD, FDS RCSEd has an employment affiliation with The University of Pennsylvania and is a consultant/advisor for Compendium of Continuing Education in Dentistry.

Eric T. Stoopler, DMD, FDS RCSEd, FDS RCSEng has an employment affiliation with The University of Pennsylvania; and is a consultant/advisor for WebMD, LLC

UNAPPROVED/OFF-LABEL USE DISCLOSURE

The EOCME requires CME faculty to disclose to the participants:

1. When products or procedures being discussed are off-label, unlabelled, experimental, and/or investigational (not US Food and Drug Administration [FDA] approved); and
2. Any limitations on the information presented, such as data that are preliminary or that represent ongoing research, interim analyses, and/or unsupported opinions. Faculty may discuss information about pharmaceutical agents that is outside of FDA-approved labelling. This information is intended solely for CME and is not intended to promote off-label use of these medications. If you have any questions, contact the medical affairs department of the manufacturer for the most recent prescribing information.

TO ENROLL

To enroll in the *Medical Clinics of North America* Continuing Medical Education program, call customer service at 1-800-654-2452 or sign up online at http://www.theclinics.com/home/cme. The CME program is available to subscribers for an additional annual fee of USD $295.

METHOD OF PARTICIPATION

In order to claim credit, participants must complete the following:
1. Complete enrolment as indicated above.
2. Read the activity.
3. Complete the CME Test and Evaluation. Participants must achieve a score of 70% on the test. All CME Tests and Evaluations must be completed online.

CME INQUIRIES/SPECIAL NEEDS

For all CME inquiries or special needs, please contact elsevierCME@elsevier.com.

Contributors

CONSULTING EDITORS

DOUGLAS S. PAAUW, MD, MACP
Professor of Medicine, Division of General Internal Medicine, Rathmann Family
Foundation Endowed Chair for Patient-Centered Clinical Education; Medicine Student
Programs, Professor of Medicine, University of Washington School of Medicine, Seattle,
Washington

EDWARD R. BOLLARD, MD, DDS, FACP
Professor of Medicine; Associate Dean of Graduate Medical Education, Designated
Institutional Official, Department of Medicine, Penn State–Hershey Medical Center,
Penn State University College of Medicine, Hershey, Pennsylvania

EDITORS

ERIC T. STOOPLER, DMD, FDS RCSEd, FDS RCSEng
Associate Professor, Department of Oral Medicine, University of Pennsylvania School of
Dental Medicine, Philadelphia, Pennsylvania

THOMAS P. SOLLECITO, DMD, FDS RCSEd
Professor; Chairman, Department of Oral Medicine, University of Pennsylvania School of
Dental Medicine, Philadelphia, Pennsylvania

AUTHORS

RAMESH BALASUBRAMANIAM, BDSc, MS
Clinical Associate Professor, School of Dentistry, University of Western Australia, Perth,
Australia

THOMAS BERARDI, DMD
Clinical Associate Professor, Department of Oral Medicine, University of Pennsylvania
School of Dental Medicine, Philadelphia, Pennsylvania

SCOTT S. DE ROSSI, DMD
Professor, Oral Medicine; Chairman, Oral Health and Diagnostic Sciences; Professor,
Dermatology; Professor, Otolaryngology/Head and Neck Surgery, Georgia Regents
University, Augusta, Georgia

ERIC J. GRANQUIST, DMD, MD
Assistant Professor, Department of Oral and Maxillofacial Surgery, Hospital of the
University of Pennsylvania, University of Pennsylvania, Philadelphia, Pennsylvania

MARTIN S. GREENBERG, DDS, FDS RCS
Professor, Department of Oral Medicine; Associate Dean, Hospital Affairs, School of
Dental Medicine, University of Pennsylvania, Philadelphia, Pennsylvania

MICHAELL A. HUBER, DDS
Professor, Department of Comprehensive Dentistry, University of Texas Health Science Center, School of Dentistry, San Antonio, Texas

GARY D. KLASSER, DMD
Associate Professor, School of Dentistry, Louisiana State University, New Orleans, Louisiana

ARTHUR S. KUPERSTEIN, DDS
Director, Oral Medicine Clinical Services; Assistant Professor, Department of Oral Medicine, University of Pennsylvania School of Dental Medicine, Philadelphia, Pennsylvania

JOEL M. LAUDENBACH, DMD
Assistant Professor, Oral Medicine and Geriatric Dentistry, College of Dental Medicine, Western University of Health Sciences, Pomona, California; Private Oral Medicine Practice, Beverly Hills, California; Medical Staff, Department of Surgery - Dentistry, Cedars-Sinai Medical Center, Los Angeles, California

FREDERICK LIU, DDS, MD
Department of Oral and Maxillofacial Surgery, School of Dental Medicine, University of Pennsylvania, Philadelphia, Pennsylvania

FARIDEH M. MADANI, DMD
Clinical Professor, Department of Oral Medicine, University of Pennsylvania School of Dental Medicine, Philadelphia, Pennsylvania

MANSOOR MADANI, DMD, MD
Chairman, Department of Oral and Maxillofacial Surgery, Capital Health System, Trenton, New Jersey; Associate Professor, Oral and Maxillofacial Surgery, Temple University, Philadelphia, Pennsylvania; Director, Center for Corrective Jaw Surgery, Bala Cynwyd, Pennsylvania

LOUIS MANDEL, DDS
Associate Dean, Clinical Professor, Department of Oral and Maxillofacial Surgery; Director, Salivary Gland Center, Columbia University College of Dental Medicine, New York, New York

PREM B. PATEL, DMD, MD
Resident, Department of Oral and Maxillofacial Surgery, Hospital of the University of Pennsylvania, University of Pennsylvania, Philadelphia, Pennsylvania

ZIV SIMON, DMD, MSc
Lecturer, Department of Continuing Education, Ostrow School of Dentistry, University of Southern California, Los Angeles, California; Private Practice Limited to Periodontics and Dental Implants, Beverly Hills, California

THOMAS P. SOLLECITO, DMD, FDS RCSEd
Professor; Chairman, Department of Oral Medicine, University of Pennsylvania School of Dental Medicine, Philadelphia, Pennsylvania

DAVID C. STANTON, DMD, MD, FACS
Associate Professor, Department of Oral and Maxillofacial Surgery, Hospital of the University of Pennsylvania, University of Pennsylvania, Philadelphia, Pennsylvania

ANDREW STEINKELER, DMD, MD
Department of Oral and Maxillofacial Surgery, School of Dental Medicine, University of Pennsylvania, Philadelphia, Pennsylvania

ERIC T. STOOPLER, DMD, FDS RCSEd, FDS RCSEng
Associate Professor, Department of Oral Medicine, University of Pennsylvania School of Dental Medicine, Philadelphia, Pennsylvania

BUNDHIT TANTIWONGKOSI, MD
Assistant Professor, Departments of Radiology and Otolaryngology, University of Texas Health Science Center San Antonio, San Antonio, Texas

Contents

> Patients will often visit their primary medical practitioner with orofacial pain complaints. Hence, it is important to recognize and have an understanding of these conditions to properly evaluate and potentially manage these disorders. If the practitioner is uncertain or uncomfortable with these conditions, then patient referral to a knowledgeable health care practitioner should be considered for further evaluation and management. In this article, the evaluation and management of various neuropathic, neurovascular, and vascular pains are discussed.

> Patients with salivary gland disease present with certain objective and/or subjective signs. An accurate diagnosis for these patients requires a range of techniques that includes the organized integration of information derived from their history, clinical examination, imaging, serology, and histopathology. This article highlights the signs and symptoms of the salivary gland disorders seen in the Salivary Gland Center, and emphasizes the methodology used to achieve a definitive diagnosis and therapy.

Foreword

Oral Medicine: A Handbook for Physicians

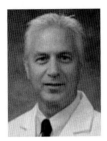

Edward R. Bollard, MD, DDS, FACP
Consulting Editor

An area of medicine that is frequently overlooked, often misunderstood, and potentially goes undertreated or untreated when signs and symptoms arise is pathology of the oral cavity and associated structures. In both ambulatory and hospital settings, diseases, dysfunction, and trauma of the teeth; periodontal tissues; bony elements; soft tissue structures; and salivary glands provide diagnostic challenges to the treating physician when she or he does not possess a thorough understanding of oral anatomy as well as oral medicine.

In June 2008, the Association of American Medical Colleges (AAMC) in collaboration with the American Dental Education Association, understanding the deficiencies in oral medicine that traditional medical school curricula contain, published a report of an expert panel as part of the *Medical School Objectives Project* entitled, "Contemporary Issues in Medicine: Oral Health Education for Medical and Dental Students."[1] This was an attempt to highlight and close the gaps in knowledge that exist in those who will be called on to evaluate the diseases of and related to the oral cavity in the practice of medicine.

In this issue of the *Medical Clinics of North America*, Dr Stoopler, Dr Sollecito, and colleagues present nine articles that also attempt to reduce this knowledge gap by emphasizing the normal anatomy, common anatomic variations, as well as relevant orofacial pathology that can be applied to our comprehensive care of the medical patient.

Edward R. Bollard, MD, DDS, FACP
Department of Medicine
Penn State–Hershey Medical Center/
Penn State University College of Medicine
Hershey, PA 17033, USA

E-mail address:
ebollard@hmc.psu.edu

Med Clin N Am 98 (2014) xv–xvi
http://dx.doi.org/10.1016/j.mcna.2014.08.022
0025-7125/14/$ – see front matter © 2014 Elsevier Inc. All rights reserved.

medical.theclinics.com

REFERENCE

1. Oral Health Educational Expert Panel. Report IX: Contemporary Issues in Medicine: Oral Health Education for Medical and Dental Students. Medical School Objectives Project, AAMC. June 2008. p. 1–24.

Preface

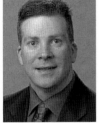

Eric T. Stoopler, DMD, FDS RCSEd, FDS RCSEng   Thomas P. Sollecito, DMD, FDS RCSEd

Editors

"Oral Medicine: A Handbook for Physicians" is designed to provide medical practitioners with clinically relevant information regarding health and disease of the oral cavity and perioral structures. While completing routine medical visits or undergoing evaluation for acute medical problems, patients often describe pain and dysfunction of the oral cavity and/or perioral structures to their physician. In fact, patients with common complaints, such as a dental abscess, ulceration of the oral mucosa, temporomandibular joint pain, and or salivary gland infections, may present to a physician rather than an oral health care provider for initial evaluation.

Physicians require in-depth knowledge of the anatomical structures of the oral cavity and perioral structures so they are equipped to distinguish normal versus pathologic findings. Many benign conditions affecting these structures may look pathologic to the untrained eye, and the physician must be able to render an accurate diagnosis. Oral cancer, a leading cause of morbidity and mortality, may present as an innocuous finding or in impressive fashion, and medical professionals need to recognize the earliest clinical signs of this frequently devastating disease.

It is incumbent upon medical practitioners to have a thorough understanding of dental and oral medicine conditions as they may have a profound effect on the patient's well-being and overall health. A wide array of systemic diseases is now well-understood to potentially affect or manifest in the oral and perioral areas. For example, the oral cavity may be a potential source of inflammation or infection, which could have a significant impact on systemic health conditions, such as diabetes. In addition, the oral cavity often provides a window to systemic health and may be the initial site of presentation of an underlying disease process. The oral cavity may even provide a more accessible location for diagnosis of certain conditions, such as hematologic, endocrine, or connective tissue diseases. When a medical practitioner evaluates the oral cavity and perioral structures, he or she must understand that local oral disease may be present or the oral condition may be a result of an underlying disorder that often requires further investigation.

In addition to considering all of these parameters, it is critical for physicians to have a basic understanding of the treatment of oral and perioral conditions. Structural problems of the dentition and facial bones are often definitively managed by the appropriate

Med Clin N Am 98 (2014) xvii–xviii

http://dx.doi.org/10.1016/j.mcna.2014.08.010

0025-7125/14/$ – see front matter © 2014 Elsevier Inc. All rights reserved.

medical.theclinics.com

oral health care provider, but it may be necessary for physicians to provide palliative care for these patients until such time occurs. Pharmacologic treatment for oral and perioral diseases often includes use of several agents in both topical and systemic formulations, such as antibiotics, antivirals, antifungals, anti-inflammatories, and corticosteroids. Medical practitioners must be able to recommend the appropriate course of therapy for oral and/or perioral diseases. In addition, physicians must be able to recognize potentially life-threatening conditions affecting these areas so they can appropriately refer the patient for urgent care.

We anticipate the information provided in this issue of *Medical Clinics of North America* will be helpful to medical practitioners to (1) enhance fundamental knowledge of the oral cavity and perioral structures, (2) recognize various common disorders affecting these structures and provisionally diagnose these conditions, (3) recognize signs and symptoms affecting these areas that may impact a known systemic disease or represent manifestation of a known or unknown systemic disease, and (4) manage these conditions until definitive care can be provided by the appropriate oral health care provider. All of the contributing authors have been carefully selected and are renowned clinicians, educators, and researchers in their respective fields. It is our hope that this issue provides valuable information to medical practitioners to improve the quality of patient care and to further substantiate the important relationship between medical and oral health care providers.

Eric T. Stoopler, DMD, FDS RCSEd, FDS RCSEng
Department of Oral Medicine
University of Pennsylvania School of Dental Medicine
240 South 40th Street
Philadelphia, PA 19104, USA

Thomas P. Sollecito, DMD, FDS RCSEd
Department of Oral Medicine
University of Pennsylvania School of Dental Medicine
240 South 40th Street
Philadelphia, PA 19104, USA

E-mail addresses:
ets@dental.upenn.edu (E.T. Stoopler)
tps@dental.upenn.edu (T.P. Sollecito)

Dedication

I dedicate this issue to my wife, Melanie, and my children, Ryan and Ethan, for their unconditional love, encouragement, and support of my academic endeavors. I also acknowledge and thank all of my mentors, colleagues, residents, students, and patients, who have contributed to my professional development.

Eric T. Stoopler, DMD, FDS RCSEd, FDS RCSEng
Department of Oral Medicine
University of Pennsylvania School of Dental Medicine
240 South 40th Street
Philadelphia, PA 19104, USA

E-mail address:
ets@dental.upenn.edu (E.T. Stoopler)

I dedicate this issue to my wife, Carolyn, and my children, Elizabeth, Peter, and Katharine, for their unconditional love and for their support of my academic pursuits. I also wish to acknowledge my mentors, colleagues, residents, students, and patients, who continually contribute to my professional development.

Thomas P. Sollecito, DMD, FDS RCSEd
Department of Oral Medicine
University of Pennsylvania School of Dental Medicine
240 South 40th Street
Philadelphia, PA 19104, USA

E-mail address:
tps@dental.upenn.edu (T.P. Sollecito)

Med Clin N Am 98 (2014) xix
http://dx.doi.org/10.1016/j.mcna.2014.08.011
0025-7125/14/$ – see front matter © 2014 Elsevier Inc. All rights reserved.

Anatomic and Examination Considerations of the Oral Cavity

Mansoor Madani, DMD, MD[a,b,c], Thomas Berardi, DMD[d],
Eric T. Stoopler, DMD, FDS RCSEd, FDS RCSEng[d,*]

KEYWORDS

- Oral anatomy • Oral examination • Oral mucosa • Dentition

KEY POINTS

- Patients often present to their physician for evaluation of dental and/or oral complaints.
- Physicians must have an understanding of basic oral anatomy and how to perform a clinical examination of the oral cavity.
- From the physical examination findings, physicians should be able to determine whether the oral cavity is in a state of health or disease.

INTRODUCTION

Comprehensive examination of the oral cavity is an area of physical diagnosis that traditionally receives decreased emphasis in the predoctoral medical curriculum and in clinical medical practice. Important information can be gained through a systematic evaluation of the oral hard and soft tissues. Although the primary objective is to distinguish between health and disease, a comprehensive oral examination, in conjunction with a thorough medical and dental history, can also provide valuable insight into the overall health and well-being of the patient. Minor changes in oral structure and function may adversely affect an individual's quality of life. In this article, anatomic considerations and clinical examination techniques of the oral cavity are discussed.

Disclosures: Dr. Stoopler receives an honorarium from WebMD for providing expert viewpoints and royalties from the American Dental Association.
[a] Department of Oral and Maxillofacial Surgery, Capital Health System, 750 Brunswick Avenue, Trenton, NJ 08638, USA; [b] Oral & Maxillofacial Surgery, Temple University, 3401 North Broad Street, Philadelphia, PA 19140, USA; [c] Center for Corrective Jaw Surgery, 15 North Presidential Boulevard, Bala Cynwyd, PA 19004, USA; [d] Department of Oral Medicine, University of Pennsylvania School of Dental Medicine, 240 South 40th Street, Philadelphia, PA 19104, USA
* Corresponding author.
E-mail address: ets@dental.upenn.edu

ANATOMIC CONSIDERATIONS

Examination of the oral cavity, in addition to the head and neck, are essential components of a patient's comprehensive physical examination. The boundary of the oral cavity is made of the lips anteriorly, the cheeks laterally, the floor of the mouth inferiorly, the oropharynx posteriorly, and the palate superiorly. The oropharynx is the area starting superiorly between the hard and the soft palate, and ends inferiorly behind the circumvallate papillae of the tongue. The hard tissue bases that these structures are attached to are the mandible and maxillae.[1,2]

Dentition and Supporting Structures

Typically, there are 32 teeth present in the oral cavity of an adult, with the first permanent tooth generally appearing by age 6 years. There are 20 primary teeth in childhood. Teeth are classified as central and lateral incisors, canines, premolars, and molars. There are no premolars or third molars in the primary dentition. Third molars appear in the mid to late teenage years, but many times do not have adequate space to erupt, often resulting in impaction, and may cause pain and/or infection. Permanent teeth may be classified according to different systems, but the most common method used in the United States is the Universal numbering system.[3,4] In this system, teeth are counted starting from the right maxilla (#1 for the right maxillary third molar) to the left maxilla (#16 for the left maxillary third molar), continuing to the left mandible (#17 for the left mandibular third molar) and ending in the right mandible (#32 for the right mandibular third molar) (**Fig. 1**). The primary teeth are labeled using the alphabet,

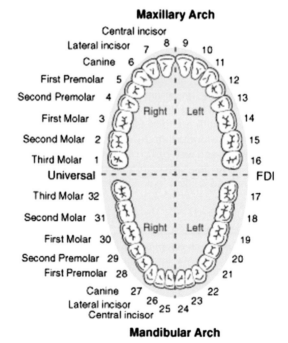

Fig. 1. Universal numbering system for permanent teeth as recommended by the Federation Dentaire Internationale (FDI). (*From* Yasny JS, Herlich A. Perioperative dental evaluation. Mt Sinai J Med 2012;79:34–45; with permission. http://dx.doi.org/10.1002/msj.21292. Available at: http://onlinelibrary.wiley.com/doi/10.1002/msj.21292/full#fig1.)

starting with the letter A for the second primary molar in the right maxilla and ending with the letter T for the second primary molar in the right mandible.[4]

Each tooth is divided into 2 parts, the crown and the root(s). The outer portion of the crown is covered by enamel, the hardest substance in the body. Dentin, which is immediately below the enamel layer, forms the bulk of the tooth and can be sensitive if the protective enamel is lost. The soft tissue containing the blood and nerve supply to the tooth (pulp) is housed within the dentin, extending from the tip of the root to the crown. A layer of cementum covers the root, which aids in attaching the tooth to the bony socket (**Fig. 2**).

Supporting structures of the teeth (periodontium) include the periodontal ligament, gingival tissue, bone, blood, and nerves. The periodontal ligament is made up of thousands of fibers, which fasten the cementum to the bony socket and alveolar bone, and act as shock absorbers for the teeth, which are subjected to heavy forces during function. These ligaments also function as sensory, nutritive, and remodeling structures surrounding the roots. Gingival tissue covers teeth and bone to protect them and provides an easily lubricated surface. The alveolar portions of the maxillary and mandibular bones contain sockets to support the roots of the teeth. Each tooth and periodontal ligament has a nerve supply, and the teeth are sensitive to a wide variety of stimuli. The blood supply is necessary to maintain the vitality of the tooth. The maxillary and mandibular divisions of the trigeminal nerve innervate the teeth and the periodontium.

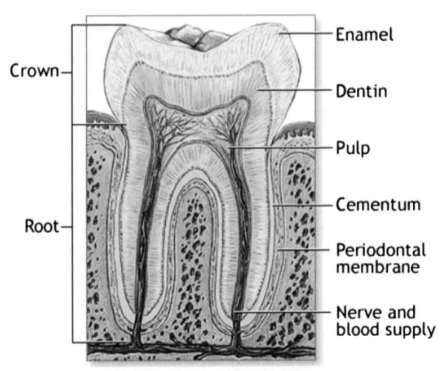

Fig. 2. Anatomy of a tooth. (*From* Yasny JS, Herlich A. Perioperative dental evaluation. Mt Sinai J Med 2012;79:34–45; with permission. http://dx.doi.org/10.1002/msj.21292. Available at: http://onlinelibrary.wiley.com/doi/10.1002/msj.21292/full#fig2.)

Lips and Oral Mucosa

The lips are musculofibrous structures that are critical to eating, swallowing, speaking, whistling, singing, expectoration, and common human behavioral communications, such as kissing, smiling, and pouting. The lips are composed of 4 tissue layers: cutaneous, muscular, glandular, and mucosa. The juncture where the lips meet the surrounding skin of the mouth is the vermillion border. The areas of the upper and lower lip meet at the corner of the mouth and are called labial commissures. The commissure is important in facial appearance, particularly during functions such as smiling. The maxillary and mandibular branches of the trigeminal nerve (V_2 and V_3, respectively) innervate the upper and lower lips. The infraorbital branches of V_2 innervate the upper lip and the surrounding skin of the face between the upper lip and the lower eyelid, except for the bridge of the nose. The mental nerve branch of V_3 innervates the lower lip, mucosa, and the labial gingival tissues anteriorly. The facial artery supplies the blood to the lips.[5–8]

Tongue and Floor of the Mouth

The tongue occupies the major part of the oral cavity and oropharynx. The tongue has several important functions, including swallowing, mastication, speech, and taste. Tongue movements also help clear food debris from the oral cavity. The major salivary glands, parotid, submandibular (or submaxillary), and sublingual glands, produce saliva to assist with swallowing. Five cranial nerves contribute to the complex innervation of this multifunctional organ. Motor innervation for all of the muscles of the tongue comes from the hypoglossal nerve (cranial nerve [CN] XII), with the exception of the palatoglossus, which is supplied by the pharyngeal plexus (fibers from the cranial root of the spinal accessory nerve carried by the vagus nerve [CN X]).

General sensation of the anterior two-thirds of the tongue is supplied by the lingual nerve, a terminal branch of V_3. Taste sensation for this portion of the tongue is carried by the chorda tympani branch of the facial nerve (CN VII). The posterior one-third of the tongue relays general sensation via the lingual-tonsillar branch of the glossopharyngeal nerve (CN IX). Some general and taste sensation from the base of tongue anterior to the epiglottis is carried by the internal laryngeal branch of the superior laryngeal nerve (CN X).

The surface of the tongue is covered by various projections of lamina propria covered with epithelium known as lingual papillae. There are 4 types of papillae: circumvallate (vallate), foliate, filiform, and fungiform. The circumvallate papillae are raised, dome-shaped structures that typically present in a V-shaped pattern in the posterior one third of the tongue. The foliate papillae are small folds of mucosa located along the lateral surface of the tongue. The filiform papillae are thin and long; they are the most numerous papillae and are located along the entire dorsum of the tongue, but are not involved in taste sensation. The fungiform papillae are mushroom-shaped and are dispersed most densely along the tip and lateral surfaces of the tongue.

The floor of the mouth forms the inferior limit of the oral cavity. In its most anterior section, the lingual frenum connects the tongue muscles to the gingival tissues. Sublingual papillae (caruncles) are present on either side of the lingual frenum. The excretory duct of the submandibular gland (Wharton's duct) is situated in the floor of the mouth along the medial border of the sublingual gland to pierce the surface of the mouth at these sublingual caruncles. In the more posterior floor of the mouth, just below the tongue, are the sublingual folds, which house the sublingual glands, with multiple small ducts to drain saliva in the mouth.

Palate and Upper Oropharynx

The palate is the U- or V-shaped arched roof of the oral cavity. The anterior section is the hard palate with oral mucosa firmly attached. The hard palate separates the oral cavity from the nasal cavities. The incisive bone, or premaxilla, and the palatine processes of the maxilla form the anterior two-thirds of the hard palate. The horizontal plates of the palatine bone form the posterior one-third of the hard palate. The midline elevated suture line of the hard palate is termed the median or palatine raphe. The transverse ridges (or rugae) make up the anterior palate.

The soft palate forms the posterior aspect of the palate; in the presence of the uvula and the movable section of the roof of the mouth, it constitutes the oropharynx and separates it from the nasopharynx. This part of the palate controls the act of swallowing and prevents food regurgitation into the nasal cavity. On the sides of the uvula, there are extensions of the soft palate in 2 directions. The anterior section connecting the soft palate to the tongue is termed the palatoglossal arch, and the posterior section connects the palate to the pharynx and is known as palatopharyngeal arch. These arches are also known as anterior and posterior palatal pillars. The palatine tonsils are generally located between these 2 arches.

During a comprehensive oral examination, it is important to evaluate the dentition, oral mucosa, gingival tissues, tongue, floor of the mouth, hard and soft palate, uvula, and tonsils for any changes in color, texture, and presence of lesions. This examination typically is of short duration, but the importance of clinical evaluation of the oral cavity in relation to systemic diseases should not be underestimated.

CLINICAL EXAMINATION CONSIDERATIONS

To perform the examination, it is best to have the patient seated in an upright position. The examiner can use one hand to support the back of the head, but the preferred position is to examine the patient in a chair with head support. Patients who are in a wheelchair can easily be examined without moving them out of the chair. Adequate lighting is essential for a proper examination of the oral cavity. For bedridden patients, the examination can take place at bedside using a tongue blade and flashlight. Placing a pillow under the patient's head will allow the examiner to have easy access to the oral cavity. In any situation, the examiner needs a flashlight or clinical examination light, tongue depressors, examination gloves, and 2 × 2 gauze sponges to dry the mucosa and/or hold the tissue structures for careful examination. It is important to develop a systematic procedure for performance of a clinical examination.

Extraoral Examination

Physicians have expertise in performing a head and neck examination, including evaluation of the cranial nerves, lymph nodes, thyroid gland, and general skeletal and facial features. This section reviews pertinent aspects of the extraoral examination with relevance to the oral cavity.

Head, face, and chin

Face the patient from front and evaluate for facial symmetry, presence of any masses, swelling, bruising, discolorations, or signs of trauma. Obvious asymmetry may be an indicator of congenital deformity, malocclusion, infection, neoplastic growths, muscle atrophy or hypertrophy, and neurologic problems. Asymmetry may also be associated with temporomandibular joint (TMJ) dysfunction. A detailed discussion of the TMJ can be found in the article by De Rossi, et al. elsewhere in this issue on temporomandibular disorders.

Salivary glands

The major salivary glands are best examined by palpation and observation of salivary flow. The parotid gland lies on the lateral surface of the mandibular ramus and folds itself around the posterior border of the mandible (**Fig. 3**). It is generally soft and is not usually palpable as a discrete gland. The anterior border of the gland may be better defined by having the patient clench the teeth together, which tenses the masseter muscle. The parotid gland lies just behind the masseter, and its consistency may be appreciated by pressing the gland on its lateral surface against the mandibular ramus.[9–13] Parotid secretions are carried to the oral cavity by Stensen's duct, which enters the oral cavity in the cheek just opposite the maxillary second molar tooth. It is visible as a small papilla in the buccal mucosa (**Fig. 4**). Careful observation of this papilla during palpation of the gland will usually reveal saliva coming from the small duct orifice. Sometimes it is helpful to dry the mucosa in the vicinity of the duct with dry gauze to visualize the flow more easily. The saliva from the parotid gland is usually clear, thin, and colorless. The clinician should look carefully for suppuration, mucus, or particulate matter in the secretion.

The submandibular gland lies just below the inferior border of the mandibular body, and is best palpated bimanually with one hand in the lateral floor of the mouth and the other on the submandibular gland (**Fig. 5**). The gland is usually soft and mobile, and should not be tender to palpation. The submandibular duct (Wharton's duct) runs superiorly and anteriorly to empty adjacent to the frenulum of the tongue. The small duct orifice is visible in the top of a papilla in this area (**Fig. 6**). Observation of salivary flow during palpation is important. The submandibular gland is more commonly associated with stone formation than the other salivary glands because (1) the secretion is more mucoid, and (2) the gland lies in a dependent position relative to the duct orifice; this may lead to stasis of secretions in the proximal duct. The sublingual glands lie just beneath the mucosa in the floor of the mouth and empty directly into the mouth or into the submandibular duct. The gland is not discretely palpable, nor are the duct openings usually visible. Salivary glands that are painful, swollen, and indurated may indicate abnormality associated with these structures. Palpation of the sublingual salivary gland, careful assessment of each duct, and the total salivary flow should be noted during the intraoral examination.

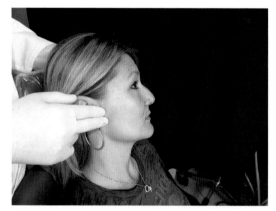

Fig. 3. Examination of the parotid gland. (*Courtesy of* Mansoor Madani, DMD, MD, Bala Cynwyd, PA; all rights reserved.)

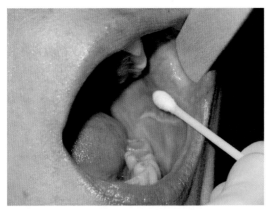

Fig. 4. Location of Stenson's duct papilla. (*Courtesy of* Mansoor Madani, DMD, MD, Bala Cynwyd, PA; all rights reserved.)

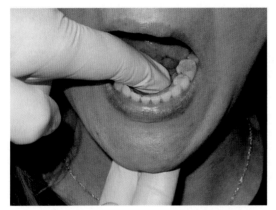

Fig. 5. Examination of the submandibular gland. (*Courtesy of* Mansoor Madani, DMD, MD, Bala Cynwyd, PA; all rights reserved.)

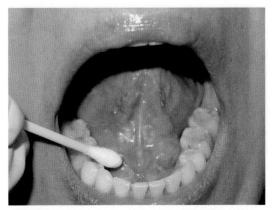

Fig. 6. Sublingual caruncle. (*Courtesy of* Mansoor Madani, DMD, MD, Bala Cynwyd, PA; all rights reserved.)

Intraoral Examination

As with any clinical examination, this portion should be completed in a systematic manner.[14–16] Tissues should be visually examined and palpated to appreciate normal and pathologic findings (if present).

Lips

Examination of the lips are an essential part of the physical evaluation. Generally, lips should be homogeneously pink in color, smooth and symmetric. The vermillion border should be clearly defined. When examining the lips, gently hold the lip between thumb and forefinger and roll it downward. Note the difference in the appearance of the normal tissue between the dry border and the wet mucous membrane. Palpate the lip for irregularities, such as submucosal nodules or areas of tenderness (**Fig. 7**). Inspect the color of the labial mucosa, and note the presence of ulcers, blisters, growths, or thickness changes. In addition, it is recommended to examine the patient's perioral areas for any signs of abnormality. There are normal variations of various conditions in the lips, such as presence of ectopic sebaceous glands and pigmentation changes related to patients' skin color, which should not be mistaken for pathologic conditions (see the article by Madani and Kuperstein elsewhere in this issue on normal variations of oral anatomy and common oral soft tissue lesions).

Labial and buccal mucosa

The labial and buccal mucosae line the inner part of the oral cavity covering the cheek and the lips. The mucosa is nonkeratinized in these regions. Clinical examination is performed by direct visualization as well as bimanual palpation of these tissues (**Figs. 8–10**). The mucosa should have a uniform consistency and appear pink in color. The parotid papilla, as previously described, should be visible bilaterally and may be confused with a pathologic condition. Any variations in color or texture, or the presence of lines or masses must be carefully evaluated and referred to a dental professional for further evaluation and management.

Tongue and floor of the mouth

The best position for examining this area is with the patient's oral cavity at eye level and the practitioner in front of or at the side of the patient. Grasp the tip of the tongue

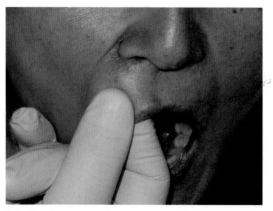

Fig. 7. Palpation of the lip. (*Courtesy of* Mansoor Madani, DMD, MD, Bala Cynwyd, PA; all rights reserved.)

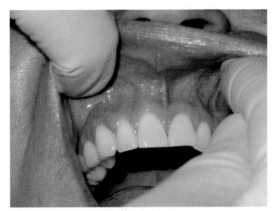

Fig. 8. Examination of the labial mucosa. (*Courtesy of* Mansoor Madani, DMD, MD, Bala Cynwyd, PA; all rights reserved.)

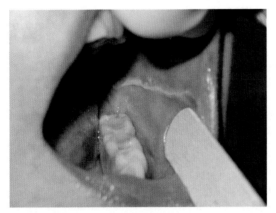

Fig. 9. Inspection of the buccal mucosa. (*Courtesy of* Mansoor Madani, DMD, MD, Bala Cynwyd, PA; all rights reserved.)

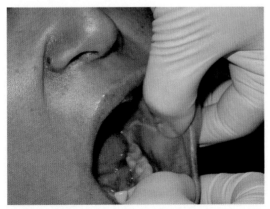

Fig. 10. Palpation of the buccal mucosa. (*Courtesy of* Mansoor Madani, DMD, MD, Bala Cynwyd, PA; all rights reserved.)

with a 2 × 2 gauze, move the tongue slightly out, and examine areas above, below, and on the sides of the tongue (**Fig. 11**). Inspect the color and texture of dorsal, ventral, and lateral surfaces. Observe for plaques, ulcerations, thickenings, and/or changes in papillae, and palpate the patient's tongue to evaluate for areas of induration and/or pain.

The floor of the mouth is also examined by direct visualization as well as bimanual palpation (**Fig. 12**). In general, ask the patient to lift their tongue and move it from side to side and note any deviation or limitation of motion. The sublingual space typically does not have highly keratinized epithelium.

The middle fold of the ventral surface of the tongue is termed the lingual frenum. Ordinarily, this frenum attaches about one-third of the way back from the tip of the tongue. At the base of the lingual frenum are the salivary ducts, which include the openings to the submandibular ducts (Wharton's duct), sublingual caruncle, and sublingual folds, as previously described (**Fig. 13**).

Near the posterior limits of the sublingual space and near the lingual border of the mandible, salivary eminences mark the superior surfaces of the sublingual glands. The remaining portion of the gland lies in the lingual fossa, which is a shallow depression in the mandible itself.

Observe the opening of Wharton's duct in the floor of the mouth and look for normal drainage of saliva from this orifice. Particular attention should be paid to the junction of the lateral border of the tongue, where the tongue base joins the anterior tonsillar pillars, as it could be easily missed on examination.

Palate and uvula

The hard palate is generally covered by very thick, keratinized, pink mucosa. Examination is by direct visualization, palpation and observing for color variation, presence of masses, swellings and ulceration (**Fig. 14**). There are several normal structures that must be noted in the hard palate. Just behind the maxillary central incisors lies the incisive papilla, a soft-tissue protuberance that covers the incisive foramen and normally appears more red in color compared to the surrounding tissues. There is a slightly elevated line extending from the incisive papilla to the soft palate, known as the midline raphe. On the sides of the raphe there are multiple corrugated ridges radiating to the sides, called palatal rugae. The exact function and reason for their

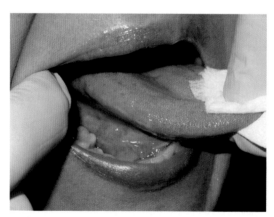

Fig. 11. Examination of the tongue. (*Courtesy of* Mansoor Madani, DMD, MD, Bala Cynwyd, PA; all rights reserved.)

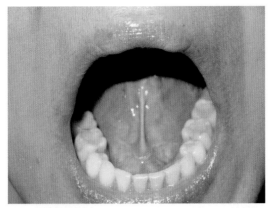

Fig. 12. Examination of the floor of mouth. (*Courtesy of* Mansoor Madani, DMD, MD, Bala Cynwyd, PA; all rights reserved.)

presence is unknown, but it is believed that rugae help with speech and pronunciation. The tori, structures representing excessive bone growth, may be present in the center of the palate. In general, palatal tori do not require removal unless the patient requires a denture and the presence of a torus interferes with denture fabrication or insertion. Any suspected abnormality should be referred to the appropriate health care provider for further evaluation and management.

The soft palate is examined using direct vision, and is normally not palpated unless necessary. Inspect for consistency of color and the presence of ulcerations, thickenings, exudates, or petechiae. Normally, this area is slightly less vascular than the oropharynx, and is usually reddish-pink in color. Observe the area as the patient says "ah." The tissue should appear loose, mobile, and symmetric during function. The tissue has a homogeneous, spongy consistency on palpation. Atypical observations include yellowish coloring from increased adipose tissue (especially in older patients), excessively long or short uvulas, and uvulas that appear slightly asymmetric at rest. Occasionally one will discover a bifid (cleft) uvula.

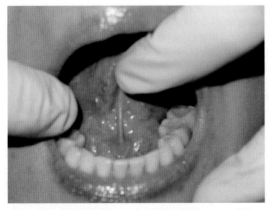

Fig. 13. Palpation of structures in the floor of mouth. (*Courtesy of* Mansoor Madani, DMD, MD, Bala Cynwyd, PA; all rights reserved.)

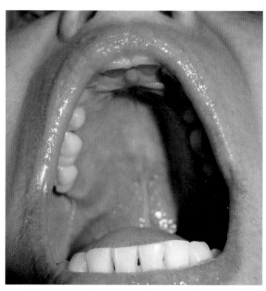

Fig. 14. Examination of the palate. (*Courtesy of* Mansoor Madani, DMD, MD, Bala Cynwyd, PA; all rights reserved.)

Tonsils

The tonsils are located on either side of the pharynx and examined by direct visualization. Tonsils often have smooth surfaces with a light pink mucosal covering, but in many instances, have rough, lobular shapes. On occasion, tonsillar crypts (cratered surfaces within the tonsil) may be observed on clinical examination. These areas are prone to collecting food debris, bacteria and calcified materials and may be a source of chronic halitosis. The anterior and posterior pillars should appear vascular, smooth, and symmetric. Examine the oropharynx by placing a mirror or tongue depressor on the dorsal surface of the tongue, applying gentle pressure without having the patient stick out the tongue. Visualize the posterior pharyngeal wall, anterior and posterior pillars, and the tonsillar crypt and tonsils, if present. These areas are normally not palpated unless there is a specific indication. The posterior pharyngeal wall is typically reddish-pink in color, smooth and may contain surface prominences (coral pink to translucent in color) that are representative of lymphoid aggregates.[17] Erythema and purulent exudate associated with pharyngitis (infection of the pharynx) may cover portions of the pharyngeal wall. Observe for ulcers, erosions, or noticeable enlargements or growths in the tonsillar region.

Dentition and occlusion

Inspect the entire dentition for number and position of teeth, tooth color, and intact surfaces (**Figs. 15** and **16**). Tooth percussion is a valuable examination technique to detect a possible dental abnormality in the absence of radiographs. The patient can often identify which tooth is the source of dental pain.[18] Multiple decayed or infected teeth, poor oral hygiene, and/or inflamed gingival tissues may be observed, in which case the patient should be referred to a dentist for further evaluation and management.

In patients with normal dental occlusion (bite relationship), the maxillary anterior teeth are positioned in front of the mandibular anterior teeth and the front cusp of

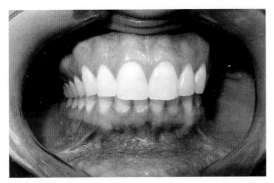

Fig. 15. Inspection of the dentition (in occlusion). (*Courtesy of* Mansoor Madani, DMD, MD, Bala Cynwyd, PA; all rights reserved.)

the maxillary first molar sits in the groove of the mandibular first molar. This type of occlusion is known as class I occlusion.[19] When a patient's jaws are malaligned, it is usually attributed to either mandibular retrognathism (lower jaw further posterior to upper jaw than usual; class II malocclusion) or mandibular prognathism (lower jaw anterior to upper jaw; class III malocclusion). In any of these situations, patients may be unable to speak properly or chew food effectively. In addition, patients with receded chin have more potential to develop sleep apnea.

Gingival and alveolar mucosa

Inspect the color and texture of the gingival and alveolar mucosa. The color of the gingival mucosa is generally pink/coral, whereas alveolar mucosa appears red because of increased vascularity. The texture of the gingiva is often smooth (although minor stippling is often present) with tight, well-defined margins, and the alveolar mucosa is consistent with other mucosal surfaces of the body. Observe for swelling, ulceration, erythema, discoloration, atrophy, recession, bleeding, and/or enlargement. Palpate any areas of enlargement to determine whether it is due to edema or an underlying bony or fibrous process.

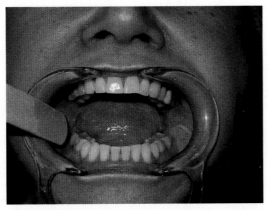

Fig. 16. Inspection of the dentition (open position). (*Courtesy of* Mansoor Madani, DMD, MD, Bala Cynwyd, PA; all rights reserved.)

SUMMARY

Many patients with dental and oral diseases present to their physician for initial evaluation. Local and systemic diseases often manifest in the oral cavity, and physicians should have an understanding of oral anatomy and the expertise to conduct a basic clinical examination of this area to provide appropriate care to patients.

REFERENCES

1. Gray H. Anatomy of the human body. Philadelphia: Lea & Febiger; 2000.
2. Hansen JT. Netter's clinical anatomy. 3rd edition. Philadelphia: Saunders; 2014.
3. Peck S, Peck L. A time for change of tooth numbering systems. J Dent Educ 1993;57:643–7.
4. Yadav SS, Sonkurla S. Sarjeev's supernumerary tooth notation system: a universally compatible add-on to the two-digit system. Indian J Dent Res 2013;24:395–6.
5. Jarvis C. Physical examination & health assessment. 5th edition. St. Louis: Elsevier Health Sciences; 2011.
6. Canaan TJ, Meehan SC. Variations of structure and appearance of the oral mucosa. Dent Clin North Am 2005;49:1–14, vii.
7. Kasper DI, Braunwald E, Fauci A, et al. Harrison's principles of internal medicine. 18th edition. New York: McGraw-Hill Publishers; 2011.
8. Jones JA. Integrating the oral examination into clinical practice. Hosp Pract 1989;24:23–7, 30.
9. Greenberg MS, Glick M, Ship JA. Burket's oral medicine. 11th edition. Hamilton: BC Decker; 2008.
10. Walker HK, Hall WD, Hurst JW, et al. Clinical methods: the history, physical, and laboratory examinations. 3rd edition. Boston: Butterworths; 1990. Chapter 129.
11. Vargas CM, Arevalo O. How dental care can preserve and improve oral health. Dent Clin North Am 2009;53:399–420.
12. Talley NJ. Clinical examination: a systematic guide to physical diagnosis. Chatswood: Churchill Livingstone; 2009.
13. Bengel W, Veltman G, Loevy HT, et al. Differential diagnosis of diseases of the oral mucosa. Chicago: Quintessence; 1988.
14. Bickley LS. Bates' guide to physical examination and history taking. 11th edition. Baltimore (MD): Lippincott Williams and Wilkins; 2012.
15. Seidel HM, Ball JW, Dains JE. Mosby's guide to physical examination. St Louis (MO): Mosby; 2002.
16. Thomas JE, Bender BS. What to look for after you say 'open wide'. A guide to examination of the oral cavity. Postgrad Med 1993;93:109–10, 113–5.
17. Burkhart NW, DeLong L. The intraoral and extraoral examination. Crest and OralB Continuing Education Course. 2012; Available at: http://www.dentalcare.com/media/en-US/education/ce337/ce337.pdf. Accessed August 28, 2014.
18. Hodgdon A. Dental and related infections. Emerg Med Clin North Am 2013;31:465–80.
19. Mitchell L. An introduction to orthodontics. 4th edition. Oxford (United Kingdom): Oxford University Press; 2013.

Common Dental and Periodontal Diseases
Evaluation and Management

 CrossMark

Joel M. Laudenbach, DMD[a,b,c],*, Ziv Simon, DMD, MSc[d,e]

KEYWORDS

- Dental caries • Dental abscess • Dental erosion • Dental attrition
- Periodontal disease • Gingivitis • Periodontal bone loss

KEY POINTS

- Dental caries is an infectious disease with multiple risk factors that can lead to pain, infection, loss of tooth structure, and loss of oral function.
- Dental abscesses can present locally surrounding a tooth with or without pain and/or swelling. Signs of an advanced dental infection may include trismus, facial paresthesia and swelling, dysphagia, odynophagia, fever, and lymphadenopathy.
- Dental erosion and attrition are considered pathologic, because each condition often negatively affects oral function and esthetics, and may be caused by a systemic condition.
- Periodontal disease is a chronic inflammatory condition of the supporting structures of teeth.
- Certain systemic conditions can manifest in the mouth in the form of periodontal disease (eg, leukemia, cyclic neutropenia).
- Uncontrolled diabetes is associated with destructive periodontitis, and improved glycemic control can positively affect periodontal disease.

INTRODUCTION

Physicians may encounter patients with dental and periodontal diseases in the context of outpatient medical practice. It is important for physicians to be aware of common

Funding sources: Colgate Oral Pharmaceuticals, Center for Oral Health (Dr J.M. Laudenbach); none (Dr Z. Simon).
Conflict of interest: None.
[a] Oral Medicine and Geriatric Dentistry, College of Dental Medicine, Western University of Health Sciences, 309 East Second Street, Pomona, CA 91766, USA; [b] Private Oral Medicine Practice, 350 S. Beverly Drive, Suite 160, Beverly Hills, CA 90212, USA; [c] Department of Surgery - Dentistry, Cedars-Sinai Medical Center, Los Angeles, California, USA; [d] Department of Continuing Education, Ostrow School of Dentistry, University of Southern California, 925 West 34th Street, Los Angeles, CA 90089, USA; [e] Private Practice Limited to Periodontics and Dental Implants, 9400 Brighton Way, #311, Beverly Hills, CA 90210, USA
* Corresponding author. College of Dental Medicine, Western University of Health Sciences, 309 East Second Street, Pomona, CA 91766.
E-mail address: jlaudenbach@westernu.edu

Med Clin N Am 98 (2014) 1239–1260
http://dx.doi.org/10.1016/j.mcna.2014.08.002
0025-7125/14/$ – see front matter © 2014 Elsevier Inc. All rights reserved.

medical.theclinics.com

dental and periodontal conditions and be able to assess for the presence and severity of these diseases. Dental caries, abscess, erosion, attrition, and periodontal disease are among the conditions in the oral cavity that physicians are readily able to recognize and for which they can initiate management and make appropriate referrals. Periodontal disease is a chronic, often painless inflammatory condition affecting the supporting tissues of teeth. If left untreated, bone and soft tissue loss can lead to mobility and eventual loss of teeth. Certain gingival conditions may present acutely in the form of a periodontal abscess, which may lead to disseminated infection and increased risk of septicemia. This article reviews common dental and periodontal conditions, their cardinal signs and symptoms, outpatient-setting assessment techniques, as well as common methods of treatment. Physicians detecting gross abnormalities on clinical examination should refer the patient to a dentist for further evaluation and management.

COMMON DENTAL DISEASES
Dental Caries

Dental caries is an infectious disease that results in tooth damage, can be associated with pain, and can lead to tooth loss. In a susceptible oral environment and/or host, dental caries occurs because of the interaction of bacteria with carbohydrates. The most common causal bacteria are *Streptococcus mutans*, *Streptococcus sobrinus*, *Lactobacillus*, and *Actinomyces* species.[1,2] Studies have shown that initial oral colonization by these bacteria often involves transmission from an infant's primary caregiver during the first 2 years of life.[3] Patients who develop dental caries must colonize causal bacteria, as well as provide food substrates and a persistent biofilm (dental plaque) environment that allows bacterial survival and proliferation. The acid generated by bacterial by-products damages the tooth structure via a demineralization process called caries (also known as tooth decay). Health care providers should screen children, adolescents, and adults for several risk factors associated with dental caries (**Boxes 1 and 2**). Providers should be aware that severe dental caries can affect the primary dentition (also known as early childhood caries and nursing bottle caries),

---

Box 1
High risk factors for dental caries in children 0 to 5 years old

- Mother/primary caregiver has active caries
- Parent/caregiver has low socioeconomic status
- Child has greater than 3 between-meal sugar-containing snacks or beverages per day
- Child is put to bed with a bottle containing natural or added sugar
- Child has special health care needs
- Child is a recent immigrant[a]
- Clinical evidence of white spot lesions or enamel defects
- Clinical evidence of visible cavities or fillings
- Clinical evidence of dental plaque on teeth

[a] Term is taken from the original article and refers to developing countries.[4]
Data from Guideline on caries-risk assessment and management for infants, children, and adolescents. In: American Academy of Pediatric Dentistry Clinical Guidelines. Reference Manual V 35|NO 6. 2013. Available at: http://www.aapd.org/media/Policies_Guidelines/G_CariesRiskAssessment.pdf. Accessed March 18, 2014.

Box 2
High risk factors for dental caries: age 6 years and older

- Patient is of low socioeconomic status
- Patient has greater than 3 between-meal sugar-containing snacks or beverages per day
- Clinical evidence of 1 or more interproximal lesions[a]
- Clinical evidence of active white spot lesions or enamel defects[a]
- Clinical evidence of low salivary flow[b]

Additional moderate risk factors include patients with special health care needs, recent immigrant[c] status, clinical evidence of defective restorations (eg, dental fillings, crowns), and patients wearing an intraoral appliance (eg, retainer, night guard).

  [a] Interproximal lesions are dental caries that occurs between two teeth that contact each other. These types of lesions are most often diagnosed by dentists with the aid of dental radiographs.
  [b] Salivary assessment can be performed by palpating and compressing the major salivary glands (parotid and submandibular) while noting any saliva that is expressed from the intraoral major salivary ducts (ie, Stensen and Wharton ducts) bilaterally.
  [c] Term is taken from the original article and refers to developing countries.[4]
  Data from Guideline on caries-risk assessment and management for infants, children, and adolescents. In: American Academy of Pediatric Dentistry clinical guidelines. Reference manual V 35|NO 6. 2013. Available at: http://www.aapd.org/media/Policies_Guidelines/G_CariesRiskAssessment.pdf. Accessed March 18, 2014.

---

as well as the adult dentition with multiple presentations and complicating risk factors (**Box 3**).[5] Healthy teeth normally appear in different shades of white with an intact and smooth enamel surface (outer layer of teeth) (**Fig. 1**A, B). Posterior teeth have developmental pits and grooves in the enamel surface (**Fig. 2**). Teeth with active dental caries have a varied clinical appearance: white-spot lesions that represent decalcified enamel; and dark, discolored, carious lesions that can vary in color from yellow to black (**Fig. 3**).[6] Clinicians may find it helpful to dry suspicious teeth with a gauze pad to better evaluate the surface appearance and texture. Symptoms and presentation of dental caries varies among patients. Signs of dental caries can be cavitation, a

---

Box 3
Other risk factors for developing dental caries

- Active dental caries within the previous 12 months
- Drug and/or alcohol abuse
- Cariogenic diet
- Chemotherapy or head/neck radiation
- Eating disorders
- Physical or mental disability with inability or unavailability of performing proper oral health care
- Salivary gland hypofunction/xerostomia: medication, radiation, or disease induced

Data from Weyant RJ, Tracy SL, Anselmo TT, et al. Topical fluoride for caries prevention: executive summary of the updated clinical recommendations and supporting systematic review. J Am Dent Assoc 2013;144(11):1279–91.

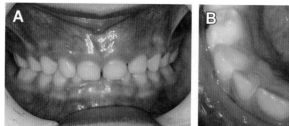
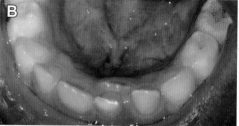

Fig. 1. (*A*) Healthy primary dentition. (*B*) Healthy primary teeth with stained grooves and newly erupting adult teeth. (*Courtesy of* [A] Dr Juan F. Yepes, Indiana University, School of Dentistry, Indianapolis, Indiana.)

fractured tooth, oral and dental pain, intraoral and facial swelling, or a combination of thereof. Dental caries is classified/diagnosed based on the affected tooth surface and location. For example, dental caries involving only the biting surface of a tooth is classified differently than caries that involves at least one proximal (side) surface of a tooth (**Fig. 4**). Clinicians should evaluate the dentition for changes in tooth surface color and texture, such as decalcification and/or gross cavitation (see **Fig. 3**). As dental caries spreads through enamel, it next penetrates the dentin layer, which is more porous than enamel and has microscopic tubules communicating with the dental pulp. Dental pulp can eventually be affected, leading to hyperemia and subsequently acute inflammation, infection, and necrosis. Dental caries can also develop on the root surfaces (cementum layer) and is more prevalent in patients with xerostomia (dry mouth) (**Fig. 5**). Exposed root surfaces caused by gingival recession can be particularly susceptible to this problem. Severity, extent and depth of dental caries are best assessed on dental radiographs. Dentists formulate a definitive diagnosis and treatment plan based on clinical and radiographic findings, as well as on patients' dental caries risk factors.[4,6]

Counseling patients about suspected dental caries and associated risk factors along with communication with the treating dentist or referral to a dentist is the first step to establish a comprehensive dental diagnosis and to initiate management. A combination of risk assessment, clinical examination, and interpretation of dental radiographs is required to determine whether dental caries extends beyond the enamel surface. When dental caries is limited to the enamel layer, remineralization techniques and control of risk factors are recommended.[2] This approach is effective in arresting

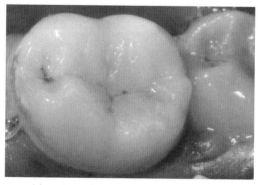

Fig. 2. Enamel grooves with stain and adjacent tooth with dark-appearing caries.

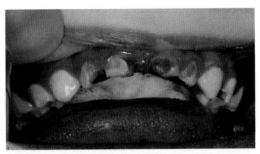

Fig. 3. Early childhood caries: primary teeth with dark yellow–appearing carious anterior teeth with cavitation and posterior teeth with white decalcification. (*Courtesy of* Dr Juan F. Yepes, Indiana University, School of Dentistry, Indianapolis, Indiana.)

the progression of dental caries in patients with low to moderate risk. However, in high-risk patients with enamel layer caries, clinical guidelines recommend that restorative intervention be initiated (soft carious lesion removed, followed by placement of a dental restoration or prophylactic sealant).[7] In addition, implementation of specific diagnostic protocols, topical fluoride regimens, and dietary counseling can be considered (**Box 4**).[2,4,5,7] These techniques include patient education (dietary avoidance of carbohydrate consumption between meals); addressing salivary flow issues, if present (increasing quantity and quality of saliva flow); increasing and improving oral hygiene measures (brushing at least twice daily with a fluoridated toothpaste and flossing all teeth at least once daily). Dentists and health care providers may choose various applications of topical fluoride (ie, varnish, toothpaste, gel and/or rinses), which are effective preventive management strategies in patients with dental caries involving enamel only. When clinical dental examination is combined with intraoral dental radiographs, clinicians are able to determine whether dental caries extends deeper into the dentin layer of teeth. Once dental caries is found in the dentin layer, restorative intervention via excavation of the affected surfaces is indicated. Physicians should refer patients with suspected dental caries to a dentist, whether based on reported pain, tooth surface color or texture changes, and/or tooth fracture. It is also important for physicians to understand the primary cause and the contributing medical conditions and medications that act as potential risk factors for dental caries. Patients' oral health can improve if collaboration between their physician and dentist is established to address the effect of certain medical conditions and medications on their oral health.

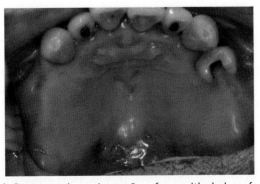

Fig. 4. Maxillary left first premolar caries on 2 surfaces with dark surface appearance and missing previous restoration.

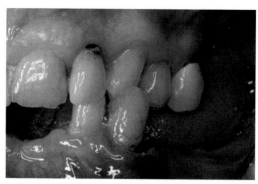

Fig. 5. Root caries on the left maxillary lateral incisor at the gingival margin.

Dental (Apical) Abscess

Patients reporting dental pain require additional questioning and a clinical intraoral examination to help practitioners differentiate between localized early odontogenic disease and advancing odontogenic infection. Dental infections often originate from extensive dental caries that introduces bacteria into the neurovascular soft tissues inside a tooth (called dental pulp). The root canal system is an enclosed space inside a tooth surrounded by tooth structure and bone at the root tip. Once colonized, this space can allow bacterial overgrowth. As the dental pulp tissues become affected by invading and replicating bacteria, patients may feel spontaneous tooth pain and/ or thermal hypersensitivity (ie, cold and/or hot liquids and foods). At this stage, the affected tooth may not be painful during mastication. Clinicians should first apply gentle finger pressure onto the biting surface of the suspected tooth involved. The next test is to use an instrument (such as a tongue blade) to apply a brief and continuous tapping pressure directly onto the biting surface of the suspected tooth (palpation). Adjacent teeth should also be tested in this fashion to see whether more than one

---

Box 4
Caries management and prevention strategies for high-risk patients 6 years of age and older

- Schedule routine dental examination appointments every 3 months
- Take new dental radiographs every 6 months
- Brush teeth twice daily with prescription-strength/home-use topical fluoride[a] (0.5% fluoride gel or paste)
- Professionally apply topical fluoride[a] every 3 to 6 months (2.26% fluoride varnish or 1.23% acidulated phosphate fluoride gel)
- Dietary counseling; recommend use of xylitol-containing products to reduce and control tooth decay
- Professionally applied dental sealants (for teeth that have deep grooves/surface anatomy or developmental defects)
- Dentist to decide which teeth should have surgical intervention/restoration (ie, early, cavitated, and/or enlarging dental caries)

    [a] Potential side effects of topical fluorides should be discussed with patients and/or parents/ caregivers (ie, nausea, emesis, and dental fluorosis while tooth enamel is developing).[5]
    Data from Refs.[2,4,5]

tooth is affected. When a symptomatic tooth is deemed nontender with palpation and percussion testing, it is likely that the dental pulp is inflamed (a diagnosis of pulpitis), with no abscess formation. This inflammation can still be reversible. Pulpitis can result from advancing dental caries and/or periodontal causes (discussed later). When a tooth has pulpitis, additional clinical tests conducted by the dentist can evaluate the status of the pulp and rule out necrosis of this tissue. Updated dental radiographs of symptomatic teeth should be obtained to evaluate for radiographic signs of deep dental caries and/or a dental abscess. Radiographic signs of dental abscess can include radiolucency (bone loss) around the root tip area. It is a combination of the patients' reported symptoms, clinical findings with regard to tooth palpation, percussion, mobility, nerve vitality testing, and radiographic findings that allow a definitive diagnosis.

As the internal dental infection progresses to a complete necrosis of the dental pulp, patients commonly report pain with chewing. Additional tests are needed to determine whether the pulpitis is irreversible or the dental pulp is necrotic. Dentists perform a vitality test by directly applying a thermal (cold) stimulus to the suspected tooth. When vitality cold testing results in no reported pain or cold sensitivity, clinicians should consider the possibility of pulpal necrosis and dental abscess. Mitigating clinical situations require further interpretation of clinical tests before making a definitive diagnosis. For example, existing dental crowns can interfere with vitality testing and radiographic assessment for dental caries. The dental pulp may be partially necrotic at the time of clinical testing, which can result in clinical suspicion of dental pulpitis without abscess, whereas dental radiographs and all other clinical signs (eg, draining fistula tract/pointing abscess; **Fig. 6**) are consistent with dental/apical abscess.

Physicians should obtain a detailed dental pain history, ask the patient to localize and identify the suspected teeth, and then perform a focused clinical examination. This process allows determination of early dental disease (suspected dental pulpitis) versus acute dental abscess. It is important for clinicians to realize that dental radiographs are required to make definitive dental diagnoses. A panoramic radiograph can assist clinicians in diagnosis as an adjunct to definitive intraoral dental radiographs.

Physicians who suspect dental pulpitis and/or a dental abscess should refer patients to a dentist in a timely fashion for a complete examination and diagnosis. Urgent referral is indicated when the following clinical signs and symptoms are present: continuous and severe spontaneous pain, pain on chewing, trismus (limited mouth opening), intraoral and extraoral soft tissue swelling, dysphagia/odynophagia, facial

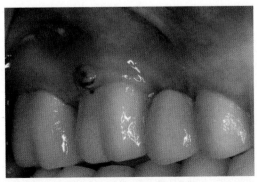

Fig. 6. Fistula swelling on the gingiva next to the right first maxillary molar, which has a crown restoration. (*Courtesy of* Dr Jay B. Laudenbach, Philadelphia, PA.)

paresthesia, fever, and/or symptomatic submandibular lymphadenopathy.[8,9] When an acute dental infection is suspected, urgent referrals may include dentists, dental specialists (often oral and maxillofacial surgeons, endodontists, and periodontists), and the local hospital emergency department. Further explanation regarding assessment of dental abscesses with a periodontal cause and common management strategies are provided later, including prescription antimicrobial regimens (**Boxes 5 and 6**).

Dental Erosion and Attrition

Enamel is the hardest substance in the human body. There are a few significant causes for enamel loss after tooth formation. Causes for enamel loss must be evaluated in the context of the patient's medical history, dental history, parafunctional history, and dietary history. The loss of enamel secondary to dental caries, its sequela, and variable management were discussed earlier. Enamel can also be lost because of chemical erosion of the tooth surface. Dental erosion is characterized by a frosted, thinned, and translucent appearance of the remaining tooth surfaces (**Fig. 7**). When salivary pH levels decrease, enamel is at risk for dissolving into the saliva, creating enamel erosion.[10,11] Chemical causes include dietary (soda, fruit juice, sport/energy drinks) and systemic disease (ie, gastroesophageal reflux disease, bulimia). As enamel erosion progresses, dentin, with its yellow color, becomes visible on inspection (**Fig. 8**A, B) and solitary dental restorations can be seen without bordering dentin and enamel. The effects of chemical-induced erosion are most often evident on the inner surfaces (facing the palate) of the maxillary anterior and posterior mandibular teeth, as well as on the biting surfaces of all teeth, appearing concave, or cupped out (**Fig. 9**).[10,11]

Enamel can also be lost from the biting surfaces of the teeth in a symmetric pattern caused by the function between the upper and lower teeth (**Fig. 10**). This type of mechanical cause resulting from occlusal forces is termed attrition. In this condition, contacting opposing teeth combined with masticatory forces and possible parafunctional habits (ie, bruxism) are keys in establishing the diagnosis.[10] Mild attrition of the enamel surfaces is considered to be a normal part of aging (wear and tear). However, attrition can become pathologic when it affects a patient's ability to chew foods and compromises the esthetic appearance.[12] Common findings are reduced tooth height,

---

Box 5
Checklist of clinical findings[a] in periodontal disease

- Dental plaque
- Calculus
- Gingival swelling
- Gingival erythema
- Gingival bleeding
- Teeth mobility
- Halitosis (bad breath)
- Suppuration
- Pathologic teeth migration (opening of spaces between teeth)

[a] When more findings are clinically evident, the presence of active periodontal disease is more likely and referral to a dentist should be strongly considered.

Box 6
Common therapeutic agents for periodontal and dental infections

Chlorhexidine gluconate 0.12%: rinse twice daily for 2 weeks (an initial adjunctive treatment with debridement)[19]

Amoxicillin/clavulanic acid 250–500 mg: 3 times a day for 10 days[20]

Metronidazole 250 mg: 3 or 4 times a day for 10 days[20]

Metronidazole 500 mg: twice a day for 1 week

Combination regimen #1 (amoxicillin 250 mg 3 times a day and metronidazole 250 mg 3 times a day for 8 days): for young and middle-aged patients[21,22]

Combination regimen #2 (ciprofloxacin 500 mg twice a day and metronidazole 500 mg twice a day for 8 days): for elderly patients and for patients in developing countries[21]

Data from Refs.[19–22]

flattened grinding surfaces, smooth and shiny dental facets corresponding with the opposing teeth, and even exposed dentin or penetration into the pulp chamber.

In certain cases, nondental external mechanical forces can cause loss of surface enamel, and the condition is then termed abrasion.[10,12] Clinical appearance of dental abrasion is most frequently isolated to the segment of the mouth where the patient is applying the external mechanical force (**Fig. 11**).

Referral to the dental professional is indicated to establish the proper diagnosis and cause for all types of enamel loss. Dentists can obtain dental radiographs and perform a clinical examination. An assessment of the causes, such as dental caries and teeth wear patterns, that indicate chemical, parafunctional/masticatory, mechanical processes can be completed. Dentists are also able to diagnose malocclusion (improper tooth relationships), which may have various causes: skeletal discrepancy, developmental defect(s) and disorders, drifting of teeth, as well as various medical conditions (eg, rheumatoid arthritis resulting in erosive condylar resorption and malocclusion; **Fig. 12**). Once a dental diagnosis is made, treatment of pathologic enamel loss can lead to full mouth rehabilitation along with control of the causes and contributing factors.

COMMON PERIODONTAL DISEASES
Periodontal Assessment

Periodontal disease is a prevalent oral disease affecting more than 90% of the population with varying severity. A patient's periodontal condition plays an important role in

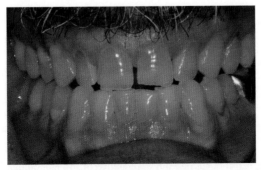

Fig. 7. Dental erosion with thinned translucent and chipped front teeth.

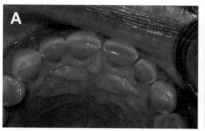
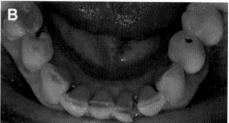

Fig. 8. (*A*) Erosion of anterior maxillary teeth with yellow dentin exposed. (*B*) Yellow dentin exposed (erosion) and fractured left central incisor with caries on mandibular teeth from erosion in a patient with gastroesophageal reflux disease, Barrett esophagus, and xerostomia.

the overall health of the oral cavity. Periodontal disease is a chronically progressing condition affecting the supporting tissues of teeth. The disease begins with bacterial, biofilm-induced inflammation of the soft tissues surrounding the teeth. This inflammation eventually causes alveolar bone deterioration and loss of teeth. Initial disease is limited to inflammation of the soft tissues and is called gingivitis (**Fig. 13**). It is characterized by swelling, redness, and bleeding of the gingiva and is considered reversible once the causal factors are controlled. Gingivitis can be present for months to years. In a susceptible patient, this chronic inflammatory state can progress into a more involved periodontal disease pattern. The second stage involves bone loss and is called periodontitis. This stage encompasses all aspects of gingivitis with varying degrees of bone loss, tooth mobility, pathologic migration of teeth, and tooth loss (see **Box 5**). A clinical and radiographic examination is necessary to establish a specific periodontal diagnosis and to formulate a treatment plan. An initial impression regarding a patient's inflammatory periodontal condition can be made based on the presence of bacterial biofilm and calculus. Bacterial biofilm, also known as dental plaque, appears in different shades of white and is combined with food debris typically found at the gingival margin bordering teeth (**Fig. 14**). Biofilm is also commonly found between teeth, where its removal requires additional efforts by using dental floss and interproximal brushes. When clinically evident, bacterial biofilm is considered the primary cause and accumulation is typically proportional to the severity of inflammation. Dental calculus is another source of periodontal inflammation. It acts as an irritant to the gingiva and also allows further retention of dental plaque. Calculus is formed by

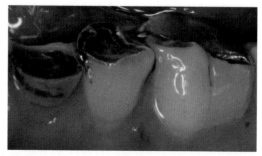

Fig. 9. Erosion and attrition: cupped-out appearance of the mandibular left premolars with staining from excess wine consumption. (*Courtesy of* Dr Jay B. Laudenbach, Philadelphia, PA.)

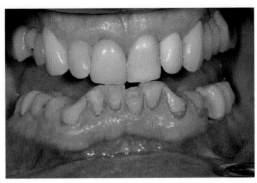

Fig. 10. Attrition is evident on the lower teeth and is caused by a combination of mastica-tory forces and porcelain (dental crowns on the upper teeth). (*Courtesy of* Dr Gary S. Solnit, DDS, MS, Beverly Hills, CA.)

calcification of dental plaque attached to a tooth surface that was not adequately removed. It can usually be detected with the naked eye and appears as white, elevated deposits on the patient's dentition at the level of the gingiva (**Fig. 15**). Calcu-lus that is below the visible level of the gingiva is most often black and can typically be removed by a dental practitioner (dentist or dental hygienist).

Initial periodontal treatment typically involves the physical removal of the biofilm, as well as calculus, and results in reduction of inflammation and improvement in the over-all periodontal condition. Dentists and periodontists may recommend additional treat-ment modalities that include surgical debridement, use of localized chemotherapeutic agents, and prescription systemic antibiotics. For a physician who suspects a severe periodontal condition, recommending an antibacterial oral rinse is often a therapeutic option, especially when based on an empiric periodontal diagnosis. This strategy al-lows for temporary management of the periodontal condition until a dentist can eval-uate the patient, establish the diagnosis, and recommend further treatment. A common antimicrobial oral rinse for bacteria-induced periodontitis is chlorhexidine gluconate 0.12%.[13] It is common to prescribe this rinse for use twice daily for a total of 2 weeks (see **Box 6**). Chlorhexidine gluconate has been established as being effec-tive against dental plaque pathogens in common forms of periodontal disease.[14] In a dental setting, chlorhexidine gluconate is rarely recommended as a sole treatment and

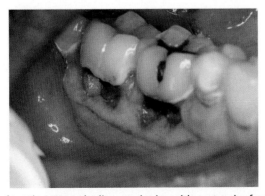

Fig. 11. Abrasion of tooth roots and adjacent gingiva with root caries from aggressive tooth brushing.

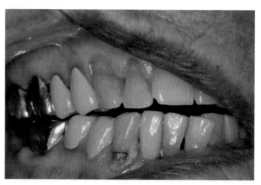

Fig. 12. Progressive anterior open bite (malocclusion) in an elderly patient subsequently diagnosed with elderly onset rheumatoid arthritis affecting both condyles of the mandible.

is typically used as an adjunct to surgical and nonsurgical treatment of bacterial plaque and calculus debridement.[15] Patients should be informed about the potential side effects, which include staining of the teeth and dorsal tongue, as well as alteration in taste sensation. Another option is to rinse with a 0.25% sodium hypochlorite solution twice weekly.[16,17] It is readily available, inexpensive, and effective in dental plaque and bleeding reduction.

Physicians are able to evaluate certain inflammatory changes in the soft tissues surrounding teeth and make an initial assessment for the clinical signs of periodontal disease. Healthy gingiva is pink and has a flat and rigid appearance. Once periodontal disease develops, typical signs of inflammation will follow: predominantly edema and erythema. It is not possible to diagnose periodontitis by visual inspection only. Periodontal diagnosis requires a thorough assessment by a dentist or a periodontist using various instruments and tests. A periodontal probe is used to measure and assess the depth of the periodontal crevice (also called pocket, located between the gingiva and tooth; **Fig. 16**). Dental radiographs are paramount to show remaining alveolar ridge bone levels, bone quality, and to assess for various patterns of bone deterioration. Conventional medical advanced imaging techniques (ie, computed tomography scan and magnetic resonance imaging) are not suitable for periodontal diagnosis. Intraoral dental radiographs are often combined with panoramic radiography in dental practice in order to make periodontal, dental, and pathologic

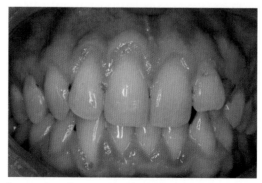

Fig. 13. Gingival inflammation characterized by gingival edema and erythema, induced by bacterial plaque.

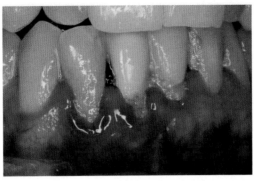

Fig. 14. Severe gingival inflammation with bleeding, teeth mobility, and initial bone loss.

diagnoses. It is also possible to obtain a microbiological sample of the bacterial biofilm and submit it to culture in aerobic and anaerobic conditions. Most periodontal pathogens are gram-negative anaerobic bacteria that can be isolated. As an alternative, saliva samples can be obtained and tested for particular bacterial DNA, thus allowing clinicians to evaluate the types of bacteria. Certain bacteria correlated with destructive periodontal disease are considered high risk and include *Porphyromonas gingivalis*, *Actinobacillus actinomycetemcomitans*, *Bacteroides forsythus*, *Prevotella intermedia*, *Campylobacter rectus*, *Treponema denticola*, *Peptostreptococcus micros*, *Fusobacterium nucleatum*, and *Eikenella corrodens*.[18] In addition, the amount of bacteria in a sample can correlate with the severity of periodontal disease and assist clinicians in determining the appropriate antibiotic regimen. Although the research on the microbiology of periodontal disease is vast, there is little consensus in the literature on the exact primary bacterial cause, and the bacterial composition can differ between affected patients. It is generally advisable to consider prescribing a broad-spectrum antibiotic (eg, amoxicillin) in conjunction with an antibiotic to target gram-negative species (eg, metronidazole). Antibiotic selection, regimen, and dosing schedules are often based on clinical judgment (see **Box 6**).

In general, 2 types of periodontal diseases can be detected clinically: chronic and aggressive. Definitive diagnosis is made with a comprehensive clinical examination by a dentist or periodontist with the appropriate instrument, tests, and radiographs. However, physicians can assess several factors in patients' oral environments and

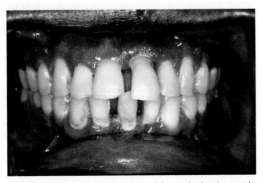

Fig. 15. Advanced chronic periodontal disease with pathologic teeth migration, calculus and plaque accumulation, and advanced mobility of teeth.

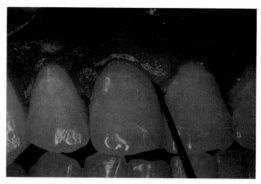

Fig. 16. A periodontal probe is placed in the gingival crevice (sulcus) to measure the depth and thereby indicate attachment level.

make initial recommendations. A retraction tool (ie, tongue depressor) allows observation of the various oral structures and retracting the cheeks, mucosa, and tongue allows direct inspection of the gingivae (**Fig. 17**). In addition, it is important to use a light source for proper inspection. At first, clinicians can evaluate the amount of dental plaque on the patient's dentition and gingiva. The amount of bacterial biofilm is typically positively and proportionally related to the amount of gingival inflammation. Typical signs of inflammation include swelling, bleeding, and redness of the gingival tissues surrounding the teeth. It is also possible to assess tooth mobility by applying horizontal pressure against the lateral and medial surfaces of teeth (**Fig. 18**). Assessment for tooth mobility can be performed using a tongue depressor alone and/or in combination with finger pressure. The extent of mobility can indicate the amount of bone support and the severity of periodontal disease. Teeth occasionally become mobile because of excessive parafunction forces (ie, bruxism). In these cases, the mobility is considered adaptive and can resolve once the excessive forces are brought under control. The presentation of malpositioned teeth with spacing, possible flaring, and accompanied by oral malodor (halitosis) are also associated with periodontal disease of chronic and aggressive patterns (**Table 1**).

Further evaluation by a dentist or a periodontist will establish a definitive diagnosis and development of the appropriate treatment plan. The chronic and aggressive periodontal disease patterns differ in several ways. Patients with aggressive periodontitis

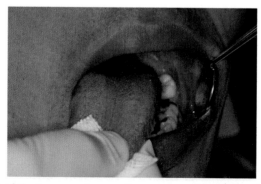

Fig. 17. Retraction of the tongue using a cotton gauze pad together with cheek retraction allows proper inspection of the gingival tissues and other oral structures.

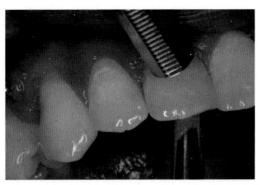

Fig. 18. The degree of tooth mobility is clinically assessed by applying back-and-forth horizontal pressure by using 2 rigid instruments.

typically present with a rapid progression of signs and symptoms, which are confirmed by dental radiographs. The amount of bacterial biofilm and calculus is not proportional to the severe destruction. These patients often have a genetic susceptibility to periodontal disease. Patients with aggressive periodontitis are likely to lose more teeth over time and at a rapid pace compared with patients with chronic periodontitis (**Fig. 19**). Some of these patients are young (from adolescents to young adults in the twentieth decade of life) and present with severe destruction of the supporting tissues. In all aggressive presentations, it is prudent to conduct a comprehensive medical evaluation to rule out systemic causes for the condition, such as immune deficiency or blood dyscrasias (**Box 7**).

Table 1
Common periodontal conditions

Condition	Localization	Characteristics
Chronic periodontitis	Localized (<30% of teeth are involved) Generalized (>30% of teeth are involved)	Periodontal pockets, bone loss, bleeding, gingival inflammation
Aggressive periodontitis	Localized (<30% of teeth are involved) Generalized (>30% of teeth are involved)	Advanced bone loss at a young age, severe teeth mobility
Abscesses of the periodontium	Gingival (limited to gingiva) Periodontal (involves the attachment) Pericoronal (around a clinical crown of a tooth)	Gingival swelling, suppuration Tooth nerve testing is typically vital (normal)
Periodontitis associated with endodontic lesion	Typically localized to a tooth with a necrotic pulp	Pain on percussion Tooth nerve testing is negative (nonvital)
Gingival hyperplasia (medication induced)	Typically generalized on all aspects of the gingiva	Gingival overgrowth covering the crown of the tooth

Data from Armitage GC. Development of a classification system for periodontal diseases and conditions. Ann Periodontol 1999;4(1):1–6.

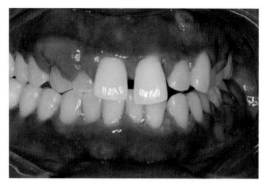

Fig. 19. Aggressive periodontitis pattern in a healthy 26-year-old woman with severe inflammation, formation of abscesses, and pathologic migration of teeth.

Patients presenting with a gradual deterioration of their periodontal conditions typically have chronic periodontitis (**Fig. 20**). These patients are often older adults with other possible risk factors (eg, smoking) and/or complicating systemic condition (eg, diabetes).

Periodontal Abscess

Localized purulent infection of the gingiva commonly occurs in patients with periodontal disease with different levels of severity (**Fig. 21**). The microorganisms that

---

Box 7
Periodontitis as a manifestation of systemic diseases

- Acquired neutropenia
- Leukemias
- Familial and cyclic neutropenia
- Down syndrome
- Leukocyte adhesion deficiency syndrome
- Papillon-Lefèvre syndrome
- Chédiak-Higashi syndrome
- Histiocytosis syndrome
- Glycogen storage disease
- Infantile genetic agranulocytosis
- Cohen syndrome
- Ehlers-Danlos syndrome (type IV and VIII)
- Hypophosphatasia
- Diabetes mellitus[a]

[a] Diabetes does not cause periodontal disease, but patients with an uncontrolled diabetic condition and poor glycemic control experience worsening of their periodontal condition. Diabetes is therefore considered a modifier of periodontal disease.

Data from Armitage GC. Development of a classification system for periodontal diseases and conditions. Ann Periodontol 1999;4(1):1–6.

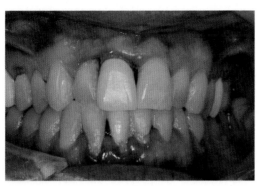

Fig. 20. Severe chronic periodontitis in a healthy 60-year-old man with gingival inflammation, as well as tissue recession, bone loss, and mobility of teeth.

colonize the abscess are predominantly gram-negative anaerobic rods[23] with a high frequency of *P gingivalis*, *P intermedia*, *F nucleatum*, *C rectus*, and *Capnocytophaga*.[24] The abscess presents with swelling of the gingival tissue that is typically localized to 1 or 2 teeth on 1 aspect only (ie, between teeth, facing the tongue or palate, or facing the cheek). There is visible erythema and discharge from the gingival sulcus or through a fistula that permits drainage. Pressing lightly on the gingival swelling in the direction of the clinical crown can be repeated multiple times until discharge is no longer visible. Because drainage can easily be achieved, systemic symptoms of infection are uncommon.

The source of the infection can vary and therefore different treatment protocols are indicated. Infections can also originate from the neurovascular bundle (dental pulp) within the teeth. The pulp is responsible for thermal, osmotic, pressure, and sensory transduction. An infection that originates from within the dental pulp is considered a primary endodontic infection and can occur because of dental caries, fractures, and/or excessive thermal stimulation (**Fig. 22**). Patients typically report severe pain that lasts for a few days and then subsides. The pain is explained by an acute infection of the dental pulp and the root canal system. Once the pulp undergoes necrosis, the pain sensation resolves. However, the necrotic dental pulp leads to infection inside the root canal system. The infection can then travel along the root canal system, progress into the alveolar bone, and cause a second occurrence of severe pain. The pain originates from an acute inflammation in bone with pressure on the adjacent structures. At

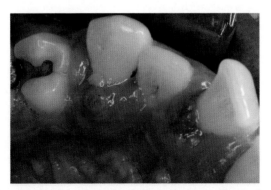

Fig. 21. A periodontal abscess on the palatal aspect with significant gingival swelling and suppuration from the sulcus that will necessitate an extraction.

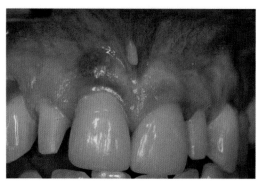

Fig. 22. Abscess formation on the gingiva of an upper incisor caused by a root fracture with associated purulent infection.

a certain point, this bone infection can perforate the alveolar bone and create drainage through the gingiva into the oral cavity (**Figs. 23–25**). This abscess presentation can remain stable for many years without any significant symptoms. Although asymptomatic, patients are in a chronic state of infection with systemic dissemination of bacteria and continuous deterioration of the bone surrounding the infected tooth. Endodontic therapy (ie, root canal therapy [RCT]) by a dentist or endodontist is the preferred treatment of these conditions. Root canal treatment accesses the infection directly through the dental crown and allows for drainage by using specialized instruments and chemotherapeutic agents for disinfection. The RCT is concluded by sealing the internal root canal, which closes off communication between the oral environment and the jawbone. In certain situations, root canal infection requires surgical intervention, debridement, and drainage of the tooth root and of the locally affected soft tissues. Infection travels through the path of least resistance, and eventually a point of drainage is created through hard and soft tissue.

Endodontic infections can also drain directly through the periodontal pocket, resulting in loss of bone and gingival support, which can ultimately lead to a compromised tooth or the need for extraction. In contrast, patients with periodontal disease present more commonly with an infection that begins in the tissues surrounding the tooth (as opposed to the internal aspect of the tooth). Abundant calculus that is under the gingiva is often associated with the periodontal abscess. In the context of a

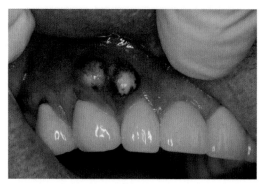

Fig. 23. Two abscesses appearing on the gingiva, each with a draining fistula where the infection originated from the dental neurovascular bundle.

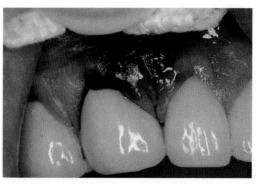

Fig. 24. The abscesses were drained by applying pressure, following administration of local anesthesia.

periodontal abscess, the dental pulp is usually healthy and tests normal because the periodontal infection is localized. Another form of a periodontal abscess emanates from a partially impacted tooth and is called a pericoronal abscess. It is a common occurrence around wisdom teeth or partially erupted teeth with an abundance of over-lying soft tissue. Food debris and bacteria can accumulate under the gingival tissues and cause infection. Oral hygiene is often compromised in these areas and an infection ensues. Patients report pain and swollen submandibular lymph nodes on the affected side, and the gingiva is visibly swollen and red. Purulence may be observed on palpation of the swollen area. The first course of treatment is prescribing broad-spectrum systemic antibiotics (see **Box 6**) and instructing the patient in home care. Irrigation with saline using a plastic syringe with a blunt end is optional and can assist with debris removal and control of the infection. On other occasions, the redundant tissue needs to be surgically removed by a dentist. If the affected tooth is a third molar, tooth extraction may be recommended. In more advanced infections, bacterial infection can spread into fascial spaces and require incision and drainage procedures as well as systemic antibiotic treatment. Infection that occupies the submandibular and submental regions can potentially jeopardize the patient's airway and become life threatening (ie, Ludwig angina). Therefore, it is important to diagnose and treat dental infections. Patients may require hospital admission, serologic evaluation, and consultation/management by an oral and maxillofacial surgeon.

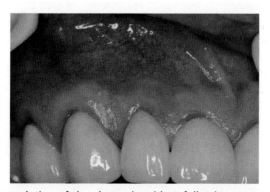

Fig. 25. Complete resolution of the abscess is evident following root canal therapy (endodontic treatment).

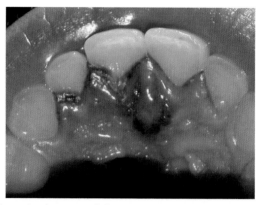

Fig. 26. NUG on the palatal aspect of the incisor teeth characterized by severe swelling, redness, gingival sloughing, and bleeding.

Necrotizing Periodontal Conditions

Necrotizing periodontal gingivitis (formally acute necrotizing ulcerative gingivitis) or periodontitis are acute, ulcerative conditions manifested in the gingiva with the potential to involve the underlying bone. The clinical presentation is pain emanating from the gingiva, necrosis of the interdental papillae (white appearance), as well as swelling and bleeding. It is often related to stress and possible malnutrition. These conditions can be aggravated by immunosuppression.

It is important for clinicians to realize that necrotizing ulcerative gingivitis (NUG) is limited to the soft tissues, whereas necrotizing ulcerative periodontitis (NUP) involves measureable bone loss. However, the necrotic and white soft tissue, oral malodor, the reported symptoms, and acute rapid onset are distinct and considered pathognomonic for NUG (**Figs. 26 and 27**). It is therefore prudent to prescribe systemic broad-spectrum antibiotics (see **Box 6**) and refer to a dentist for further evaluation. The treatment involves localized debridement with local anesthesia. This condition resolves completely in cases of NUG, and with residual bone loss in cases of NUP. The resolution is typically rapid (similar to the onset) and immediate treatment is necessary to minimize irreversible supporting bone damage. When NUG and/or NUP are suspected, clinicians should also rule out systemic diseases, such as human

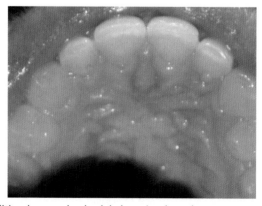

Fig. 27. NUG condition has resolved solely by using broad-spectrum, systemic antibiotics.

immunodeficiency virus/acquired immunodeficiency syndrome, other immunodeficiencies, and malnutrition.

SUMMARY

Common dental diseases can cause orofacial symptoms, loss of function, poor esthetics, and/or tooth damage. Periodontal conditions and diseases affect supporting tissues around the teeth and can lead to eventual tooth loss. Physicians may encounter patients with chronic and acute periodontal conditions, which may be related to local destruction in the oral environment as well as systemic manifestation/dissemination. Proper initial diagnosis, medical work-up to rule out potentially associated systemic disease, treatment, and a timely referral to a dentist are advised when physicians encounter common dental and periodontal conditions in medical practice.

REFERENCES

1. Tanner AC, Mathney JM, Kent RL, et al. Cultivable anaerobic microbiota of severe early childhood caries. J Clin Microbiol 2011;49(4):1464–74.
2. García-Godoy F, Hicks MJ. Maintaining the integrity of the enamel surface: the role of dental biofilm, saliva and preventive agents in enamel demineralization and remineralization. J Am Dent Assoc 2008;139(Suppl):25S–34S.
3. Protecting all children's teeth (PACT): a pediatric oral health training program for physicians. American Academy of Pediatrics Oral Health Initiative; 2014. Available at: http://www2.aap.org/oralhealth/pact/ppt/Caries.ppt. Accessed March 18, 2014.
4. Guideline on caries-risk assessment and management for infants, children, and adolescents. In: American Academy of Pediatric Dentistry clinical guidelines. Reference Manual V 35|NO 6. 2013. Available at: http://www.aapd.org/media/Policies_Guidelines/G_CariesRiskAssessment.pdf. Accessed March 18, 2014.
5. Weyant RJ, Tracy SL, Anselmo TT, et al. Topical fluoride for caries prevention: executive summary of the updated clinical recommendations and supporting systematic review. J Am Dent Assoc 2013;144(11):1279–91.
6. Laudenbach JM. Dental caries. In: Laudenbach JM, Ship JA, editors. American Academy of Oral Medicine clinician's guide to oral health in geriatric patients. 3rd edition. Edmonds (WA): American Academy of Oral Medicine; 2010. p. 10–1.
7. Ramos-Gomez F, Ng MW. Into the future: keeping healthy teeth caries free: pediatric CAMBRA protocols. J Calif Dent Assoc 2011;39(10):723–33.
8. Flynn TR. Principles of management and prevention of odontogenic infections. In: Hupp JR, Ellis E, Tucker MR, editors. Contemporary oral and maxillofacial surgery. 6th edition. St Louis (MO): Elsevier Mosby; 2014. p. 296–318.
9. Flynn TR. Complex odontogenic infections. In: Hupp JR, Ellis E, Tucker MR, editors. Contemporary oral and maxillofacial surgery. 6th edition. St Louis (MO): Elsevier Mosby; 2014. p. 319–33.
10. Harpenau LA, Noble WH, Kao RT. Diagnosis and management of dental wear. J Calif Dent Assoc 2011;39(4):225–31.
11. Noble WH, Donovan TE, Geissberger M. Sports drinks and dental erosion. J Calif Dent Assoc 2011;39(4):233–8.
12. Neville BW, Damm DD, Allen CM, et al. Abnormalities of teeth. In: Neville BW, Damm DD, Allen CM, et al, editors. Oral and maxillofacial pathology. 3rd edition. St Louis (MO): Saunders; 2009. p. 61–5.

13. Goutham BS, Manchanda K, Sarkar AD, et al. Efficacy of two commercially available Oral Rinses - Chlorohexidine and Listrine on Plaque and Gingivitis - A Comparative Study. J Int Oral Health 2013;5(4):56–61.

14. Addy M. Chlorhexidine compared with other locally delivered antimicrobials. A short review [review]. J Clin Periodontol 1986;13(10):957–64.

15. Zanatta FB, Antoniazzi RP, Rösing CK. The effect of 0.12% chlorhexidine gluconate rinsing on previously plaque-free and plaque-covered surfaces: a randomized, controlled clinical trial. J Periodontol 2007;78(11):2127–34.

16. Galván M, Gonzalez S, Cohen CL, et al. Periodontal effects of 0.25% sodium hypochlorite twice-weekly oral rinse. A pilot study. J Periodontal Res 2013. http://dx.doi.org/10.1111/jre.12151.

17. De Nardo R, Chiappe V, Gómez M, et al. Effects of 0.05% sodium hypochlorite oral rinse on supragingival biofilm and gingival inflammation. Int Dent J 2012; 62(4):208–12.

18. Haffajee AD, Socransky SS. Microbial etiological agents of destructive periodontal diseases. Periodontol 2000 1994;5:78–111.

19. Persson GR, Yeates J, Persson RE, et al. The impact of a low-frequency chlorhexidine rinsing schedule on the subgingival microbiota (the TEETH clinical trial). J Periodontol 2007;78(9):1751–8.

20. Walker C, Karpinia K. Rationale for use of antibiotics in periodontics. J Periodontol 2002;73(10):1188–96.

21. Slots J. Low-cost periodontal therapy. Periodontol 2000 2012;60(1):110–37.

22. Zandbergen D, Slot DE, Cobb CM, et al. The clinical effect of scaling and root planing and the concomitant administration of systemic amoxicillin and metronidazole: a systematic review. J Periodontol 2013;84(3):332–51.

23. Newman MG, Sims TN. The predominant cultivable microbiota of the periodontal abscess. J Periodontol 1979;50(7):350–4.

24. Hafström CA, Wikström MB, Renvert SN, et al. Effect of treatment on some periodontopathogens and their antibody levels in periodontal abscesses. J Periodontol 1994;65(11):1022–8.

Common Dental and Orofacial Trauma
Evaluation and Management

Prem B. Patel, DMD, MD*, David C. Stanton, DMD, MD, FACS,
Eric J. Granquist, DMD, MD*

KEYWORDS

- Dental trauma • Facial wounds • Maxillofacial trauma

KEY POINTS

- Preservation and restoration of normal function and normal aesthetics is of paramount importance in the treatment of orofacial and dental trauma.
- Injuries can be limited to the soft tissue, or be complex multisystem trauma; however, the fundamental approach and goals are the same.
- Consideration of the basic principles discussed in this article will help promote successful outcomes and patient satisfaction when managing trauma to the head and face.

COMMON DENTAL AND OROFACIAL TRAUMATIC INJURIES ENCOUNTERED BY THE GENERAL PHYSICIAN

Fundamental abilities such as vision, speech, mastication, and respiration, in addition to appearance, can be affected by traumatic injuries to the head and face; therefore, a primary goal is to preserve and restore normal function and aesthetics. As with any traumatic injury, the patient must be assessed according to Advanced Trauma Life Support guidelines before receiving oral and maxillofacial surgery care. Life-threatening problems involving the maxillofacial region may be encountered, such as excessive bleeding and airway compromise, and should be promptly addressed.[1] The neck should be temporarily immobilized until cervical spine injuries have been ruled out. Once the patient is stabilized, it is important to obtain an adequate history and a mechanism of injury for proper evaluation and management. A focused Head, Ears, Eyes, Nose, Throat (HEENT) examination and neurologic examination are especially important in head and facial injuries. Any significant neurologic change from baseline warrants immediate assessment and management.

Department of Oral and Maxillofacial Surgery, Hospital of the University of Pennsylvania, University of Pennsylvania, 5th Floor White Building, Philadelphia, PA 19104, USA
* Corresponding authors.
E-mail addresses: Prem.Patel@uphs.upenn.edu; Eric.Granquist@uphs.upenn.edu

Med Clin N Am 98 (2014) 1261–1279
http://dx.doi.org/10.1016/j.mcna.2014.08.003
0025-7125/14/$ – see front matter Published by Elsevier Inc.
medical.theclinics.com

Soft-Tissue Injuries

Facial soft-tissue injuries are common, and can vary considerably in type and severity. Because soft-tissue injuries can be associated with more extensive underlying trauma, a thorough physical examination should be performed.[2] In general, soft-tissue injuries can be subdivided into abrasions, contusions, lacerations, and avulsions. Specific considerations and treatment depend on anatomic location of injury.

Abrasions

Description An abrasion is a wound caused by superficial damage to the skin, usually limited to the epidermis, but may occasionally involve the dermis. Patients may also present with mucosal abrasions inside the mouth. Abrasions occur as a result of friction between exposed skin and an object, such as scraping. Abrasions demonstrate denuded epithelium and can be painful because they may involve terminal nerve fiber endings; however, bleeding is usually minor. Abrasions that involve and extend into the subcutaneous layer are considered avulsions.

Treatment The abraded area should be cleansed thoroughly with saline irrigation to remove foreign debris. Local anesthetics and, possibly, a scrub brush may be required for deeper abrasions. Topical antibiotic ointment to keep the wound moist with an optional bandage is sufficient, and topical anesthetics may be applied for pain control. Systemic antibiotics are usually not indicated, and nonprescription pain medications may be used based on severity of symptoms. Intraoral mucosal abrasions usually require no treatment besides routine oral hygiene. Within a week, superficial epidermal abrasions will usually scab and reepithelialize without scarring. Abrasions that extend into deeper tissues will likely result in scar formation. For deep abrasions with the potential for significant soft-tissue deformity or questionable involvement of other structures in proximity, referral to a maxillofacial surgeon is recommended.

Contusions

Description A contusion, commonly referred to as a bruise, is a hematoma of the tissue without a break in the surface. Contusions occur by physical compression from blunt trauma. Contusions may appear to be simply a soft-tissue hemorrhage; however, examination for any underlying osseous and dentoalveolar injuries is warranted.

Treatment Contusions will usually self-resolve. Ice or pressure dressings can help decrease swelling. The body will resorb the hematoma over time, and during the healing process the bruise may change colors, appear to spread, and mistakenly appear worse. One must be wary of systemic symptoms, which may indicate more serious underlying injury or infection. Because contusions generally resolve on their own, referral is not necessary unless the hematoma is expanding, in which case emergent surgical intervention may be required.

Lacerations

Description Any tear in the soft tissue (skin or mucosa) is considered a laceration (**Fig. 1**). Skin lacerations are very common. Lacerations result from sharp-edged objects, such as a knife, razor, or glass, but also from underlying bony fractures. Lacerations may appear linear, jagged, or stellate depending on the mechanism of injury. Damage to deeper structures (based on anatomic location), such as nerves, vessels, ducts, muscles, and glands, should be ruled out.

Treatment Treatment of lacerations will vary based on depth and location of the laceration (eg, skin, mouth, ear, eyelid, lips), but similar principles apply to the initial

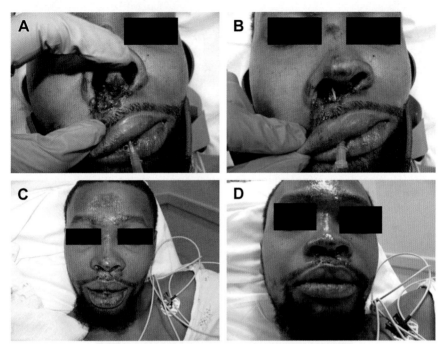

Fig. 1. (*A*) Laceration of the upper lip and base of nose. (*B*) angiocatheter demonstrating communication of the laceration with the oral cavity. This through-and-through laceration requires layered closure of the oral mucosa, muscle, and skin. (*C, D*) Closure of laceration demonstrating tension-free closure of the skin and wound reapproximation. Note the application of petroleum ointment the abrasions and laceration. Photographs *courtesy of Dr Diamantis, Lowell MA.*

treatment. The area should be thoroughly cleansed with copious saline irrigation to remove foreign debris. Local anesthetics and, possibly, a scrub brush may be required. Any notable devitalized tissue should be debrided. Ensure hemostasis before closure. Small lacerations may only require adhesive rather than sutures. If sutures are needed, determine if layered closure is appropriate, and assure proper positioning of the tissue and anatomic landmarks. Lacerations should be closed from the inside out. For example, a through-and-through laceration of the lip should be closed in the following order: (1) oral mucosa first to seal off the oral flora; (2) muscle tissue; (3) subcutaneous tissue; (4) skin. Some grossly contaminated wounds may be left partially open to allow for potential drainage. Different types of sutures, such as resorbable versus nonresorbable, may be used based on clinician preference and tissue layer involved. Resorbable sutures are ideal for intraoral lacerations and lacerations in children to help avoid a second procedure for suture removal. Nonresorbable sutures are often used on the face for improved cosmetic results. Most facial skin sutures will require removal after 5 to 7 days. Topical antibiotic ointment may be used to keep the wound moist, and systemic antibiotics may be needed in deep lacerations and certain lacerations communicating with the oral cavity. Appropriate wound care should be discussed, and the patient's tetanus status should be up to date. Many lacerations on the face will exhibit surrounding erythema, which will gradually fade over time. Although most lacerations will lead to a scar, proper closure can significantly improve cosmetic results. Deep lacerations, lacerations in close

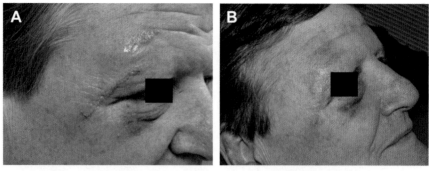

Fig. 2. (A) Laceration repaired with nonresorbable suture. Note slight eversion of the skin edges. (B) Wound following suture removable. Nonresorbable sutures are removed between 5 and 7 days after repair.

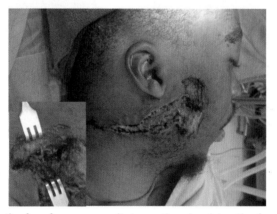

Fig. 3. Wound to the face from an assault. Lacerations involving the face posterior to the lateral canthus of the eye and anterior to the auricle require evaluation of the facial nerve before repair. This patient suffered transection of the facial nerve, which required exploration and primary anastomosis (inset).

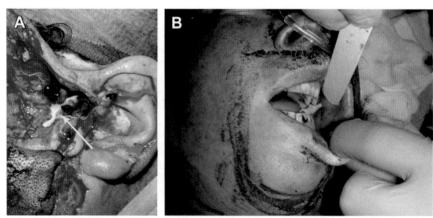

Fig. 4. (A) Laceration of the face involving the malar region required evaluation of Stenson duct. (B) Integrity of the Stenson duct can be evaluated by cannulating the duct and injecting a sterile agent. Here, propofol is used because it is sterile, easily identified in the soft tissue, and readily available in the operating room. Note extravasation of propofol into the soft tissue (arrow in A), suggesting laceration or transection of the duct that requires repair.

proximity to important neurovascular or ductal structures, inadequate hemostasis, and underlying osseous or complex dentoalveolar injuries should be referred, as thorough surgical intervention may be required. Lacerations involving the eyelid, vermilion border of the lip, or ear warrant appropriate referral for evaluation and treatment (**Figs. 2–4**).

Soft-tissue avulsions

Description An injury in which a structure is forcibly detached from its normal point of insertion is an avulsion. With regard to soft-tissue injury, an avulsion is an extensive abrasion involving all layers of the skin. Avulsions commonly occur with motor vehicle accidents, bites, and falls. Avulsion injuries to the face can involve many structures including the skin, ears, eyelids, lips, and teeth, all of which will lead to exposure of underlying structures. Pain and bleeding are usually present.

Treatment Initial management of avulsions consists of hemostatic control with direct pressure and alleviation of pain, followed by copious saline irrigation to help determine the severity of the injury. Minor avulsions can be treated like abrasions, although sutures may be required. More significant avulsion injuries should be appropriately referred. Avulsed structures should be handled in a clean manner (avoid cleaning the avulsed segment) and wrapped in gauze, then placed in a plastic bag surrounded by ice. Direct contact with ice may cause tissue damage. Relevant information for management includes tetanus status, information regarding the animal in the case of bite injuries, and time of avulsion. Avulsions will generally result in scar formation. Depending on the severity, soft-tissue deformity can result and reconstructive surgery may be required. Most avulsions will require referral to a maxillofacial surgeon. Immediate referrals can help improve prognosis, especially with potential reattachment of avulsed segments.

Dentoalveolar Injuries

Dentoalveolar refers to the teeth and their associated soft and hard tissues, including the gingiva and alveolar sockets of the maxilla and mandible (**Fig. 5**).[3] Dentoalveolar injuries can result from many types of trauma, such as falls, fights, sporting injuries, motor vehicle accidents, and abuse. Direct and indirect injury to the teeth can be associated with soft-tissue injuries, and may lead to considerable pain and anxiety. Also noteworthy is that with any dentoalveolar injury, specifically tooth fractures and tooth

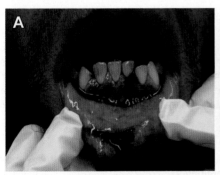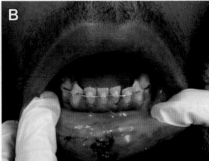

Fig. 5. (*A*) Dentoalveolar fracture. Note the laceration of gingiva and malposition of multiple teeth. (*B*) Bony segment repositioned and stabilized with a splint. These splints are required to be in place until bone union has occurred (typically 4–6 weeks).

avulsions, aspiration can occur, and a chest radiograph should be performed if clinically indicated. Dental injuries can involve any teeth, but the anterior teeth are most commonly involved and are of primary concern to patients for reasons of aesthetics. Primary teeth and permanent teeth are often managed similarly; however, any differences will be discussed. It is usually the lack of cooperation from a child that results in treatment compromises (ie, extraction of teeth).

Proper and timely assessment, diagnosis, and management can significantly affect outcomes. Many dentoalveolar injuries will require a referral to a dentist or dental specialist, who have expertise in treating these injuries and also the access to radiographs to aid in diagnosis. However, it is important for the physician to recognize how these injuries should be managed, and to be able to discuss expectations and goals with patients. Most dentoalveolar injuries will require commitment from patients, such as adhering to a soft diet, maintaining good oral hygiene, avoidance of additional trauma, and serial follow-up examinations. Also required is an understanding that some treatment modalities may not be successful or that more extensive dental treatment may subsequently be required, such as root canal therapy and/or extraction. For example, it is important that patients understand that even though the natural tooth may be saved, root canal therapy may be required at a later time.

Crown fracture

Description Crown fractures, which affect the coronal portion of the teeth, can be limited to the enamel or involve the dentin and/or the pulp.

Treatment The depth of the tooth fracture primarily dictates the treatment of crown fractures. Fractures involving only the enamel do not require acute treatment or, indeed, any treatment. A simple enamel smoothing may be all that is required. Deeper fractures into the enamel or into the dentin will likely require restorative treatment and referral to a dentist.[4] Crown fractures extending into the pulp will require special restorative materials and possibly root canal therapy, and should be referred to a dentist or endodontist (root canal specialist). In general, the deeper the tooth injury, the sooner a patient should be seen in an attempt to maintain pulp vitality. Typically in the primary dentition exposed pulp often leads to extraction, but pediatric dentists may be able to provide alternative treatments to help the patient retain the affected primary tooth.

Crown-root fracture

Description Crown-root fractures involve both the crown and root of the tooth, but may or may not involve the pulp.

Treatment Fractures that do not involve the pulp and do not extend far apically into the root may be restorable by a dentist. If the pulp is involved and the fracture is limited, root canal therapy by a dentist or endodontist will likely be required. Fractures that extend far into the root will require extraction by a dentist or oral surgeon. On occasion, if the crown-root fracture deems the tooth nonrestorable and there is also a bony alveolus fracture, the removal of the tooth can be delayed for several weeks to allow the bony fracture to heal.[5]

Root fracture

Description Root fractures involve the root or roots of the teeth. Clinically these may be difficult to detect without radiologic examination.

Treatment Treatment is based on the level of root fracture and the willingness and commitment of the patient. Root fractures situated near the crown may be restored with root canal therapy, post and core, and a crown. Root fractures located in the middle to apical third of the root may be properly repositioned, if needed, and immobilized for 2 to 4 months in hopes that the fracture will heal. Apical root fractures will likely involve removal of the tooth; however, the apical fragment may be left in the socket to resorb physiologically and/or avoid alveolus damage with surgical extraction.

Tooth concussion
Description Tooth concussion is sensitivity of the teeth to touch or percussion without tooth mobility or displacement.

Treatment In general, no acute treatment is necessary for tooth concussion. Symptomatic relief may be possible by relieving occlusal contact off the sensitive tooth via enameloplasty on the opposing tooth. Periodic follow-up examinations by a dentist are recommended.

Tooth subluxation
Description Subluxation is tooth mobility or looseness without tooth displacement.

Treatment The level of tooth mobility will dictate treatment. Minimally mobile teeth can be treated similarly to tooth concussion with occlusal contact relief. Significantly mobile teeth will likely require splinting and immobilization, applied by a dentist, for 7 to 10 days.

Tooth displacement
Description Teeth can be displaced in any direction, most commonly in a buccal-lingual direction but also in a mesiodistal direction, and may also be intruded (displacement into the socket) or extruded (displacement out of the socket). Tooth displacements may likely involve alveolar wall fractures.

Treatment Prognosis and treatments vary depending on the direction of displacement.

Labial, palatal/lingual, and lateral displacement These displacements are more common and more likely to be associated with alveolar bone fractures. Regardless of the direction of displacement, the teeth will require manual repositioning along with splinting and immobilization for about 2 weeks. Concurrent alveolar bone fractures will also need to be repositioned and similarly splinted and immobilized for approximately 4–6 weeks to allow for osseous healing. Significant gingival lacerations should be copiously irrigated and sutured. Antibiotics for approximately 7 days are often advised for significant bony and soft-tissue injury. Multiple tooth displacements with significant alveolar bone fractures may necessitate referral to an oral and maxillofacial surgeon (OMFS).

Intrusion Intrusions usually involve the maxillary teeth. Occasionally the intrusion may be so severe that the tooth appears to be missing. Intrusions tend to have the worst prognosis. Treatment is somewhat controversial, and affected patients should be referred and managed on a case-by-case basis. Some clinicians suggest surgical repositioning and splinting, some recommend leaving intruded teeth alone and allowing them to reerupt, and others favor immediate orthodontic forces to aid in reeruption and prevent tooth-to-bone ankylosis. With regard to intruded deciduous (primary) teeth, proximity and involvement of the associated succedaneous (permanent) tooth/follicle are important, with the primary goal of ensuring the health of the succedaneous tooth. If there is no disruption to the succedaneous tooth/follicle, the deciduous tooth may be observed and allowed to reerupt. However, if there is disruption or any doubt, the deciduous tooth should be atraumatically extracted.

Extrusion Extruded teeth can generally be pushed back into the appropriate position within their sockets, and will require splinting and immobilization for about 2 weeks. Because of disruption of the dental nerves and vessels at the apical foramen, these teeth will likely need subsequent root canal therapy.

Tooth avulsion

Description Tooth avulsion is a complete displacement of the tooth out from its alveolar socket; hence, pulpal health and periodontal health may be significantly compromised.

Treatment The prognosis for avulsed teeth can vary greatly depending on many factors, including out-of-alveolus (extra-alveolar) time, the current periodontal state, the presence of large dental restorations, alveolar socket disruption, gross contamination, and the method of preservation before reimplantation. Deciduous (primary) avulsed teeth generally should not be reimplanted. Patients should be advised and appropriately guided before clinical evaluation.

Extra-alveolar time The goal is to reimplant the avulsed tooth as soon as possible. Teeth reimplanted within 20 minutes have the best prognosis.[6] Out-of-alveolus time exceeding 2 hours often has poor results.[7]

Preservation and handling Patients should be promptly directed on how to handle and preserve the avulsed tooth to improve prognosis. The tooth should only be handled by the crown and not by the root, because the periodontal ligament (PDL) cells on the root surface must remain vital for successful reimplantation. The tooth should gently be rinsed (not scrubbed or brushed) with the best available medium to free the tooth of any gross debris. Many storage and cleansing mediums exist, of which the most ideal are Hanks balanced salt solution (HBSS) or saline solution. However, these solutions may not be available unless the patient is in a school or ambulance. The best accessible medium is milk, which has been shown to maintain vitality of the PDL cells.[8] The patient's saliva (keeping the tooth in vestibule of the mouth) is the next best medium, although this maneuver is not recommended if there is concern for a head injury, or difficulty with protecting the airway as it may pose an aspiration risk. Water is the least recommended medium owing to its hypotonicity, causing PDL cell lysis. Once gently rinsed, the patient should attempt to reimplant the tooth into its socket and hold it in place while en route to the dentist or emergency room. If the tooth cannot be placed into the socket, it should be placed in the best available medium until care is available.

Clinical evaluation If the patient arrives with the tooth in an appropriate position, it should be radiographed (if possible) and splinted in place. If the patient arrives with a tooth that has been out of alveolus for longer than 20 minutes regardless of the preserving medium, the tooth should be placed in HBSS for 30 minutes and then in doxycycline (1 mg/20 mL saline) for 5 minutes. This solution inhibits bacteria and seems to reduce ankylosis. Certain avulsed teeth may not be appropriate or favorable for reimplantation, such as in patients with advanced periodontal disease, severely crowded teeth, significant alveolar socket disruption, and large dental restorations.

Stabilization Reimplanted teeth can be stabilized via acrylic, wire and composite, arch bars, interdental wiring, and splints in an attempt to recreate the patient's prior occlusion. Wire (orthodontic wire or even a paperclip) and composite (acid-etched composite system) is most often used for stabilization, owing to ease of application and removal and the ability of patients to cleanse easily. Stabilization need not be absolutely rigid, as some physiologic movement promotes fibrous attachment and prevents osseous ankylosis. In general, splinting 1 or 2 teeth on either side of the reimplanted tooth is sufficient. The duration of stabilization depends on the maturity of the avulsed tooth. Mature teeth (complete root formation, small apical foramen) should be immobilized for 7 to 10 days. Immature teeth (incomplete root formation, wide apical foramen) should be immobilized for 3 to 4 weeks because of the more favorable prognosis for pulpal survival and revascularization.

Adjuvant treatment Antibiotics directed against oral flora (ie, penicillin, clindamycin) are usually appropriate for 7 to 10 days. Also, one must confirm that the patient is up to date with his or her tetanus booster. Regular and frequent follow-up will be required. Patients must adhere to a soft diet and maintain good oral hygiene to minimize the inflammatory response.

Expected outcomes Patients should be advised that reimplantation will likely require future root canal therapy, which may not always be successful. Root resorption, ankylosis, infection, tooth mobility, occlusal differences, and loss of the tooth can occur.[9] However, whenever feasible, an attempt should be made to salvage the natural tooth. Some patients may prefer to avoid reimplantation and later proceed with other dental treatment, such as a partial denture or dental implant.

Alveolar bone fracture
Description Alveolar bone fractures involve injury to the alveolar process in the presence or absence of teeth. These fractures usually are accompanied by other injuries such as tooth displacement, crown fractures, root fractures, and soft-tissue injuries.

Treatment The goal of treatment of alveolar process fractures is proper repositioning and stabilization. Repositioning may be accomplished manually or may require surgical manipulation with the help of an OMFS. Immobilization for 4–6 weeks to facilitate osseous healing will be required by wire splint, acrylic splint, or arch bar ligation. Copious irrigation and soft-tissue suturing should be performed as appropriate (**Fig. 5**).

Orofacial Bony Injuries

Orofacial trauma can result in a wide range of injuries, from mild soft-tissue and dentoalveolar injuries to significant facial bony fractures (**Fig. 6**). The major components of the maxillofacial skeleton affected in trauma include the orbital complex, nasal bones, nasoorbital-ethmoid (NOE) complex, zygomaticomaxillary complex (ZMC), maxilla, and mandible.[10] Facial fractures can occur through any trauma significant enough to cause skeletal compromise. Falls, altercations, sporting injuries, motor vehicle accidents, work-related injuries, and abuse are the more common mechanisms of injury to the face.[11]

Trauma patients should be immediately assessed and treated for critical life-threatening emergencies. Once stabilized, a thorough history and physical examination should be performed. Physical evaluation should include a thorough HEENT and neurologic examination, keeping in mind the underlying structures that may be affected. Many of these patients will require radiologic evaluation and likely an OMFS consult. Imaging should be obtained to confirm clinical findings and determine the extent of injury. The OMFS can recommend which studies may be indicated, such

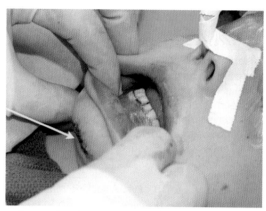

Fig. 6. A pediatric patient with a fracture involving the temporomandibular joint. Note the laceration to the chin (*arrow*). A laceration to the chin and malocclusion is suggestive of a fracture of the mandible, and requires imaging.

as (1) plain films with multiple views, (2) panoramic films, and/or (3) noncontrast computed tomography (CT) scans with or without 3-dimensional reconstruction.[12] In general, a noncontrast head CT is usually performed to rule out neurologic injury, and can therefore include a maxillofacial CT to access the facial skeleton as well. If CT of the head is not warranted, clinical history, clinical examination, and hospital capabilities should dictate additional imaging. In general, midface (maxilla, zygoma, NOE, and the temporomandibular joint) injuries warrant dedicated CT imaging. Suspected fractures of the mandible may be evaluated with an orthopantomogram (if available) or mandible series (plain films).[13]

Fractures can be classified in different ways depending on the specific bone involved. All fractures can be divided into open or closed fractures. Closed fractures are those whereby the skin and mucosa remain intact. Open fractures are those whereby the fracture is in communication with the external or oral environment. In maxillofacial injuries, external environment communication can exist through mucosal and skin lacerations, gingival tears, and sinus lining communication. Any jaw fracture within a tooth-bearing segment is considered an open fracture. Open fractures carry higher risks of infection; therefore, antibiotics are usually warranted. Other considerations in fracture classification are the displacement and angulation of the fractured segments.

Certain facial emergencies require immediate attention, including loss of airway, retrobulbar hematomas, and nasal septal hematomas. Given that most facial fractures are not emergent surgical cases, treatment can be delayed or postponed for several days in lieu of other nonfacial injuries that require earlier intervention or until facial swelling improves. Certain fractures may not require surgical repair, or patients may choose to avoid repair if no functional or cosmetic deformity exists. Discussions should be held with the patient regarding benefits, risks, and complications with and without repair.[14] Patients should be informed that many jaw fractures will require nutritional modifications (full liquid or soft diet) for several weeks. Many mandible fractures will also involve periods of intermaxillary fixation (wired jaw), which may require changes in the delivery of common medications (tablet-to-liquid). Fractures involving the sinuses will require patients to adhere to sinus precautions (no nose blowing, open mouth sneezing and coughing, no sucking, no straws, no smoking) for at least 2 weeks.

General goals of therapy for most facial fractures are to restore normal function (ocular, nasal, and masticatory), obtain stable occlusion, regain full range of motion, restore speech, prevent growth disturbances, and maintain aesthetics. Basic fracture repair principles include proper and adequate anatomic reduction, fixation for bony immobilization, and minimization of adverse effects. Surgical approaches for facial fractures vary, although many can be modified to use existing soft-tissue injuries. Bony fracture repair should generally precede soft-tissue injury repair, although this depends on the timing of fracture treatment. If fracture repair will be delayed, one should proceed with soft-tissue repair.

Orbital fractures

Description Orbital complex fractures may include fractures of the medial and lateral orbital walls, orbital roof and floor, and orbital rim. Clinical findings may include maxillary (midface) V2 paresthesia, periorbital edema, subconjunctival hemorrhage, diplopia, and impaired extraocular movements (**Fig. 7**). Direct orbital trauma can cause visual acuity and pupillary changes, but these signs and symptoms can also signify intracranial trauma and bleeding, in which case consultation with Neurosurgery should be considered. Irregular, asymmetric pupils can be caused by globe rupture, and Ophthalmology should be consulted as necessary.

Treatment Orbital fracture repair is usually indicated with enopthalmus greater than 2 mm, diplopia, floor defect greater than 1 cm, and ophthalmoplegia. Orbital floor and wall treatment involves restoring original orbital volume using autogenous grafts or alloplastic materials.[15] Orbital rim fractures can be repaired via internal fixation. Several surgical approaches exist, including transconjunctival, subciliary, subtarsal, and infraorbital. Patients with orbital fractures in communication with the sinuses should be advised to follow sinus precautions.

Retrobulbar hematoma Although rare, a retrobulbar hematoma is an emergency and presents following blunt orbital trauma. It occurs from bleeding posterior to the globe that can increase intraocular pressure (IOP) and result in vascular damage to the optic nerve. Irreversible blindness can occur within 2 hours if not treated.[16] Clinical findings may include proptosis, chemosis, change or loss of vision, increased IOP, ophthalmoplegia, and severe pain. Diagnosis can be made by clinical presentation of superior orbital fissure syndrome (loss of forehead sensation, loss of corneal reflex, ptosis, fixed dilated pupil, and exophthalmos) or orbital apex syndrome (superior orbital fissure syndrome plus visual changes from optic nerve involvement), ophthalmic tonometry, and thin-sectioned CT scan. Therapy is based on orbital decompression via lateral canthotomy under local anesthesia. Scissors are used to carefully dissect between the eyelids laterally down to the orbital rim and lateral fornix. The lateral canthus is then identified and released.

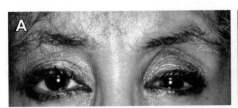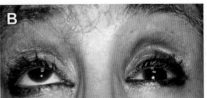

Fig. 7. (A) A patient with fracture of the left orbital floor and muscle entrapment. (B) The patient demonstrates entrapment of the extraocular muscle (inferior rectus). Note the lack of upward gaze of the left eye.

Nasal fractures

Description Nasal bone fractures are generally diagnosed by physical examination. Clinical findings may include nasal edema, ecchymosis, epistaxis, septal deviation, mobility, crepitus, and nasal deformity. CT scans and plain films may be useful for further evaluation.

Treatment Nasal fracture repair is optimal within 1 to 2 days; however, if treatment within this time frame is not possible, waiting 7 to 10 days is recommended to allow for resolution of soft-tissue swelling. After swelling resolution, patients may choose not to undergo repair if no functional or cosmetic deformity exists. If repair is desired, most nasal fractures can be treated via closed reduction with a nasal splint for 5 to 7 days and intranasal packing for 2 to 3 days. Open reduction may be required with compound fractures or with nasal bones or septa that cannot be reduced with a closed technique.[17]

Septal hematoma A septal hematoma is an emergency and can occasionally accompany nasal trauma. Clinical findings may include bulging of the nasal septal tissue, pain, and airflow obstruction. If a septal hematoma is present, it must be evacuated to prevent underlying cartilage necrosis. Evacuation can be performed under local anesthesia and a large-bore needle or blade to create dependent drainage. Nasal compression packing should be placed to prevent reformation of a hematoma.

Nasoorbital-ethmoid fractures

Description NOE fractures can be determined by physical examination alone, but CT imaging may be beneficial. The condition of the medial canthal tendon (MCT) is an important structural consideration, and its status can be assessed via maneuvers such as the Bowstring test. This test involves lateral pull on the eyelid with a gloved digit, which should result in the medial canthus angle becoming more acute. No change in the angle of the medial canthus or lateral movement suggests a fracture of the underlying bone or avulsion of the tendon. Clinical findings may include loss of nasal projection, periorbital ecchymosis, epistaxis, telecanthus, visual disturbance, and cerebrospinal fluid (CSF) leak. The classification of NOE fractures is based on the attachment of the MCT to the bone and the status of the bone.[18] In type I NOE, the MCT is attached to a large bony segment without comminution. Type II NOE is a comminuted fracture with the MCT still attached to the bone. Type III NOE is a severely comminuted fracture with detachment of the MCT from the bone.

Treatment Treatment options for NOE fractures are closed reduction, open reduction with internal fixation, or transnasal canthopexy. Multiple surgical approaches exist, such as via lower eyelid, coronal, transcaruncular, or proceeding through an existing laceration.[19]

Zygomaticomaxillary complex fractures

Description All ZMC fractures involve the orbital floor, as opposed to an isolated zygomatic arch fracture. Clinical findings may include loss of cheek projection, step deformity, trismus, chemosis, and periorbital edema (**Fig. 8**). Maxillofacial CT is useful to detail the extent of the fracture. For isolated zygomatic arch fractures, a submental vertex view is usually sufficient.

Treatment ZMC fractures should be surgically repaired when there is trismus, significant displacement, and loss of malar projection. If no functional or cosmetic deficit exists, surgery usually is not indicated. Multiple surgical approaches exist, such as

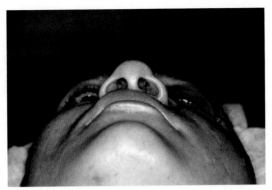

Fig. 8. Worm's-eye view of a patient with a fracture of the zygoma and associated structures. Note the lack of projection of the left malar region.

via intraoral vestibule, lower eyelid, upper eyelid, Gillies (preauricular), coronal, or transcaruncular.[20]

Maxillary fractures

Description Maxillary fractures can be divided into LeFort I, II, and III, depending on the extent of the midfacial fractures.[21] LeFort I fractures extend horizontally through the maxillary sinuses and nasal floor, separating the maxilla from the pterygoid plates, zygoma, and nasal structures. LeFort II fractures extend across the nasal bones and septum and involve the medial orbital wall and inferior orbital rim, separating the maxilla and attached nasal complex from the orbital and zygomatic structures. LeFort III fractures extend more superiorly and involve both the medial and lateral orbital walls, resulting in complete midface dysjunction and separation of the NOE complex and ZMC from the cranial base. Clinical findings may include malocclusion, maxillary and midface mobility, edema, orbital ecchymosis, and potential CSF leaks. Maxillofacial CT with thin sections is the recommended imaging study.

Treatment Maxillary LeFort fractures are usually treated with open reduction and internal fixation.[22] Maxillomandibular fixation (MMF) may be required for fracture reduction. Patients should be instructed to follow sinus precautions and to maintain a soft diet.

Mandibular fractures

Description The anatomic distribution of mandibular fractures is based on injury type, force, and direction of trauma (**Figs. 9–11**). Mandibular fractures occur in multiple locations, the most common of which are the condyle (29.1%), angle (24.5%), symphysis (22%), and body (16%).[23] Mandibular fractures can also be classified as greenstick (incomplete fracture with flexible bone), simple (complete transection), comminuted (multiple fractured segments), and compound (open to external or oral environment) fractures. These fractures can also be referred to as favorable (muscle pull resists displacement) or unfavorable (muscle pull results in displacement) based on vector of muscle pull.[24] Clinical examination findings may include malocclusion, trismus, jaw deviation, jaw segment mobility, step defects, mandibular V3 and mental nerve paresthesia, pain, gingival lacerations, ecchymosis, and tooth mobility. In children, one should assess for condylar fractures when a patient presents with chin lacerations. Panoramic radiographs are the imaging modality of choice if available, although CT can also be performed (**Figs. 12–14**).

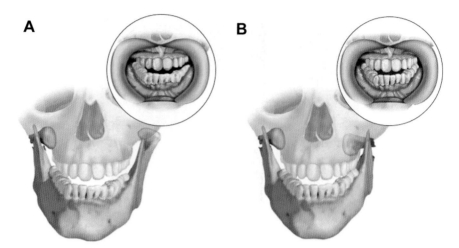

Fig. 9. (*A*) Unilateral fracture of the subcondylar region of the mandible. Physical findings (*inset*) will include premature contact of the posterior teeth on the ipsilateral side of the fracture. (*B*) Bilateral subcondylar fractures of the mandible. Patients often present with new anterior open bite of the dental occlusion (*inset*).

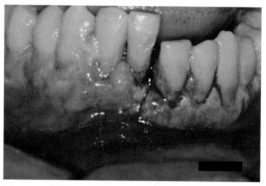

Fig. 10. Fracture of the mandible. Note the laceration of the gingiva and abrupt "step-off" in the occlusion or level of the teeth.

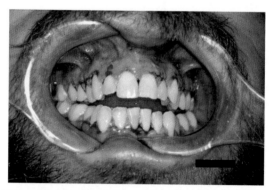

Fig. 11. New anterior open bite. Note the wear on the front teeth suggesting previous contact. This appearance suggests a bilateral subcondylar fracture (see **Fig. 7**B).

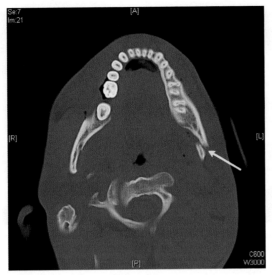

Fig. 12. Axial computed tomography (CT) demonstrating a left angle fracture of the mandible (*arrow*).

Treatment Mandibular fractures can be treated via open or closed reduction. Closed reduction entails MMF for approximately 2 to 6 weeks. Shorter fixation times are common for younger patients and noncomplex condylar fractures. Closed reduction can be achieved in several ways with arch bars, IMF (intermaxillary fixation) screws, Ivey loops, and gunning splints (prostheses for edentulous patients). Open reduction entails surgical incisions via a variety of approaches including intraoral, submandibular, retromandibular, preauricular, and face lift. Open reduction is indicated for unstable or

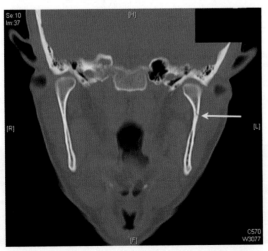

Fig. 13. Coronal CT of a patient with a nondisplaced subcondylar fracture of the mandible (*arrow*). This fracture can often be treated with a short period (2 weeks) of maxillomandibular fixation.

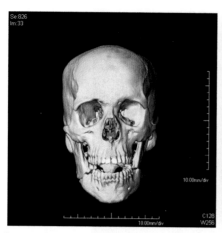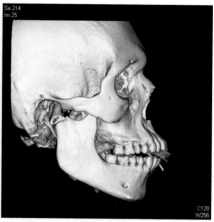

Fig. 14. Three-dimensional reconstructions showing fractures of the mandible. Such reconstructions are often used for surgical planning.

unfavorable fractures, panfacial fractures, patients who cannot tolerate MMF, and complex condylar fractures.[25] Patients should be educated on diet modifications, especially with MMF and fractures not requiring treatment (**Fig. 15**).

Temporomandibular Joint Trauma

Any trauma to the mandible can direct the force of impact to either or both temporomandibular joints (TMJs). Falls on the chin, fists to the mandible, sporting injuries, motor vehicle accidents, and even dental treatment and/or oral surgery can all cause TMJ trauma. Clinical findings may include TMJ pain, limited range of motion, trismus, clicking, popping, or locking. Most acute trauma patients will likely have a CT scan to identify head and facial bony injuries. Fractures are treated as described previously.

Alternatively, isolated TMJ pain after trauma should be treated conservatively, and does not immediately warrant extensive imaging.[26] Panorex imaging can be useful to help rule out any referred pain elicited from dentoalveolar trauma. Management of TMJ trauma includes reassurance, moist heat, jaw rest (no gum chewing, bracing yawns, avoiding foods requiring wide opening), soft diet, nonsteroidal anti-inflammatories (if tolerable), and possibly a short course of steroids. Prolonged and worsening TMJ pain for several weeks warrants referral to an OMFS, who can better aid in classifying and diagnosing the TMJ symptoms, assist in appropriate imaging, and recommend further therapy including occlusal splints or surgical interventions.

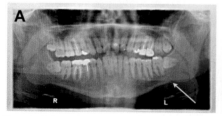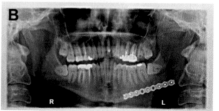

Fig. 15. (A) Preoperative Panorex of a patient with a fracture of the left mandibular body (arrow). (B) Postoperative film following open reduction and internal fixation of the fracture.

Physical Abuse

Physical, sexual, or child abuse can result in orofacial and dental trauma, and thorough craniofacial and intraoral examinations should be performed and documented. Physicians are obligated to report suspected cases of abuse to social services or law enforcement agencies, which can help prevent escalation of abuse. Accidental and unintentional injuries do occur and must be carefully distinguished from abuse. If the patient's history, mechanism of injury, and timing are inconsistent, and if there are multiple injuries and/or injuries in different stages of healing, there should be increased suspicion for abuse.[27] Physical abuse can generally result in any soft-tissue, dentoalveolar, or bony injury.

Head, face, and neck injuries occur in 50% to 85% of cases of physical child abuse.[28] Common orofacial injuries include fractured teeth, frenulum tears, burns and lacerations, bruising of the pharynx, and facial bony fractures. In children, commonly used items for abuse are utensils, forced baby bottles, abuser's fingers, and scalding liquids. Lips are most commonly injured in children, followed by the mucosa, teeth, gingiva, and tongue.[29] Bruises in infants younger than 8 months who are not as mobile are uncommon, as "babies who don't cruise will rarely bruise."[30] Suspected victims of child abuse younger than 2 years should have a full skeletal survey. Head imaging in suspected abuse cases must be obtained in infants younger than 6 months and in infants younger than 1 year with orofacial injuries. Child sexual abuse frequently may involve the mouth, although visible oral injuries are rare. Palatal petechiae may be evidence of forced oral sex.

Another distinguishing sign of abuse, if present, are bite marks. Contusions, abrasions, or lacerations in an oval or elliptical pattern are the characteristic bite-mark pattern.[31] Human bites generally compress tissue, whereas animal bites tend to lacerate or avulse tissue. Bite marks can be a clue in identifying the perpetrator. Forensic dentists are available to help collect evidence. No matter how minimal the injury, there is always the possibility of abuse. As health care providers, physicians must use their best clinical judgment to determine abuse potential and reach out to the proper authorities to protect patients.

SUMMARY

Preservation and restoration of normal function and normal aesthetics is of paramount importance in the treatment of orofacial and dental trauma. Injuries can be limited to the soft tissue or be complex multisystem trauma; however, the fundamental approach and goals are the same. Consideration of the basic principles mentioned in this article will help promote successful outcomes and patient satisfaction when managing trauma to the head and face.

REFERENCES

1. Bagheri SC, Bell RB, Khan HA. Current therapy in oral and maxillofacial surgery. St Louis (MO): Elsevier; 2012.
2. Hupp JR, Ellis E III, Tucker MR. Contemporary oral and maxillofacial surgery. 5th edition. St Louis (MO): Mosby; 2008.
3. Andreasen JO, Bakland LK, Flores MT, et al. Traumatic dental injuries: a manual. 3rd edition. Ames (IA): Wiley Blackwell; 2011.
4. Rauschenberger CR, Hovland EJ. Clinical management of crown fractures. Dent Clin North Am 1995;39:25.

5. Donley KJ. Management of sports-related crown fractures. Dent Clin North Am 2000;44:85.
6. Andreasen JO, Adreasen FM. Textbook and color atlas of traumatic injuries to the teeth. 3rd edition. Copenhagen (Denmark): Wiley; 1994.
7. Andreasen JO, Hjorting-Hansen E. Radiographic and clinical study of 110 human teeth replanted after accidental loss. Acta Odontol Scand 1966;24:263.
8. Trope M. Clinical management of the avulsed tooth. Dent Clin North Am 1995; 39:93.
9. Andreasen JO. Etiology and pathogenesis of traumatic dental injuries. Scand J Dent Res 1970;78:339.
10. Fonseca RJ, Walker RV, Betts NJ, et al. Oral and maxillofacial trauma. 3rd edition. Philadelphia: Saunders; 2004.
11. Batters AA, Doherty T, Lewen G. Facial fractures and concomitant injuries in trauma patients. Laryngoscope 2003;113:102.
12. Saigal K, Winokur RS, Finden S, et al. Use of three-dimensional computerized tomography reconstruction in complex facial trauma. Facial Plast Surg 2005; 21:214.
13. Gerlock AJ, Sinn DP, McBride KL. Clinical and radiographic interpretation of facial fractures. Boston: Little, Brown; 1981.
14. Afzelius L, Rosen C. Facial fractures: a review of 368 cases. Int J Oral Surg 1980; 9:25.
15. Koornneef L. Current concepts on the management of orbital blow-out fractures. Ann Plast Surg 1982;9:185.
16. Gerbino G, Ramieri GA, Nasi A. Diagnosis and treatment of retrobulbar haematomas following blunt orbital trauma: a description of eight cases. Int J Oral Maxillofac Surg 2005;34:127.
17. Ziccardi VB, Braidy H. Management of nasal fractures. Oral Maxillofac Surg Clin North Am 2009;21:203.
18. Sargent LA, Rogers GF. Nasoethmoid orbital fractures: diagnosis and management. J Craniomaxillofac Trauma 1999;5:19.
19. Papadopoulos H, Salib NK. Management of naso-orbital-ethmoidal fractures. Oral Maxillofac Surg Clin North Am 2009;21:221.
20. Ellis E, Kittidumkerng W. Analysis of treatment for isolated zygomaticomaxillary complex fractures. J Oral Maxillofac Surg 1996;54:386.
21. Bagheri SC, Holmgren E, Kademani D, et al. Comparison of the severity of bilateral LeFort injuries in isolated midface trauma. J Oral Maxillofac Surg 2005;63:1123.
22. Manson PM, Hoopes JE, Su CT. Structural pillars of the facial skeleton: an approach to the management of LeFort fractures. Plast Reconstr Surg 1980;60:54.
23. Olson RA, Fonseca RJ, Zeitler DL, et al. Fractures of the mandible: a review of 580 cases. J Oral Maxillofac Surg 1985;43:417.
24. Ellis E 3rd. Management of fractures through the angle of the mandible. Oral Maxillofac Surg Clin North Am 2009;21:163.
25. Ochs MW, Tucker MR. Current concepts in management of facial trauma. J Oral Maxillofac Surg 1993;51:42.
26. Okeson JP. Management of temporomandibular disorders and occlusion. 6th edition. St Louis (MO): Mosby; 2007.
27. Fenton SJ, Bouquot JE, Unkel JH. Orofacial considerations for pediatric, adult, and elderly victims of abuse. Emerg Med Clin North Am 2000;18:601.
28. Simon P. Orofacial Trauma of Child Abuse/Neglect. Penn Dent J 2001;117(10): 21–32.

29. O'Neill JA Jr, Meacham WF, Griffin JP, et al. Patterns of injury in the battered child syndrome. J Trauma 1973;13:332.
30. Sugar NF, Taylor JA, Feldman KW. Bruises in infants and toddlers. Arch Pediatr Adolesc Med 1999;153:399.
31. Kellogg N. Oral and dental aspects of child abuse and neglect. Pediatrics 2005; 116:1565.

Normal Variations of Oral Anatomy and Common Oral Soft Tissue Lesions

Evaluation and Management

Farideh M. Madani, DMD[a], Arthur S. Kuperstein, DDS[b],*

KEYWORDS

- Leukoedema • Fordyce granules • Linea alba • White sponge nevus • Ankylogossia
- Lingual thyroid • Hairy tongue • Fissured tongue

KEY POINTS

- Physicians should be able to recognize normal variations of oral and oropharyngeal anatomy.
- Physicians should be able to recognize common soft tissue lesions of the oral and oropharyngeal structures.
- Physicians should be able to determine if referral to an oral health care provider for further evaluation and management is warranted based on physical examination findings.

BUCCAL AND LABIAL MUCOSA
Cheek Biting (Morsicatio Buccarum)

Habitual, repetitive, parafunctional masticatory activity against the delicate nonkeratinized buccal mucosal tissue may result in a whitish, ragged surface and irregularly textured area of varying size known as morsicatio buccarum (chronic cheek biting).[1–4] These areas are found unilaterally or bilaterally, in the vicinity of and lateral to the occlusal surfaces of the dentition. Histologic appearance is consistent with hyperkeratosis.

Management
Typically, there is no treatment other than reassurance, but use of an occlusal guard may be indicated to protect the buccal mucosa from chronic trauma (**Fig. 1**).[5–7]

Disclosures: No disclosures to be made.
[a] Department of Oral Medicine, University of Pennsylvania School of Dental Medicine, 240 South 40th Street, Philadelphia, PA 19104, USA; [b] Oral Medicine Clinical Services, Department of Oral Medicine, University of Pennsylvania School of Dental Medicine, 240 South 40th Street, Philadelphia, PA 19104, USA
* Corresponding author.
E-mail address: arthurk@dental.upenn.edu

Med Clin N Am 98 (2014) 1281–1298
http://dx.doi.org/10.1016/j.mcna.2014.08.004
0025-7125/14/$ – see front matter © 2014 Elsevier Inc. All rights reserved.

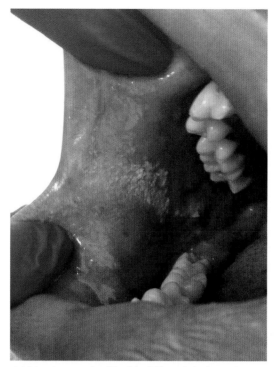

Fig. 1. Chronic cheek biting has resulted in this diffuse right buccal mucosal lesion. (*Courtesy of* A. Kuperstein, DDS, Philadelphia, PA.)

Leukoedema

Leukoedema is a common benign mucosal alteration of unknown cause that is considered to be a normal variation. It is usually discovered as an incidental finding during routine oral examination. In the United States it is present in about 70% to 90% of African-American adults and 50% of African-American children. It is observed less frequently in whites, and overall is commonly seen in males.[8–10]

Leukoedema is characterized by accumulation of the fluid within the epithelial cells of the buccal mucosa. Leukoedema usually start to appear around age 2 to 5; however, it is not often noticeable until adulthood.[11] Clinically leukoedema presents as an asymptomatic, grayish white semitransparent mucosal alteration, located in the buccal mucosa bilaterally. Occasionally, folds or white lines crisscross the affected area.

The buccal mucosa is the most common site for leukoedema; however, it can extend to the labial mucosa, floor of the mouth, and pharyngeal areas. Other mucosal surfaces can be affected, such as vagina and larynx. Leukoedema cannot be wiped off; however, it can be eliminated temporarily by stretching of the mucosa, which is referred to as clinical stretch test.[12–17] Differential diagnoses of leukoedema include white sponge nevus, smoker's tobacco, frictional keratosis, candidiasis, lichen planus, and hereditary benign intraepithelial dyskeratosis. Leukoedema can be easily diagnosed clinically by not being temporarily eliminated.

Management

Leukoedema is considered to be a normal variation; therefore, no treatment is required for this condition. There is no relationship between leukoedema and dysplasia and malignancy (**Fig. 2**).[18]

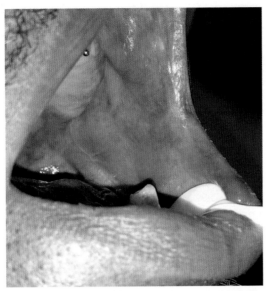

Fig. 2. A classic manifestation of leukoedema of the left buccal mucosa. Stretching the mucosa causes the grayish coloring to temporarily disappear. (*Courtesy of* F. Madani, DMD, Philadelphia, PA.)

Fordyce Granules

Fordyce first described these ectopic sebaceous glands or sebaceous choristomas (normal tissue in abnormal location) within the oral mucosa in 1896.[19] Normally, sebaceous glands are seen within the skin, in association with hair follicles; however, Fordyce granules do not exhibit any association with hair structures in the oral cavity. The condition is considered to be a variation of normal and is seen in approximately 80% to 90% of the adult population. Clinically, they present as multiple asymptomatic, slightly elevated, yellowish or yellowish white maculopapular structures that measure 1 to 2 mm in diameter. The lesions generally are symmetrically distributed and the sites of predilection include the buccal mucosa and the vermilion of the upper lip. They tend to become obvious after puberty, possibly because of hormonal changes and the number usually increases with age. Fordyce granules are asymptomatic and are often discovered incidentally by the patient or by the practitioner during a routine oral examination. Fordyce granules are neither related to smoking nor systemic atherosclerosis, and there is no race or gender predilection for these lesions.[20–22]

Management

No treatment is indicated for this particular condition and because the clinical appearance is virtually diagnostic, no biopsy is usually required. Fordyce granules on the vermilion border of the upper lip may require surgical removal for esthetic reasons. Rare cases of pseudocysts and sebaceous cell hyperplasia and adenoma have been reported.[23] Differential diagnosis of Fordyce granules includes pseudomembranous candidiasis. However, these conditions can be differentiated easily because Fordyce granules do not wipe off, whereas plaques associated with pseudomembranous candidiasis can be easily removed (**Fig. 3**).

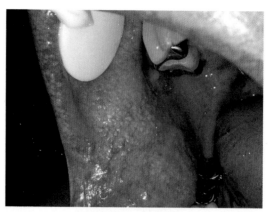

Fig. 3. The patient's right buccal mucosa is covered by a diffuse collection of Fordyce granules. (*Courtesy of* F. Madani, DMD, Philadelphia, PA.)

Linea Alba

Linea alba is a white, linear elevation of buccal mucosa at the level of occlusal plane of the teeth. It usually extends from the angle of the mouth toward the pterygomandibular raphe and terminates at the most posterior teeth that are in occlusion. The hyperkeratotic area is associated with repetitive pressure, frictional trauma, or other parafunctional habits from buccal surfaces of the dentition. The clinical appearance is typically diagnostic.

Management
No treatment is required for linea alba, which may disappear if the offending source of friction is mitigated (**Fig. 4**).[7]

Traumatic Ulcer

A solitary ulcer of the mucosa may be the direct result of a physical, mechanical, chemical, or thermal injury. It is not uncommon for patients to inadvertently bite their lips or buccal mucosa while eating or after a dental visit if local anesthesia was

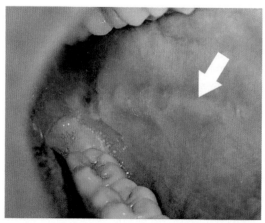

Fig. 4. Located along the occlusal line of the patient's left maxilla and mandible is the linear white line (*arrow*) of linea alba. (*Courtesy of* A. Kuperstein, DDS, Philadelphia, PA.)

administered. A traumatic ulcer may be caused by repetitive biting, secondary to orthodontic or other oral appliances, or malpositioned or irregularly contoured or fractured teeth. A traumatic ulcer of the palate is commonly caused by thermal injury from eating or drinking extremely hot foods or beverages. Unintentional application of caustic medicaments and/or chemicals during dental treatment or inappropriate topical use of aspirin, by the patient, may cause a burn. However, nonresolving mucosal ulcerations may imply underlying infection, systemic disease, immunocompromised status, or even a neoplasm.[24–26]

Management
Typically, palliative care is sufficient for management of a traumatic ulcer. If the ulcer is refractory to palliative care and is present for greater than 2 weeks, further investigation including biopsy is warranted (**Fig. 5**).

TONGUE
Ankyloglossia

Ankyloglossia, or "tongue-tie," is a developmental anomaly characterized by an abnormally short and anteriorly positioned lingual frenum that results in restricted tongue movement. Ankyloglossia can range in severity from mild cases with little clinical significance (common) to complete ankyloglossia, in which the tongue is anatomically attached to the floor of the mouth. Complete ankyloglossia is rare and occurs in two to three cases of every 10,000 births.[27]

Complications associated with complete ankyloglossia may include eating problems (particularly during infancy, such as breastfeeding or sucking problems), periodontal problems caused by high mucogingival attachment of the lingual frenum, speech defects, and mandibular midline diastema.

Management
Treatment ranges from no treatment to lingual frenectomy, if it causes functional or periodontal problems (**Fig. 6**).[28–36]

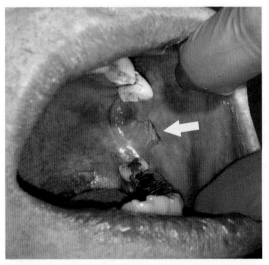

Fig. 5. A large, deep traumatic ulcer of the left buccal mucosa (*arrow*), secondary to chronic repetitive mechanical trauma from fractured sharp teeth. (*Courtesy of* A. Kuperstein, DDS, Philadelphia, PA.)

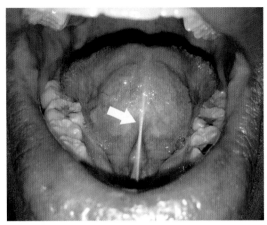

Fig. 6. Ankyloglossia. Note the stretched shortened lingual frenum (*arrow*) as the tongue is retracted posteriorly. (*Courtesy of* A. Kuperstein, DDS, Philadelphia, PA.)

Lingual Thyroid

Lingual thyroid tissue is a rare anomaly characterized by the development of a submucosal mass of thyroid tissue on the midposterior dorsum of the tongue. Embryologically, the thyroid gland anlage arises at the site of foramen cecum and migrates inferiorly along the thyroglossal tract to its ultimate destination in the anterior neck. If all or part of the thyroid anlage fails to migrate, remnants of thyroid tissue can develop along its path of migration. A lingual thyroid nodule represents a thyroid remnant in the region of the thyroid gland's origin. Of all ectopic thyroids, 90% are found in this region.[11] Microscopic examination of human tongues removed at autopsy reveals that despite the absence of a clinically apparent thyroid nodule, as many as 10% exhibited remnants of thyroid tissue within the tongue.[37,38] Lingual thyroid occurs more commonly among females and may range from a small asymptomatic nodule to a large mass that can obstruct the airway. The most common clinical symptoms are dysphagia, dysphonia, and dyspnea.

Hypothyroidism has been reported in up to 33% of patients with lingual thyroid, possibly as a secondary phenomenon to compensate for thyroid hypofunction, and as many as 75% of patients with infantile hypothyroidism have some ectopic thyroid tissue.[39–43]

The clinical appearance is variable. Diagnosis is best established by thyroid scan using iodine isotope or technetium 99m.[44] Computed tomography and magnetic resonance imaging can be helpful in delineating the size and the extent of the lesion.[45,46] Biopsy is often avoided because of risk of hemorrhage due to the vascular nature of these lesions and because the mass may represent the patient's only functioning thyroid tissue. However, in some cases, incisional biopsy might be indicated to confirm the diagnosis and to rule out malignant changes.

Management

No treatment except for periodic follow-up is required for asymptomatic lingual thyroid. In symptomatic patients the use of suppressive hormonal therapy with levothyroxine[47] may reduce the size of the lesion. If hormone therapy does not eliminate symptoms, surgical removal or ablation with radioactive iodine-131 can be performed. If the mass is surgically excised, autotransplantation to another body site can be attempted to maintain functional thyroid tissue and to prevent hypothyroidism. Rare examples of carcinoma arising from lingual thyroid have been reported (**Fig. 7**).[5]

Hairy Tongue

Hairy tongue is a consequence of the elongation of the filiform papillae on the dorsum of the tongue resulting in hairlike appearance. It is related to marked accumulation of keratin on the filiform papillae caused by increase in keratin production or decrease in normal keratin desquamation. The elongated papillae are generally confined to the posterior third of the dorsal tongue, but may include the middle third in lesser amounts. The color ranges from white to yellow, brown, and black as a result of overgrowth of pigment-producing bacteria or staining from food or tobacco. The cause of hairy tongue is unknown in most of cases; however, most patients are heavy smokers. Other predisposing factors for this condition include neglected oral hygiene, dryness of the oral cavity, antibiotics, immunosuppressive drugs, systemic diseases, radiation treatment, excess use of mouthwashes containing peroxidase, and candidiasis.[48] The condition is typically asymptomatic, although patients may complain of a gagging sensation or bad taste.[49–52] Diagnosis is made by clinical appearance and biopsy is unnecessary. Hairy tongue is found in about 0.5% of adults.[53]

Management

Treatment of hairy tongue is focused on reduction or elimination of predisposing factors and excellent oral hygiene should be encouraged. Desquamation of the hyperkeratotic papillae can be promoted by periodic (gentle) scraping or brushing with a toothbrush or tongue scraper. This condition is often mistakenly diagnosed as oral candidiasis, and patients are often prescribed antifungal agents unnecessarily. If the clinician suspects a diagnosis of oral candidiasis, further investigations should be conducted (ie, exfoliative cytology) to rule this out as a cause for the patient's condition (**Fig. 8**).

Fissured Tongue

Fissured tongue is relatively common and affects 2% to 5% of the overall population.[54] It is characterized by deep grooves and fissures on the dorsal surface of the tongue. It can be seen in children and adults; however, severity and prevalence increases with age. There is a strong association between fissured tongue and geographic tongue,

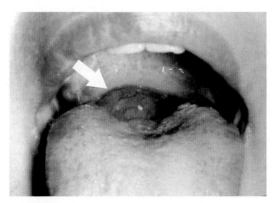

Fig. 7. Lingual thyroid presenting as a large mass behind the tongue or area near the foramen cecum (*arrow*). Patient complained of constant dysphagia. (*Courtesy of* A. Kuperstein, DDS, Philadelphia, PA.)

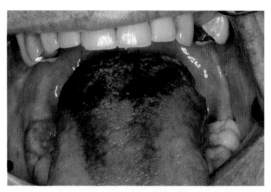

Fig. 8. Black hairy tongue is represented in this photograph. Patient is a smoker with poor oral hygiene. (*Courtesy of* Dr A. Houston, Philadelphia, PA.)

and most individuals have both of these conditions at the same time.[55] The cause of fissured tongue is uncertain but heredity seems to play an important role.[56] Aging and local environmental factors may contribute to its development. Fissured tongue is usually asymptomatic, although some patients may complain of burning sensation or mild soreness, particularly after eating hot or spicy foods. Fissured tongue has been seen more in individuals with Down syndrome than the general population.[57] Fissured tongue is a component of Melkerson-Rosenthal syndrome, characterized by the classic triad of facial palsy, facial swelling, and fissured tongue.[56,58–60] Fissured tongue is a benign condition and no specific treatment is indicated. Patients should be encouraged to brush the tongue, because food or debris entrapped in the grooves may act as a source of irritation. If the patient is symptomatic, clinicians may consider use of topical anesthetics for palliative treatment. There is a report of fissured tongue responding to biologics during the treatment of psoriasis (**Fig. 9**).[61]

Geographic Tongue (Benign Migratory Glossitis–Erythema Migrans)

Geographic tongue, which is also called benign migratory glossitis or erythema migrans, is a common condition that primarily affects the tongue. This condition is usually recognized as an incidental finding on routine oral examination. It affects 1% to 3% of the population, and females are affected more commonly than males by a 2:1 ratio.[62] The cause of geographic tongue is unknown, yet heredity and environmental factors may play a role in pathogenesis of geographic tongue. There is a strong association between geographic tongue and fissured tongue.[63–66]

Geographic tongue is primarily located on the dorsal anterior two-thirds of the tongue. The lesions appear as well-demarcated red zones secondary to atrophy of the filiform papillae. The erythematous zones are completely or partially surrounded by a slightly elevated white serpentine or scalloped border. The peripheral zone disappears after some time, and healing of the erythematous area begins. The lesions can appear on the lateral or ventral surface of the tongue; however, in most patients, it is accompanied by similar lesions on the dorsal surface of the tongue. This condition can also affect other oral mucosal surfaces, such as labial mucosa, buccal mucosa, soft palate, and gingiva.

Management

Geographic tongue is usually asymptomatic and no treatment is required; however, some patients may complain of a burning sensation or sensitivity to hot or spicy foods.

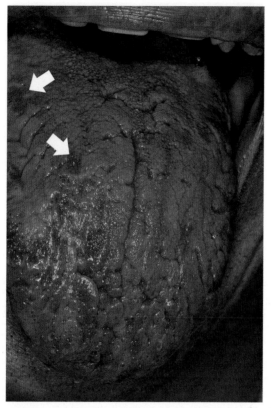

Fig. 9. Fissured tongue of the dorsal surface. Tongue also presents with an associated benign migratory glossitis distributed over the dorsal surface (selectively indicated by *arrows*). (*Courtesy of* T. Musbah, BDS, Philadelphia, PA.)

In those patients, topical steroids and/or anesthetic may be beneficial in some cases. Patients should be assured of the benign nature of their condition (**Fig. 10**).[54,65,67,68]

Lateral Lingual Tonsil

Lateral lingual tonsil is an aggregate of lymphoid tissue that is located at the posterior lateral portion of the tongue, related to foliate papillae. Coloration of the nontender submucosal masses is often red-yellow. They usually are bilateral, generally asymptomatic, and discovered on routine oral examination.[11]

Management

Typically they require no treatment except for reassurance of the patient. However, asymmetrical presentation may be suggestive of lymphoma and further evaluation and management, including biopsy, may be warranted (**Fig. 11**).[69–72]

Oral Varicosities (Varices)

Oral varicosities or varices are abnormally dilated or tortuous veins, with an unknown cause. This condition is rare among children so it is thought to represent a physical manifestation of the aging process. Lingual varicosities appear as tortuous, blue, red, and purple elevations that course over the ventrolateral surface of the tongue. They represent a degenerative change in the adventitia of the venous wall and are

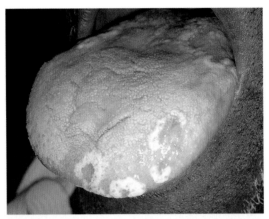

Fig. 10. Benign migratory glossitis distributed on the ventral and lateral borders of the tongue. Note the circumferential white borders surrounding the atrophic central regions. (*Courtesy of* A. Kuperstein, DDS, Philadelphia, PA.)

of no clinical consequence.[68,73–75] They are painless and are not thought to be subject to rupture and/or hemorrhage.[76]

A focal dilatation of a vein or group of venules is known as varix. These lesions also tend to occur in elderly persons and are primarily located on the lower lip, appearing as a focal raised blue, red, or purple nodule.

Management

These conditions do not require any treatment unless they become calcified or create an esthetic problem **Fig. 12**.

Crenation of Lateral Tongue

Crenations or scalloping of the lateral border, and occasionally the tip of the tongue, is a common finding. It may be associated with stress-related chronic pressure exerted

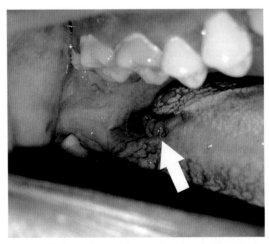

Fig. 11. Lateral lingual tonsil tissue (*arrow*) located at the right posterior tongue. (*Courtesy of* F. Madani, DMD, Philadelphia, PA.)

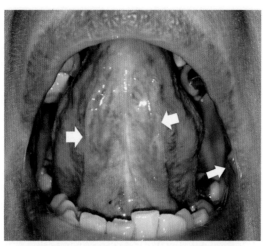

Fig. 12. Bilateral lingual varicosities along the ventral tongue (*large arrows*). Labial varix of lower lip at the left commissure (*small arrow*). (*Courtesy of* A. Kuperstein, DDS, Philadelphia, PA.)

by the tongue musculature against the curved lingual surfaces of the dentition, imparting the scalloped margin. Occasionally, it may be associated with systemic disease, such as macroglossia associated with acromegaly. There have been some indications of association with obstructive sleep apnea.[77–79]

Management
Typically no treatment is necessary (**Fig. 13**).

GINGIVA
Amalgam Tattoo

An amalgam tattoo represents an exogenous pigmentation, which may be identified on the buccal mucosa, gingiva, ventral tongue, floor of mouth, or hard palate. The color may vary from a light gray to a dark blue-black hue. The cause is inadvertent embedding or migration of amalgam restorative material into the mucosa. Over time the foreign material may disperse into surrounding tissue, which may lighten the area's color. Amalgam tattoo must be differentiated from other pigmented lesions including malignant melanoma.[79–81]

Management
No treatment is required for suspected amalgam tattoos. However, if there is clinical suspicion for other etiologies of the pigmented lesion, referral to a dentist for further evaluation and management is recommended (**Fig. 14**).

Physiologic Pigmentation

The oral mucosa may present with variations in physiologic pigmentation. Association with varying skin color seems to be variably related with oral physiologic pigmentation. The spectrum of pigmentation, from light to a darker brown, typically presents on the labial gingiva, but also may be observed on the dorsum of the tongue, the gingival surfaces, lips and palate, and buccal mucosa.

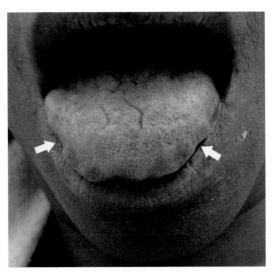

Fig. 13. Crenations, scalloping of the lateral borders and tip of the tongue (*arrows*). (*Courtesy of* A. Kuperstein, DDS, Philadelphia, PA.)

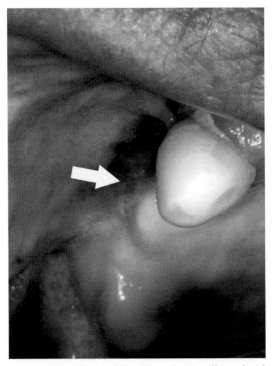

Fig. 14. Amalgam tattoo (*arrow*) located buccal to the maxillary alveolar ridge at the site of a previously extracted and amalgam restored molar. (*Courtesy of* A. Kuperstein, DDS, Philadelphia, PA.)

Management
Physiologic pigmentation is often observed in infancy, young children, and adolescence with pubertal darkening. If adult onset is noted, a biopsy may be indicated, because the presentation may represent underlying systemic disease, neoplasm, trauma, and/ or reactive pigmentation. Endocrinopathies, such as Addison disease, may present with oral mucosal pigmentation.[82] The clinical presentation of endocrinopathy-associated pigmentation in the oral cavity is usually a diffuse but dappled melanosis of multiple mucosal surfaces. A medical work-up including biopsy, serum cortisol, and electrolyte levels should be performed if endocrinopathy-associated pigmentation is suspected **(Fig. 15)**.[83,84]

PALATE, ALVEOLAR PROCESS
Tori, Exostoses

These osseous structures have a relatively high frequency of presentation and the manner in which they impact the overlying oral mucosa. Tori are nonneoplastic, exophytic, often nodular, dense cortical bony structures that may be located in the midline of the hard palate (torus palatinus), typically bilaterally along the lingual cortical plate of the mandible (torus mandibularis), and beneath the buccal and labial alveolar mucosa (exostoses). Typically thin oral mucosa overlies the underlying bony mass giving the mucosa a pale yellow-white coloration, when actually its translucency permits the bone color to be visualized through it. Nevertheless, the practitioner should be cognizant of the potential for the bony expansion associated with dentoalveolar infection, Paget disease, or the fibro-osseous lesions of fibrous dysplasia.

Management
Typically no treatment is indicated unless there is persistent trauma to the overlying mucosa or dental prosthetic are indicated. In cases in which dental prostheses are indicated, the exophytic osseous growths may need to be excised or recontoured to accommodate the restoration **(Figs. 16–18)**.[68,85,86]

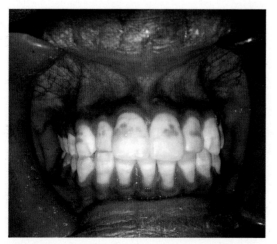

Fig. 15. Physiologic melanotic pigmentation of the maxillary and to a lesser degree, mandibular labial gingiva. (*Courtesy of* A. Kuperstein, DDS, Philadelphia, PA.)

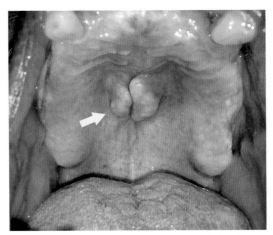

Fig. 16. Torus palatinus. Note two-lobed structure of the bony mass (*arrow*). The translucency of the mucosa can be readily observed. (*Courtesy of* F. Madani, DMD, Philadelphia, PA; and A. Kuperstein, DDS, Philadelphia, PA.)

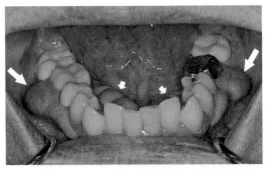

Fig. 17. Bilateral torus mandibularis (*small arrows*) and buccal exostoses (*large arrows*). The translucency of the mucosa can be observed. (*Courtesy of* T. Musbah, BDS, Philadelphia, PA.)

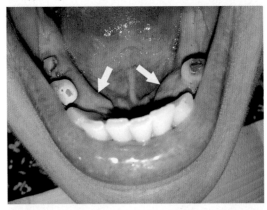

Fig. 18. Torus mandibularis. Typical bilateral presentation of the bony exophytic mass (*arrows*). The translucency of the mucosa can be observed as on the palatal lesion. (*Courtesy of* J. Thoppay, BDS, Philadelphia, PA.)

SUMMARY

This article highlights the importance of recognizing common variations of normal oral anatomy and clinical findings that may suggest association with systemic, psychological, and behavioral health conditions. Physicians should have an understanding of these findings to provide appropriate patient care.

REFERENCES

1. Vargas CM, Arevalo O. How dental care can preserve and improve oral health. Dent Clin North Am 2009;53(3):399–420.
2. Lankarani KB, Sivandzadeh GR, Hassanpour S. Oral manifestation in inflammatory bowel disease: a review. World J Gastroenterol 2013;19(46):8571–9.
3. Padovani MC, Barbosa PS, Baeder F, et al. Oral manifestations of systemic alterations in early childhood. J Contemp Dent Pract 2013;14(2):327–31.
4. Islam NM, Bhattacharyya I, Cohen DM. Common oral manifestations of systemic disease. Otolaryngologic Clinics of North America 2011;44(1):161–82.
5. Greenberg MS, Ship JA, Glick M. Burket's oral medicine. 11th edition. Hamilton (Canada): BC Decker; 2011.
6. Woo SB, Lin D. Morsicatio mucosae oris: a chronic oral frictional keratosis, not a leukoplakia. J Oral Maxillofac Surg 2009;67(1):140–6.
7. Neville BW, Damm DD, Allen CM, et al. Physical and chemical injuries. In: Oral and maxillofacial pathology. 3rd edition. St Louis (MO): WB Saunders; 2009.
8. Martin JL, Crump EP. Leukoedema of the buccal mucosa in children and youth. Oral Surg Oral Med Oral Pathol 1972;34(1):49–58.
9. Axéll T, Henricsson V. Leukoedema: an epidemiologic study with special reference to the influence of tobacco habits. Community Dent Oral Epidemiol 1981;9(3):142–6.
10. Martin JL. Leukoedema: an epidemiological study in white and African American. J Tenn Dent Assoc 1997;77:18–21.
11. Bouquot BW, Neville DD, Damm CM, et al. Oral & maxillofacial pathology. 2nd edition. Philadelphia: WB Saunders; 2002.
12. Sandstead HR, Lowe JW. Leukoedema and keratosis in relation to leukoplakia of the buccal mucosa in man. J Natl Cancer Inst 1953;14(2):423–37.
13. Durocher RT, Thalman R, Fiore-Donno G. Leukoedema of the oral mucosa. J Am Dent Assoc 1972;85(5):1105–9.
14. Bánóczy J. Oral leukoplakia and other white lesions of the oral mucosa related to dermatological disorders. J Cutan Pathol 1983;10(4):238–56.
15. Martin JL. Nutrition: a non-factor in leukoedema. Ann Dent 1977;36(1):24–8.
16. Waitzer S, Fisher BK. Oral leukoedema. Arch Dermatol 1984;120(2):264–6.
17. Van Wyk CW, Ambrosio SC, van der Vyver PC. Abnormal keratohyalin-like forms in leukoedema. J Oral Pathol 1984;13(3):271–81.
18. Scully C. Oral and maxillofacial medicine: the basis of diagnosis and treatment. Edinburgh (United Kingdom): Churchill Livingstone; 2013. p. 388.
19. Fordyce J. A peculiar affection of the mucous membrane of the lip and oral cavity. J Cutan Genito-Urin Dis 1896;14:413–9.
20. Miles AE. Sebaceous glands in the lip and cheek mucosa of man. Br Dent J 1958;105:235–9.
21. Miller AS, McCrea MW. Sebaceous gland adenoma of the buccal mucosa. J Oral Surg 1968;26:593–5.
22. Scully C. Oral and maxillofacial medicine: the basis of diagnosis and treatment, vol. 170. Edinburgh (United Kingdom): Churchill Livingstone; 2013. p. 392.

23. Gorsky M, Buchner A, Fondoianu-Dayan D, et al. Fordyce's granules in the oral mucosa of adult Israeli Jews. Community Dent Oral Epidemiol 1986;14:231–2.
24. Compilato D, Cirillo N, Termine N, et al. Long-standing oral ulcers: proposal for a new 'S-C-D classification system'. J Oral Pathol Med 2009;38(3):241–53.
25. Bascones-Martínez A, Figuero-Ruiz E, Esparza-Gómez GC. Oral ulcers. Med Clin (Barc) 2005;125(15):590–7 [in Spanish].
26. Hegde ND, Hegde MN, Puri A, et al. Differential diagnosis of long term tongue ulcers. Int Res J Pharm 2012;3(8):145–8.
27. Messner AH, Lalakea ML. The effect of ankyloglossia on speech in children. Otolaryngol Head Neck Surg 2002;127(6):539–45.
28. Messner AH, Lalakea ML. Ankyloglossia: controversies in management. Int J Pediatr Otorhinolaryngol 2000;54:123–31.
29. Lalakea M, Lauren M, Anna H. Frenotomy and frenuloplasty: if, when, and how. Operative Techniques in Otolaryngol Head Neck Surg 2002;13:93.
30. Wallace H, Clarke S. Tongue-tie division in infants with breast-feeding difficulties. Int J Pediatr Otorhinolaryngol 2006;70(7):1257–61.
31. Ruffoli R, Giambelluca MA, Scavuzzo MC, et al. Ankyloglossia: a morphofunctional investigation in children. Oral Dis 2005;11(3):170–4.
32. Breward S. Tongue tie and breastfeeding: assessing and overcoming the difficulties. Community Pract 2006;79(9):298–9.
33. Lalakea ML, Messner AH. Ankyloglossia: does it matter? Pediatr Clin North Am 2003;50(2):381–97.
34. Yoon PJ. Tongue-tie (ankyloglossia): current diagnosis and treatment: pediatrics. 20th edition. New York: McGraw-Hill; 2011. p. 485.
35. Messner AH, Lalakea L, Aby J, et al. Ankyloglossia: incidence and associated feeding difficulties. Arch Otolaryngol Head Neck Surg 2000;126(1):36–9.
36. Ricke LA, Baker NJ, Madlon-Kay DJ, et al. Newborn tongue-tie, prevalence and effect on breast-feeding. J Am Board Fam Pract 2005;18(1):1–7.
37. Baik SH, Choi JH, Lee HM. Dual ectopic thyroid. Eur Arch Otorhinolaryngol 2002;259:105–7.
38. Paludetti G, Galli J, Almadori G, et al. Ectopic thyroid gland. Acta Otorhinolaryngol Ital 1991;11:117–33.
39. Chanin LR, Greenberg LM. Pediatric upper airway obstruction due to ectopic thyroid: classification and case reports. Laryngoscope 1988;98:422–7.
40. Hazarika P, Siddiqui SA, Pujary K, et al. Dual ectopic thyroid: a report of two cases. J Laryngol Otol 1998;12:393–5.
41. Huang TS, Chen HY. Dual thyroid ectopia with a normally located pretracheal thyroid gland: case report and literature review. Head Neck 2007;29:885–8.
42. Mussak EN, Kacker A. Surgical and medical management of midline ectopic thyroid. Otolaryngol Head Neck Surg 2007;136:870–2.
43. Alderson DJ, Lannigan FJ. Lingual thyroid presenting after previous thyroglossal cyst excision. J Laryngol Otol 1994;108:341–3.
44. Willinsky RA, Kassel EE, Cooper PW, et al. Computed tomography of lingual thyroid. J Comput Assist Tomogr 1987;11(1):182–3.
45. Shah HR, Boyd CM, Williamson M, et al. Lingual thyroid: unusual appearance on computed tomography. Comput Med Imaging Graph 1988;12(4):263–6.
46. Takashima S, Ueda M, Shibata A, et al. MR imaging of the lingual thyroid. comparison to other submucosal lesions. Acta Radiol 2001;42(4):376–82.
47. Pinto A, Glick M. Management of patients with thyroid disease: oral health considerations. J Am Dent Assoc 2002;133(7):849–58.
48. Nally F. Diseases of the tongue. Practitioner 1991;235(1498):65–71.

49. Redman RS. Prevalence of geographic tongue, fissured tongue, median rhomboid glossitis, and hairy tongue among 3,611 Minnesota schoolchildren. Oral Surg Oral Med Oral Pathol 1970;30(3):390–5.

50. Kostka E, Wittekindt C, Guntinas-Lichius O. Tongue coating, mouth odor, gustatory sense disorder: earlier and new treatment options by means of tongue scraper. Laryngorhinootologie 2008;87(8):546–50.

51. Lawoyin D, Brown RS. Drug-induced black hairy tongue: diagnosis and management challenges. Dent Today 2008;27(1):60, 62–3.

52. Pigatto PD, Spadari F, Meroni L, et al. Black hairy tongue associated with long-term oral erythromycin use. J Eur Acad Dermatol Venereol 2008;22(10): 1269–70.

53. Thompson DF, Kessler TL. Drug-induced black hairy tongue. Pharmacotherapy 2010;30(6):585–93.

54. Reamy BV, Derby R, Bunt CW. Common tongue conditions in primary care. Am Fam Physician 2010;81(5):627–34.

55. Liu R, Yu S. Melkersson-Rosenthal syndrome: a review of seven patients. J Clin Neurosci 2013;20(7):993–5.

56. Eidelman E, Chosack A, Cohen T. Scrotal tongue and geographic tongue: polygenic and associated traits. Oral Surg Oral Med Oral Pathol 1976;42(5):591–6.

57. Dar-Odeh NS, Hayajneh WA, Abu-Hammad OA, et al. Orofacial findings in chronic granulomatous disease: report of twelve patients and review of the literature. BMC Res Notes 2010;3(1):37.

58. Stein SL, Mancini AJ. Melkersson-Rosenthal syndrome in childhood: successful management with combination steroid and minocycline therapy. J Am Acad Dermatol 1999;41:746–8.

59. Alioglu Z, Caylan R, Adanir M, et al. Melkersson-Rosenthal syndrome: report of three cases. Neurol Sci 2000;21(1):57–60.

60. Nakane T, Hatakeyama K, Nakamura K, et al. Melkersson-Rosenthal syndrome with isolated immunoglobulin E hypogammaglobulinaemia. J Int Med Res 2007; 35(6):922–5.

61. D'Erme AM, Agnoletti AF, Prignano F. Fissured tongue responding to biologics during the treatment of psoriasis: the importance of detecting oral involvement of psoriasis. Dermatol Ther 2013;26(4):364–6.

62. Neville BW, Damm DD, Allen CA, et al. Oral & maxillofacial pathology. 2nd edition. Philadelphia: WB Saunders; 2002. p. 677–9.

63. Greenberg MS, Glick M, Ship JA. Burket's oral medicine. 11th edition. BC Decker; 2008. p. 103–4.

64. Scully C. Oral and maxillofacial medicine: the basis of diagnosis and treatment. 2nd edition. Edinburgh: Churchill Livingstone; 2013. p. 205–6.

65. Shulman JD, Carpenter WM. Prevalence and risk factors associated with geographic tongue among US adults. Oral Dis 2006;12(4):381–6.

66. Zhu JF, Kaminski MJ, Pulitzer DR, et al. Psoriasis: pathophysiology and oral manifestations. Oral Dis 1996;2(2):135–44.

67. Ching V, Grushka M, Darling M, et al. Increased prevalence of geographic tongue in burning mouth complaints: a retrospective study. Oral Surg Oral Med Oral Pathol Oral Radiol 2012;114(4):444–8.

68. Canaan TJ, Meehan SC. Variations of structure and appearance of the oral mucosa. Dent Clin North Am 2005;49:1–14.

69. Kenna MA, Amin A. Anatomy and physiology of the oral cavity. In: Snow JB, Wackym PA, editors. Ballenger's otorhinolaryngology head and neck surgery. 17th edition. Shelton (CT): BC Decker Inc; 2009. p. 769–74.

70. Wiatrak BJ, Woolley AL. Pharyngitis and adenotonsillar disease. Cummings otolaryngology head and neck surgery. 3rd edition. London: Mosby; 1998. p. 188–215.

71. William JL, Lawrence SS, Steven P, et al. Human embryology. 3rd edition. Philadelphia: Elsevier; 2001. p. 375–6.

72. Robb PJ. The adenoid and adenoidectomy. Gleeson's otorhinolaryngology, head and neck surgery. 7th edition. London: Hodder Arnold; 2008. p. 1094–101.

73. Neville BW, Damm DD, Allen CM, et al. Oral & maxillofacial pathology. Philadelphia: Saunders; 2002. p. 337–69.

74. Kleinman HZ. Lingual varicosities. Oral Surg Oral Med Oral Pathol 1967;23:546–8.

75. Colby RA, Kerr DA, Robson HB. Color atlas of oral pathology. 2nd edition. Philadelphia: JBLippincott Company; 1961. p. 125.

76. Viswanath V, Nair S, Chavan N, et al. Caviar tongue. Indian J Dermatol Venereol Leprol 2011;77(1):78–9.

77. Zonato AI, Martinho FL, Bittencourt LR, et al. Head and neck physical examination: comparison between nonapneic and obstructive sleep apnea patients. Laryngoscope 2005;115(6):1030–4.

78. Patel M. Amyloidosis, not to be taken lightly. Society of Hospital Medicine [abstracts]. J Hosp Med 2012;7:1.

79. Al-Mobeeriek A. Oral health status among psychiatric patients in Riyadh, Saudi Arabia. West Indian Med J 2012;61(5):549–54.

80. Tran HT, Anandasabapathy N, Soldano AC. Amalgam tattoo. Dermatol Online J 2008;14:19.

81. Lewandowski B, Niedziela W. Amalgam staining of the oral mucosa as a simulation of melanoma. Family Medicine and Primary Care Review 2010;12(4): 1095–8.

82. Eisen D. Disorders of pigmentation in the oral cavity. Clin Dermatol 2000;18(5): 579–87.

83. Alawi F. Pigmented lesions of the oral cavity: an update. Dent Clin North Am 2013;57:699–710.

84. Lawson W. Pigmented oral lesions: Clues to identifying the potentially malignant. Consultant 2012;52(5):347–52.

85. Antoniades DZ, Belazi M, Papanayiotou P. Concurrence of torus palatinus with palatal and buccal exostoses: case report and review of the literature. Oral Surg Oral Med Oral Pathol Oral Radiol Endod 1998;8(5):552–7.

86. Sawair FA, Shayyab MH, Al-Rabab'ah MA, et al. Prevalence and clinical characteristics of tori and jaw exostoses in a teaching hospital in Jordan. Saudi Med J 2009;30(12):1557–62.

Oral and Oropharyngeal Cancer

Michaell A. Huber, DDS[a],*, Bundhit Tantiwongkosi, MD[b,c]

KEYWORDS

- Squamous cell carcinoma • Oropharynx • Oral cavity • Biopsy • Tobacco • Alcohol
- HPV • Areca nut

KEY POINTS

- Major risk factors for oral and oropharyngeal cancer (OPC) are exposure to tobacco, alcohol, areca nut, and human papillomavirus 16.
- OPCs usually arise from a preexisting potentially malignant disorder such as leukoplakia, erythroplakia, oral submucous fibrosis, actinic cheilosis, and oral lichen planus.
- Common signs and symptoms include the presence of a persistent mass, nodule, or indurated ulcer, as well as pain, dysphagia, otitis, weight loss, fixation, trismus, and paresthesia or anesthesia.
- Evidence to support oral cancer screening is sparse, but clinicians are encouraged to perform an oral soft tissue examination.
- Persistent oral lesions should be referred for further assessment or undergo biopsy.
- A biopsy is required to establish the diagnosis of OPC and the value of adjunctive devices and tests purported to increase diagnostic yield and accuracy remains undetermined.
- Potential morbidities associated with therapeutic interventions include disfigurement, trismus, speech impairment, dysphagia, pain, infection, mucositis, salivary dysfunction, and bone necrosis.

INTRODUCTION AND EPIDEMIOLOGY

Cancer affecting the oral cavity[1] and oropharyngeal[2] space is a complex and often relentless malignancy prone to local invasion and dissemination. For convenience, "oral and oropharyngeal cancer" (OPC) is used in this article as an inclusive term to

Disclosures: None.
[a] Department of Comprehensive Dentistry, University of Texas Health Science Center, School of Dentistry, 7703 Floyd Curl Drive, Mail Code 7919, San Antonio, TX 78229, USA; [b] Department of Radiology, University of Texas Health Science Center San Antonio, 7703 Floyd Curl Drive, Mail Code 7800, San Antonio, TX 78229, USA; [c] Department of Otolaryngology, University of Texas Health Science Center San Antonio, 7703 Floyd Curl Drive, Mail Code 7800, San Antonio, TX 78229, USA
* Corresponding author.
E-mail address: huberm@uthscsa.edu

refer to cancers of both the oral cavity and oropharyngeal space (**Table 1**). Approximately 89% of OPCs are of the squamous cell type.[3] Other cancers potentially presenting in this area include salivary gland tumors, lymphomas, and sarcomas. This article focuses on squamous cell–derived OPC. Therapeutic interventions to treat OPC are complex and often associated with significant debilitating side effects that often negatively affect the patient's quality of life. The cost of treating OPC may be among the highest of all cancers in the United States.[4]

As with most cancers, diagnosis at an early stage is associated with the best opportunity for cure. However, only 31% OPCs are diagnosed at a localized stage; in contrast, 40% of colorectal cancers are diagnosed at a localized stage.[5] Some clinicians express concern that practitioners fail to recognize early disease by not accomplishing a thorough soft tissue examination on a routine basis.[6] However, patient apathy may contribute to diagnostic delay, because more than 35% of patients acknowledge not seeing an oral health care provider on a routine basis and wait until symptoms develop before seeking care.[7,8]

Most OPCs are thought to arise from a preexisting potentially malignant disorder (PMD). Common PMDs are summarized in **Table 2** and include leukoplakia (**Figs. 1** and **2**), erythroplakia (**Figs. 3** and **4**), oral lichen planus (discussed elsewhere in this issue), oral submucous fibrosis, actinic cheilosis (**Fig. 5**), and snuff patch (**Fig. 6**).[9–14] Leukoplakia and erythroplakia are descriptive clinical terms used to imply concern.

- The original 1978 definition of leukoplakia is, "A white patch or plaque that cannot be characterized clinically or pathologically as any other disease and is not associated with any physical or chemical causative agent except use of tobacco." In 2007, a workshop coordinated by the World Health Organization Collaborating Centre for Oral Cancer and Precancer amended the definition to, "White plaques

Table 1
Site definitions for OPC

Oral Cavity Space[a]	Oropharyngeal Space[b]
The oral cavity extends from the skin-vermilion junctions of the lips to the junction of the hard and soft palates above and to the line of circumvallate papillae below to include the following specific areas: • Lip • Anterior two-thirds of tongue • Buccal mucosa • Floor of mouth • Upper and lower gingiva • Retromolar trigone • Hard palate	The oropharynx is located between the soft palate superiorly and the hyoid bone inferiorly; it is continuous with the oral cavity anteriorly and communicates with the nasopharynx superiorly and the supraglottic larynx and hypopharynx inferiorly. The oropharynx is divided into the following sites: • Base of the tongue, which includes the pharyngoepiglottic folds and the glossoepiglottic folds • Tonsillar region, which includes the fossa and the anterior and posterior pillars • Soft palate and uvula • Posterior and lateral pharyngeal walls

[a] *Data from* National Cancer Institute. PDQ® Lip and Oral Cavity Cancer Treatment. Bethesda (MD): National Cancer Institute; 2012. Available at: http://cancer.gov/cancertopics/pdq/treatment/lip-and-oral-cavity/HealthProfessional. Accessed February 5, 2014.
[b] *Data from* National Cancer Institute. PDQ® Oropharyngeal Cancer Treatment. Bethesda (MD): National Cancer Institute; 2013. Available at: http://cancer.gov/cancertopics/pdq/treatment/oropharyngeal/HealthProfessional. Accessed February 5, 2014.

Table 2 PMDs	
PMD	**Comment**

Leukoplakia	• Most common PMD (80% of PMD cases)
	• Overall prevalence of 0.5%
	  o Homogeneous form is characterized as being thin, flat, and possibly cracked
	  o Nonhomogeneous form typically has a red component and is often described as speckled and nodular
	  o Verrucous leukoplakia is clinically indistinguishable from verrucous carcinoma
	• Malignant transformation rate is low for homogeneous form, higher for nonhomogeneous forms
	• Highest-risk sites are the floor of the mouth and ventral/lateral tongue

Proliferative verrucous leukoplakia	• Multiple, simultaneous leukoplakias • Typically affects elderly women • History of tobacco use is often absent • High rate of malignant transformation
Erythroplakia	• Highest-risk PMD • Low prevalence (0.02%–0.83%) • Most commonly observed as a solitary lesion on the ventral and lateral aspects of the tongue, the retromolar trigone–soft palate complex, and the floor of the mouth • Characterized as being flat with a smooth or granular surface • Most (~90%) erythroplakias represent severe dysplasia or frank carcinoma at discovery
Oral submucous fibrosis	• Strong association with areca nut exposure • Early findings include burning sensation, mucosal blanching, and leathery mucosa • Later findings include stiffening of the oral cavity and oropharynx, fibrous bands, and trismus • Annual malignant transformation rate of about 0.5%
Oral lichen planus	• Commonly occurring chronic oral lesion • Risk of malignant transformation is low, but higher than controls • Mandates frequent monitoring (every 3–6 mo)
Actinic cheilosis	• Sunlight-induced keratosis affecting the lip vermilion • Prevalence unknown, but likely high • Characterized by chronic chapping, loss of elasticity, loss of definition of the vermilion-cutaneous border, mottling, erosion, and ulceration
Snuff patch	• Characteristic white lesion directly attributable to smokeless tobacco placement • Risk of malignant transformation is considered low

Data from Refs.[9–14]

of questionable risk having excluded (other) known diseases or disorders that carry no increased risk for cancer."[14]

• Erythroplakia is defined as, "A fiery red patch that cannot be characterized clinically or pathologically as any other definable disease."[15]

PMDs should be biopsied to establish a histologic diagnosis. Leukoplakia and erythroplakia can show some degree of epithelial dysplasia characterized as being

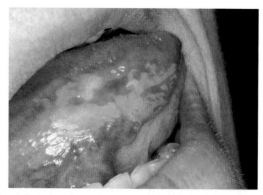

Fig. 1. Leukoplakia: right ventrolateral tongue of a 67-year-old woman.

mild, moderate, or severe. Although the presence of severe dysplasia seems to correlate well with future progression to malignancy, the presence of a PMD does not predict that such progression will occur. Only a small number of PMDs ultimately progress to cancer, although most either remain noncancerous or even regress.[16]

Cancers are characterized by self-sufficiency in growth signals, insensitivity to growth-inhibitory signals, evasion of programmed cell death, immortality or unlimited replicative potential, sustained angiogenesis, and tissue invasion and metastasis.[17] They arise clonally from transformed cells that have undergone specific genetic and epigenetic alterations within a clonal population of cells.[16] These alterations may occur as a consequence of genomic instability from chromosomal rearrangement, amplification, deletion, methylation, and mutation. Progression to malignancy typically occurs over time and requires the accumulation of multiple genetic alterations. In contrast with a malignancy such as chronic myeloid leukemia, which is attributed to a specific reciprocal chromosomal translocation, numerous cumulative causal events seem to underlie the development of OPC.[18] As a consequence, OPC is characterized by substantial molecular, pathologic, and phenotypic heterogeneity.[16,19]

Ongoing research into the molecular pathogenesis of OPC has resulted in the identification of numerous biological markers whose altered activity seems to be associated with PMD and OPC initiation and progression.[16,17,19–24] A brief characterization of some of the biological markers under investigation is presented in **Table 3**. (**Fig. 7**) shows putative linear models of progression correlating histologic changes with potential underlying molecular changes. Although not absolutely predictive,

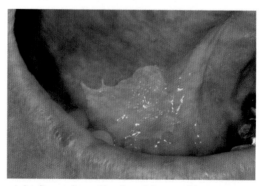

Fig. 2. Leukoplakia: right floor of mouth of an 84-year-old woman.

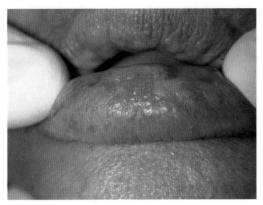

Fig. 3. Erythroplakia: lower lip vermilion of a 58-year-old man.

such models serve as guides for ongoing research. It is presumed that future research to identify consistent patterns or signatures of biological marker expression predictive of PMDs or OPC progression will lead to both better prognostic modeling and the development of targeted therapeutic interventions.

RISK FACTORS

Risk factors (**Table 4**) implicated as potential initiators and/or promoters of oral cancer and OPC include tobacco,[25–28] alcohol,[25,27–29] ultraviolet radiation,[13,30] human papillomavirus (HPV),[31–35] immunosuppression,[30,36] areca nut (betel nut or quid),[10,25,28] maté,[37] and socioeconomic status.[38] Concurrent exposure to some of these factors, such as smoking and alcohol, synergistically results in a higher risk than the simple addition of either's individual risk.[26,27,29] Individuals who consume 2 or more packs of cigarettes and more than 4 alcoholic drinks per day have a 35-fold increased risk for developing OPC.[39] Individuals who use tobacco, alcohol, and betel quid have more than a 120-fold increased risk of developing OPC.[40]

Because many of these risk factors are behavioral, health care professionals have an opportunity to identify patients at increased risk and introduce appropriate preventive and behavioral modification measures.[25,28] An estimated 75% of OPCs could be prevented by the elimination of tobacco smoking and a reduction in alcohol consumption.[41] Within 1 to 4 years of smoking cessation, the risk of OPC is reduced by 35%.[42]

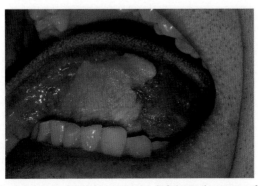

Fig. 4. Erythroplakia distal to leukoplakia: anterior left lateral tongue of a 61-year-old man.

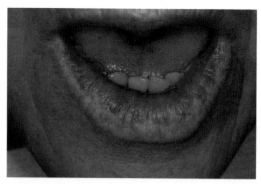

Fig. 5. Actinic cheilosis in a 66-year-old woman.

After 20 years of smoking cessation, the risk of OPC equals that of never-smokers. Cessation of alcohol consumption for more than 20 years is associated with a 40% decreased risk of OPC.[42] Prudent sun exposure and the use of protective lip balms reduces the risk of actinic cheilosis and lip cancer.[13] Preliminary research has shown that vaccination against HPV-16 may be effective in reducing the burden of oral HPV[43]; however, current Food and Drug Administration recommendations do not recognize this specific indication (**Table 5**).[44,45] Vaccination is only effective when provided before natural exposure and the development of counseling programs addressing high-risk sexual behaviors seem warranted.[46]

INCIDENCE

In 2012, there were an estimated 303,373 new cases and 145,328 deaths attributable to OPC worldwide.[47] For 2014, an estimated 42,440 patients (30,220 men, 12,220 women) in the United States were diagnosed with OPC. During the same period an estimated 5730 men and 2660 women succumbed to the disease, a rate of 1 death per hour.[5] The current prevalence of OPC in the United States is estimated to be 275,193.[48]

The incidence of OPC has wide geographic variation (**Table 6**) and largely depends on risk factor exposure.[47] Age-standardized incidence rates for 2012 varied from 0.3 per 100,000 for Cape Verde to 25 per 100,000 for Papua New Guinea. Several

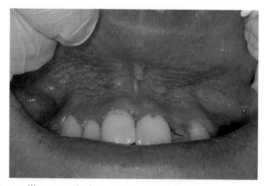

Fig. 6. Snuff patch maxillary vestibule in a 31-year-old man.

Table 3
Some biological markers associated with PMDs and OPC

Aneuploidy	• Marker of chromosomal instability and imbalanced DNA content
	• Present in 50%–60% of OPCs
	  ○ Associated with higher risk of local recurrence and lymph node metastasis
	• Present in 20%–45% of oral dysplasias
	  ○ Conflicting evidence regarding usefulness as predictive tool for progression

miRNA	• Noncoding RNA sequences of 20–22 nucleotides that functionally may act as tumor suppressors or oncogenes
	• More than 1000 identified
	  ○ miRNAs with tumor suppressor activity include let-7a/b, miR-16, miR-29a, miR-125a/b, miR-143, miR-145, miR-148b, miR-194, miR-200a/b/c, and miR-203
	  ○ miRNAs with oncogene activity include miR-17, miR-21, miR-31, miR-134, miR-154, miR-181b/c, miR-184, miR-200b, miR-222, miR-762
	• Dysregulation of miRNAs observed in PMDs and OPC
	• Value as predictive markers undetermined

AI	• Indicates the gain or loss (ie, loss of heterozygosity) of 1 copy of a polymorphic marker (with 2 slightly different alleles) • Occurs across the genome at low frequency • Higher occurrence noted at 3p, 9p21, 17p13 • AI at 3p and 9p under investigation as marker of dysplastic progression in PMDs
Hypermethylation	• Aberrations of DNA methylation contribute to tumorigenesis • Hypermethylation within the CpG islands within promoter regions of many tumor suppressor genes has been observed in PMDs and OPC • Value as a predictive marker undetermined
Proliferation markers	• Increased suprabasilar expression of the proliferation marker Ki-67 may correlate with increasing grades of dysplasia • Other markers under investigation include PCNA and MCM2 • Specificity and value as predictive maker undetermined
Telomerase regulation	• Increased telomerase activity noted in PMDs and OPC • Facilitates cell immortalization • Value as predictive maker undetermined

Tumor suppressor genes	• Tumor suppressor gene mutations are often observed in dysplasia and OPC
	  ○ p53 maps to chromosome 17p13.1
	  ○ p63 maps to chromosome 3q27–29
	  ○ p73 maps to chromosome 1p36
	  ○ p21maps to chromosome 6p21.2
	  ○ p16 maps to chromosome 9p21–22
	• Value as predictive markers undetermined

Receptor kinase pathways	• Alterations of signal transduction pathways network are frequently observed in PMDs and OPC
	  ○ Receptor tyrosine kinase (EGFR/TGF-α) pathway
	  ○ PI3K/AKT pathway
	  ○ The extracellular-signal regulated kinases (ERK/MAPKs) pathway
	  ○ Cyclin D1 pathway
	  ○ VEGF pathway
	• Value as predictive markers undetermined

Abbreviations: AI, allelic imbalance; EGFR, epidermal growth factor receptor; ERK, extracellular-signal regulated kinase; MAPK, mitogen-activated protein kinase; MCM2, minichromosome maintenance complex component 2; miRNA, microRNA; PCNA, proliferating cell nuclear antigen; PI3K, phosphoinositide 3-kinase; TGF-α, transforming growth factor alpha; VEGF, vascular endothelial growth factor.
   Data from Refs.[16–24]

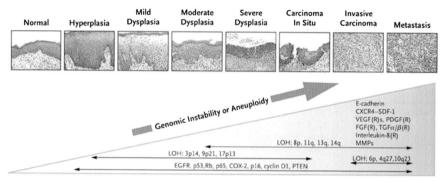

Fig. 7. Head and neck cancer is considered to progress through a multistep process from normal histologic features to hyperplasia, mild dysplasia, moderate dysplasia, severe dysplasia, carcinoma in situ, invasive carcinoma, and metastasis. Underlying genetic instabilities including the loss of heterozygocity (LOH) of certain chromosomes (3p14, 9p21, 17p13, 8p, 11q, 13q, 14q, 6p, 4q27, and 10q23) and amplification or deletion or up-regulation or down-regulation of certain oncogenes or tumor-suppressor genes, including epidermal growth factor receptor (EGFR), p53, Rb, p65, cyclooxygenase 2 (COX-2), p16, cyclin D1, and phosphatase and tensin homolog (PTEN) have been identified as genetic alterations in each of the pathological stages of this disease. Several genes — including those encoding E-cadherin (CDH1), chemokine (C-X-C motif) receptor–stromal-cell–derived factor (CXCR4–SDF-1), vascular endothelial growth factor (VEGF), platelet-derived growth factor (PDGF), fibroblast growth factor (FGF), transforming growth factor α and β (TGF-α and TGF-β), interleukin-8, and the respective receptors, along with matrix metalloproteinase (MMP) — are involved mainly in the progression of metastasis and in early stages of tumor progression. (*From* Haddad RI, Shin DM. Recent advances in head and neck cancer. N Engl J Med 2008;359(11):1143–54; with permission. Copyright ©2008 Massachusetts Medical Society.)

important trends pertaining to the increasing burden of HPV infection have become evident over the past few decades:

- From 1973 to 2004, oral cavity cancer (typically associated with tobacco and/or alcohol exposure) incidence declined by 1.9% each year in the United States, likely attributable to decreased tobacco usage rates.[49]
- During the same period, annual OPC rates increased 1.3% for base of tongue and 0.6% for tonsils, likely attributable to increased HPV infection. Similar increases in HPV-associated cases of OPC have been noted in Sweden, the United Kingdom, and the Netherlands.[49]
- Patients with HPV-associated OPC tend to be young and often relate minimal tobacco/alcohol exposure.[49]
- By 2020, the number of cases of HPV-associated OPC is predicted to exceed the number of cases of invasive cervical cancer.[31]

SIGNS AND SYMPTOMS

Overt OPC presents as a persistent mass, nodule, or indurated ulcer (**Figs. 8–11**). Color changes are common and consist of red or red and white hues. Most OPCs originate from nonkeratinized mucosa (eg, the freely moveable, nonattached mucosa). Symptoms are often absent in early stage disease but become frequent with advanced local invasion. Findings consistent with more advance disease include pain, dysphagia, otitis, weight loss, fixation, and trismus. The findings of paresthesia and anesthesia, in the absence of a history of trauma, strongly suggest an invasive malignancy.

Table 4
Risk factors for OPC

Risk Factor	Comment

Tobacco	• Predominant risk factor for OPC
	• Observed in 74% of all cases
	  ○ 80% for men
	  ○ 61% for women
	• Smoking generally considered higher risk than oral tobacco use (eg, dipping, snuff, chew)

Alcohol	• Risk increases with exposure
	  ○ ~1.7-fold increased risk with 1–2 drinks/d
	  ○ ~2.3-fold increased risk with 3–4 drinks/d
	  ○ ~5.5-fold increased risk with 5 or more drinks/d

UVR	• Prime cause for actinic cheilosis and lip cancer • UVR is capable of inducing both direct and indirect tissue damage • UVR exposure accelerates premature skin aging and increases risk of developing carcinoma

HPV	• Predominant cause of oropharyngeal site cancers; 15-fold increased risk compared with controls
	• HPV-16 involved in >85% of HPV-associated cases
	  ○ Estimated oral prevalence of 1.0% in the United States
	  ○ Oncoprotein E6 targets multiple cellular pathways to interfere with transcription, cytokine signaling, chromatin remodeling, protein degradation, cell polarity, and apoptosis, leading to genomic instability
	  ○ Oncoprotein E7 can induce keratinocyte immortalization

Immunosuppression	• Chronic states of immunosuppression increases risk of developing OPC
	  ○ Drug induced (eg, antirejection drugs for HSCT)
	  ○ Disease induced (eg, HIV)

Areca nut (betel nut)	• Predominant contributor to oral submucous fibrosis
	• Estimated 700 million users worldwide
	• Areas of high exposure include India, southeast Asia
	  ○ BQ (paan): betel leaf wrapped around mix of areca nut, slaked lime, condiments
	    ■ Gutkha: BQ with tobacco
	    ■ Paan masala: BQ without tobacco
	  ○ Supari: sun-dried or cured forms of areca nut
	  ○ Tambul: wet fermented areca nut
	• Components (eg, alkaloids, tannins, trace elements) contribute to carcinogenesis

Maté	• Hot aqueous infusion of *Ilex paraguariensis* herb • Commonly consumed in Latin America • Estimated 2-fold increased risk of OPC compared with controls
Socioeconomic status	• Individuals with low income have a 2.4-fold increased risk of developing OPC

Abbreviations: BQ, betel quid; HIV, human immunodeficiency virus; HPV, human papillomavirus; HSCT, hematopoietic stem cell transplantation; UVR, ultra violet radiation.
  Data from Refs.[13,26,29–31,33,34,36–38]

Metastatic dissemination occurs through the submandibular, cervical, and jugular lymphatic pathways and distant metastases most commonly target the lung.

Oral cavity cancers are usually readily discoverable when accomplishing a visual and tactile examination; however, OPCs are often not readily or easily observed until

Table 5
Approved indications for available HPV vaccines

Gardasil (Merck Sharp and Dohme)[a]	Cervarix (GlaxoSmithKline Biologicals)[b]

• Prevention of vulvar and vaginal cancer
• Vaccination in female patients 9–26 y of age for prevention of the following diseases caused by HPV types 6, 11, 16, and 18:
  ○ Cervical cancer
  ○ Genital warts (condyloma acuminata) and the following precancerous or dysplastic lesions:
    ■ Cervical AIS
    ■ CIN grade 2 and grade 3
    ■ VIN grade 2 and grade 3
    ■ VaIN grade 2 and grade 3
    ■ CIN grade 1
• Vaccination in boys and men 9–26 y of age for the prevention of genital warts caused by HPV types 6 and 11
• Vaccination in people aged 9–26 y for the prevention of anal cancer and associated precancerous lesions caused by HPV types 6, 11, 16, and 18
	• Prevention of cervical cancer, CIN grade 2 or worse and AIS, and CIN grade 1 caused by oncogenic HPV types 16 and 18, in women 9–25 y of age

Abbreviations: AIS, adenocarcinoma in situ; CIN, cervical intraepithelial neoplasia; VaIN, vaginal intraepithelial neoplasia; VIN, vulvar intraepithelial neoplasia.
[a] *Data from* Food and Drug Administration. Gardasil [package insert]. Available at: http://www.fda.gov/downloads/BiologicsBloodVaccines/Vaccines/ApprovedProducts/UCM111263.pdf. Accessed February 5, 2014.
[b] *Data from* Food and Drug Administration. Cervarix [package insert and patient information]. Available at: http://www.fda.gov/downloads/BiologicsBloodVaccines/Vaccines/ApprovedProducts/UCM186981.pdf. Accessed February 5, 2014.

extensive growth or local spread has occurred (**Figs. 12** and **13**). Further confounding discovery is the insidious nature of OPC and early signs and symptoms (eg, sore throat, hoarseness, lymphadenopathy, otitis) that often mimic common benign conditions such as pharyngitis or tonsillitis. Persistence of such signs and symptoms should be referred for a thorough medical work-up by an otolaryngologist (ear, nose, and throat).[50]

DIAGNOSTIC DILEMMAS

Numerous benign conditions (**Figs. 14–19, Table 7**) may mimic a PMD or OPC.[11,50] Most of these conditions may be diagnosed through a careful correlation of the history, pattern of presentation, and, when indicated, response to therapy. Any finding deemed suspicious or equivocal should be referred either for further assessment or immediate biopsy.

DIAGNOSIS

The diagnosis of OPC is established by histologic assessment. Suspected PMDs should also be biopsied as necessary to determine the presence of dysplasia or carcinoma. A variety of adjunctive products are currently marketed with the stated goal of improving the practitioner's ability to identify mucosal abnormalities such as PMDs and OPC (**Table 8**).[51–53] Studies addressing the efficacy of these products when

Table 6
Selected regional and country age-standardized OPC incidence rates

	Male	Female
Eastern Africa	4.5	2.8
Middle Africa	3.5	1.8
Northern Africa	2.8	1.8
Southern Africa	6.3	2.3
Western Africa	1.7	1.4
Caribbean	4.8	1.8
Central America	2.6	1.7
South America	5.3	2.4
North America	7.2	3.2
Eastern Asia	2.4	1.1
South-Eastern Asia	4.0	2.5
South-Central Asia	9.9	4.7
Western Asia	2.7	1.6
Central and Eastern Europe	9.1	2.0
Northern Europe	5.9	3.1
Western Europe	7.9	3.2
Australia and New Zealand	8.3	3.7
Papua New Guinea	30.3	21.1

Age-standardized rate incidence per 100,000.
Data from World Health Organization, International Agency for Research on Cancer. GLOBOCAN 2012: Latest world cancer statistics. Available at: http://globocan.iarc.fr/Default.aspx. Accessed February 5, 2014.

used in clinical practice are limited and often conflicting. The usefulness of these products in the clinical setting to discriminate between PMDs and OPCs against the milieu of benign mucosal lesions remains unknown.[54] These devices are not a substitute for tissue biopsy.

STAGING

Staging is useful for treatment planning, prognostication, and comparison of treatment outcomes. Once diagnosed, all OPCs are clinically staged using the TNM (tumor,

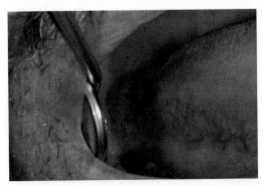

Fig. 8. Squamous cell carcinoma of the right base of tongue in a 69-year-old man.

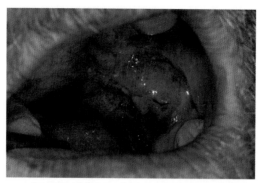

Fig. 9. Large squamous cell carcinoma of the left soft palatal complex in a 62-year-old man.

node, metastasis) classification system.[55] T refers to the size of the primary neoplasm, N refers to the extent of lymph node involvement, and M refers to the presence of distant metastasis. The differentiation of localized disease (stages I and II) from more advanced disease (stages III and IV) remains an essential determination for treatment planning.[56] Imaging techniques such as computed tomography (CT), magnetic resonance imaging (MRI), and positron emission tomography are useful in further assessing tumor size, nodal involvement, and dissemination.[57] CT has long been regarded as the imaging modality of choice for assessing the size, location, and spread (both in soft tissue and regional lymph nodes) of the primary tumor. MRI technology offers potential advantages in terms of superior soft tissue contrast, multiplanar imaging capability, lack of ionizing radiation, and freedom from metallic artifacts from dental restorations. However, none of the imaging techniques are accurate enough on their own and a combination of clinical and multiple imaging techniques offers the best results in assessing OPC.[57]

The major limitation of the TNM classification system is its inability to account for the unique biological behavior of a given OPC.[22,58] Other important parameters to consider in tumor assessment include (1) tumor volume, (2) histologic grade, (3) the level of nodal metastasis (eg, upper/middle/lower jugular), (4) growth pattern, (5) extracapsular spread, and (6) field cancerization.

Field cancerization refers to the approximately 10% of patients presenting with OPC who manifest more than 1 independent area of malignancy.[59] This phenomenon is observed in other cancers such as cancers of the esophagus, lungs, cervix, vulva, anus, colon, breast, bladder, and skin. It is postulated that exposure to carcinogens

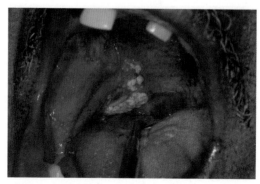

Fig. 10. Squamous cell carcinoma of the right soft palatal complex in a 73-year-old man.

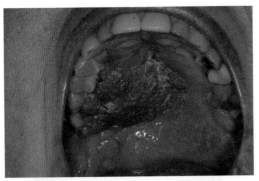

Fig. 11. Large squamous cell carcinoma of the right palate in an 83-year-old woman with a 20-year history of lichen planus.

such as tobacco and alcohol promote anaplastic changes throughout the area of exposure. There are 2 prevailing theories to explain the manner in which field cancerization occurs. One theory holds that ongoing carcinogenic insult leads to the development of independent malignant clones, whereas the other theory proposes that a single malignant clone may spread or migrate to new sites.[59]

Perhaps the most intriguing criterion to consider in the near future will be the tumor's biological signature (see **Table 3**). Shiraki and colleagues[23] measured the expression of 3 biological markers associated with OPC (p53, cyclin D1, and EGFR) in 140 resected tumors. The expression of p53, cyclin D1, and epidermal growth factor receptor (EGFR) was noted in 64 cases (46%), 54 cases (39%), and 54 cases (39%), respectively, but no interrelationship between any 2 markers was noted. Although EGFR expression independently was significantly associated with poor differentiation and invasive growth, it had no significant impact on survival. However, the coexpression of all 3 markers was significantly associated with

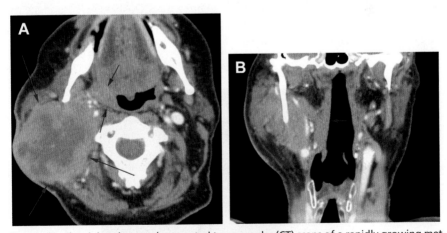

Fig. 12. (A, B) Axial and coronal computed tomography (CT) scans of a rapidly growing metastatic right-side neck mass in a 68-year-old man. The patient noted the mass about 6 weeks earlier and it was initially assessed as an abscess. He denied sore throat, dysphagia, or hoarseness. Physical examination showed a hard and tender right level II solid neck mass without evidence of a readily visible oropharyngeal lesion. Note the mild thickening of the right palatine tonsil (*red arrow*) and solid neck mass with internal necrosis (*blue arrows*).

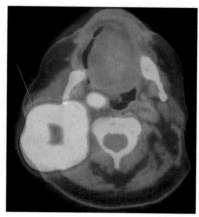

Fig. 13. Axial positron emission tomography/CT of the same patient revealed that the right level II mass is hypermetabolic, representing metastatic lymphadenopathy from the primary right palatine tonsil tumor, which proved to be an HPV-positive squamous cell carcinoma. Red arrow, right palatine tonsil; blue arrow, solid neck mass with internal necrosis.

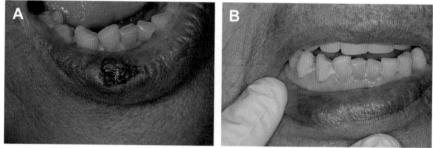

Fig. 14. (*A*) Overzealous scrubbing by a 77-year-old woman of lip irritation, which resolved 5 weeks after the habit was discontinued (*B*).

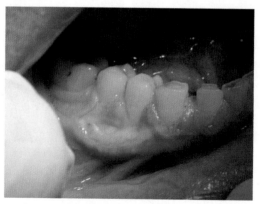

Fig. 15. Chemical burn from inappropriate use of self-applied over-the-counter whitening strips.

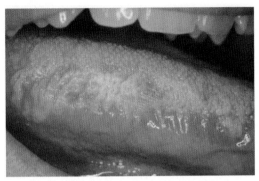

Fig. 16. Oral hairy leukoplakia of the right lateral tongue in a 27-year-old man.

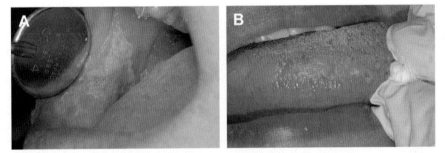

Fig. 17. Chronic cheek (A) and tongue (B) biting habit 49-year-old man.

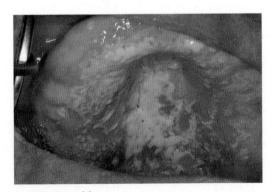

Fig. 18. Candidiasis in a 52-year-old man.

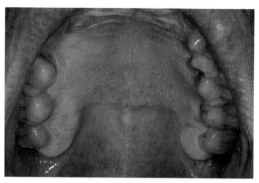

Fig. 19. Nicotine stomatitis in a 54-year-old man.

invasive growth and shortened survival. The investigators concluded that coexpression of p53, cyclin D1, and EGFR may prove to be useful in stratifying patients into low-risk or high-risk groups.[23] The challenge for ongoing and future research is to determine which panel or mix of the numerous biological markers available for consideration will show the highest predicative value for clinical use.[16,22]

MANAGEMENT

OPC is typically treated by 1 or a combination of 3 principal therapeutic modalities: surgery, radiotherapy, and chemotherapy. The use of one treatment protocol or regimen rather than another depends not only on the size, location, and stage of the primary tumor but also on the patient's comorbidities, nutritional status, ability to tolerate treatment, and desires.[58] The delivery of care is best coordinated by a multidisciplinary team that may include a head and neck surgeon, a general and/or oral and maxillofacial pathologist, a radiation oncologist, a medical oncologist, oral health care providers, a nutritionist, a nurse specialist, a speech pathologist, and a tobacco cessation counselor. The direct and indirect costs of OPC therapy render it one of the most costly of all cancers to treat.[4]

Surgical excision is the preferred modality for most well-defined and accessible solid tumors; however, its use to manage inaccessible or advanced tumors showing lymph node involvement and/or metastasis is limited. For such cases, radiotherapy may be either an effective alternative to surgery or a valuable adjunct to surgery

Table 7 Conditions that may mimic a PMD or OPC	
Traumatic irritations	Chemical injury
Leukoedema	White sponge nevus
Oral hairy leukoplakia	Chronic cheek/tongue biting
Candidiasis	Nicotine stomatitis
Chronic ulcerations	Sore throat

Data from Cleveland JL, Junger ML, Saraiya M, et al. The connection between human papillomavirus and oropharyngeal squamous cell carcinomas in the United States: implications for dentistry. J Am Dent Assoc 2011;142(8):915–24; and van der Waal I. Potentially malignant disorders of the oral and oropharyngeal mucosa; terminology, classification and present concepts of management. Oral Oncol 2009;45(4–5):317–23.

Table 8 Available adjunctive diagnostic aids	
Cytopathology	OralCDx Brush Test
Toluidine blue vital staining	ViziLite Plus with TBlue OraBlu Oral Lesion Marking System
Visualization adjuncts	ViziLite Plus with TBlue Microlux VELscope Vx Sapphire Plus Identafi DOE Oral Exam System OralID

Data from Refs.[51–53]

and/or chemotherapy in the locoregional treatment of malignant head and neck tumors. Although the benefit of neoadjuvant (induction) chemotherapy remains a topic of debate,[60,61] several studies have shown that concomitant chemoradiotherapy improves both locoregional control and survival.[62–64]

Patients with OPC frequently experience both acute and chronic adverse complications related to therapy (**Table 9**).[65,66] Surgical complications include disfigurement, trismus, speech impairment, and dysphagia. Chemotherapy complications tend to be acute and resolve after cessation of therapy, whereas radiotherapy often incurs permanent site-specific damage to structures within the beam. Adverse therapeutic complications often negatively affect the patent's quality of life. Specific therapeutic efforts to reduce the burden of adverse effects include the use of transoral robotic surgery, transoral laser microscopy, microsurgical reconstruction, altered fractionation, intensity modulated radiotherapy, stereotactic radiotherapy, the free radical oxygen scavenger amifostine during radiotherapy, and submandibular salivary gland transfer surgery.[19,65,67]

The burden of oral complications, in terms of both risk and severity, seems to be increased for patients who have poor oral health going into cancer therapy. A comprehensive dental examination should be obtained as part of the patient's comprehensive medical work-up before the initiation of cancer therapy. Necessary dental care should be accomplished as early as possible in the medical treatment planning phase.

Table 9 Common complications of OPC treatment	
Acute	**Chronic**
Functional impairment/disfigurement	Functional impairment/disfigurement
Mucositis	Damaged mucosa
Salivary dysfunction	Salivary dysfunction (xerostomia)
Pain	Pain (chemosensory, neuropathic)
Infection	Infection
Dysgeusia	Dysgeusia
	Increased dental disease (caries, periodontitis)
	Necrosis (osteonecrosis, soft tissue)

Data from National Cancer Institute. PDQ® oral complications of chemotherapy and head/neck radiation. Bethesda (MD): National Cancer Institute; 2013. Available at: http://cancer.gov/cancertopics/pdq/supportivecare/oralcomplications/HealthProfessional. Accessed February 5, 2014.

Predictable protocols to manage PMDs do not exist and current efforts focus on risk factor elimination (eg, tobacco and alcohol exposure), ablation if possible (surgery, laser, cryotherapy, chemical), and regular monitoring for progression.[41,68,69] PMDs showing mild dysplasia tend to be monitored (so-called watchful waiting), whereas more severe dysplasia is usually excised.[70] Holmstrup and colleagues[71] followed 269 lesions (188 homogeneous leukoplakia, 66 nonhomogeneous leukoplakias, 15 erythroplakias) treated with surgical excision or scheduled monitoring for a period of 1.1 to 20.2 years (**Table 10**). Following excision there were 12 instances of recurrence and ultimately 11 lesions (1 homogeneous leukoplakia, 9 nonhomogeneous leukoplakias, 1 erythroplakia) developed carcinoma after a mean follow-up period of up to 7.5 years. Of the lesions undergoing monitoring without surgical intervention, 28 lesions disappeared and 7 lesions developed carcinoma after a mean observation period of 6.6 years. The risk of malignant transformation was most strongly associated with nonhomogeneous leukoplakia (odds ratio [OR], 7) and lesions greater than 200 mm^2 in size (OR, 5.4). In considering other variables such smoking habit, lesion site and demarcation, and the characterization of epithelial dysplasia, none were statistically significant factors for progression to malignancy. The investigators concluded that surgical intervention does not prevent PMD progression to malignancy and the uniform use of surgical management remains unproven.[71]

Chemoprevention protocols to manage PMDs using agents such as epidermal growth factor, retinoids, receptor kinase inhibitors, cyclooxygenase-2 inhibitors, green tea extract, and peroxisome proliferator–activated receptor-gamma agonists are currently being studied for potential application in clinical practice.[72]

Table 10
Long-term outcomes of 269 cases of leukoplakia and erythroplakia monitored or surgically excised

	Percentage Dysplasia 0–2[a] (n)	Percentage Dysplasia 3–4[a] (n)	Percentage Recurred[b] (n)	Percentage Carcinoma[c] (n)
Lesions Excised				
Homogeneous leukoplakia (n = 39)	97 (38)	3 (1)	5 (2)	3 (1)
Nonhomogeneous leukoplakia (n = 46)	73 (34)	27 (12)	17 (8)	20 (9)
Erythroplakia (n = 9)	56 (5)	44 (4)	22 (2)	11 (1)
Lesions Monitored				
Homogeneous leukoplakia (n = 149)	—	—	—	3 (4)
Nonhomogeneous leukoplakia (n = 20)	—	—	—	15 (3)
Erythroplakia (n = 6)	—	—	—	0

[a] Characterization of dysplasia on excision: 0, none; 1, mild dysplasia; 2, moderate dysplasia; 3, severe dysplasia; 4, carcinoma in situ.
[b] Three nonhomogeneous and 2 homogeneous leukoplakias had 2 recurrences and 1 nonhomogeneous and 1 homogeneous leukoplakia had 3 recurrences during the follow- up period.
[c] Carcinoma developed during follow-up period (mean 7.5 years for excised lesions; mean 6.6 years for monitored lesions).
Data from Holmstrup P, Vedtofte P, Reibel J, et al. Long-term treatment outcome of oral premalignant lesions. Oral Oncol 2006;42(5):461–74.

Table 11 HPV-associated tumor tendencies	HPV Negative	HPV Positive
Histology	Keratinized	Nonkeratinized
Stage at diagnosis	Variable	III/IV
Risk factors	Tobacco/alcohol	Sexual behavior
p53	Mutated	Not mutated
Survival	Unchanged	Improved

Data from Marur S, D'Souza G, Westra WH, et al. HPV-associated head and neck cancer: a virus-related cancer epidemic. Lancet Oncol 2010;11(8):781–9; and Rautava J, Syrjanen S. Biology of human papillomavirus infections in head and neck carcinogenesis. Head Neck Pathol 2012;6 Suppl 1:S3–15.

PROGNOSIS

The number of oral cancer survivors in the United States exceeds 275,000.[48] Five-year survival rates for localized, regional, and distant staged OPC are 83%, 59%, and 36% respectively.[5] Lifelong surveillance is mandatory, because up to 30% of treated patients develop a second primary tumor at some point in the future.[73] Continued smoking and heavy alcohol consumption after OPC therapy contributes to reduced treatment efficacy; increased posttherapy complications, recurrence, and additional disease; and reduced quality of life and survival.[74] Up to one-third of survivors continue to smoke after therapy and one-half continue to consume alcohol.[27] Smoking cessation treatment should follow the standards of practice such as those set forth in the US Department of Health and Human Services publication *Treating Tobacco Use and Dependence: 2008 Update - Clinical Practice Guideline*.[75]

Patients with HPV-16–positive tumors and low rates of tobacco exposure show distinct biological characteristics and an improved response to therapy compared with patients with HPV-16–negative tumors and high rates of tobacco/alcohol exposure (**Table 11**).[34,35,49] Postulated reasons for this improved outcome include reduced exposure to tobacco/alcohol, absence of field cancerization, lower comorbidity burden, and the presence of functional unmutated p53.[33,49]

Patients with adverse side effects induced by therapy or disease should be strongly encouraged to obtain necessary dental care. Most survivors of OPC who have undergone radiotherapy as part of their treatment experience some degree of chronic oral compromise that adversely affects their quality of life. The patient should be placed on a frequent maintenance recall schedule with an oral health care provider (every 3–4 months) to monitor for, and manage, therapy-related complications (eg, compromised mucosa, salivary dysfunction, infection, altered taste, pain, caries, and osteonecrosis) and to assess the patient's commitment and compliance with oral hygiene. Scheduled examinations by the oral health care provider also serve as another surveillance check point to monitor for recurrent or new disease.

SUMMARY

OPC is a relentless and debilitating cancer, the burden of which is significant and growing. Despite advances in the understanding of OPC and improved therapeutic interventions, it continues to be diagnosed at an advanced stage and the survival rate remains poor. Geographic incidence rates for OPC vary widely and correlate well with exposure to established risk factors such as tobacco, alcohol, areca nut, and HPV infection. Health care providers can be instrumental in both reducing the incidence of OPC and improving on its early diagnosis by understanding its capricious nature, identifying patients at highest risk through risk factor assessment, providing preventive education, and diligently performing a disciplined physical examination. Findings deemed suspicious or equivocal should be referred for further assessment or undergo immediate biopsy, whereas findings deemed innocuous should be reevaluated within 2 to 3 weeks and referred for further assessment or undergo biopsy if still present.

REFERENCES

1. National Cancer Institute. PDQ® lip and oral cavity cancer treatment. Bethesda (MD): National Cancer Institute; 2012. Available at: http://cancer.gov/cancer topics/pdq/treatment/lip-and-oral-cavity/HealthProfessional. Accessed February 5, 2014.
2. National Cancer Institute. PDQ® oropharyngeal cancer treatment. Bethesda (MD): National Cancer Institute; 2013. Available at: http://cancer.gov/cancertopics/pdq/treatment/oropharyngeal/HealthProfessional. Accessed February 5, 2014.
3. Cooper JS, Porter K, Mallin K, et al. National Cancer Database report on cancer of the head and neck: 10-year update. Head Neck 2009;31(6):748–58.
4. Jacobson JJ, Epstein JB, Eichmiller FC, et al. The cost burden of oral, oral pharyngeal, and salivary gland cancers in three groups: commercial insurance, Medicare, and Medicaid. Head Neck Oncol 2012;4:15.
5. Siegel R, Ma J, Zou Z, et al. Cancer statistics, 2014. CA Cancer J Clin 2014;64(1):9–29.
6. Mignogna MD, Fedele S, Lo Russo L, et al. Oral and pharyngeal cancer: lack of prevention and early detection by health care providers. Eur J Cancer Prev 2001;10(4):381–3.
7. Gomez I, Warnakulasuriya S, Varela-Centelles PI, et al. Is early diagnosis of oral cancer a feasible objective? Who is to blame for diagnostic delay? Oral Dis 2010;16(4):333–42.
8. Pleis JR, Ward BW, Lucas JW. Summary health statistics for U.S. adults: National Health Interview Survey, 2009. Vital Health Stat 10 2010;(249):1–207.
9. Greer RO Jr. Oral manifestations of smokeless tobacco use. Otolaryngol Clin North Am 2011;44(1):31–56, v.
10. Sharan RN, Mehrotra R, Choudhury Y, et al. Association of betel nut with carcinogenesis: revisit with a clinical perspective. PLoS One 2012;7(8):e42759.
11. van der Waal I. Potentially malignant disorders of the oral and oropharyngeal mucosa; terminology, classification and present concepts of management. Oral Oncol 2009;45(4–5):317–23.
12. van der Waal I. Potentially malignant disorders of the oral and oropharyngeal mucosa; present concepts of management. Oral Oncol 2010;46(6):423–5.
13. Vieira RA, Minicucci EM, Marques ME, et al. Actinic cheilitis and squamous cell carcinoma of the lip: clinical, histopathological and immunogenetic aspects. An Bras Dermatol 2012;87(1):105–14.
14. Warnakulasuriya S, Johnson NW, van der Waal I. Nomenclature and classification of potentially malignant disorders of the oral mucosa. J Oral Pathol Med 2007;36(10):575–80.
15. Pindborg JJ, Reichart PA, Smith CJ, et al. Histological typing of cancer and pre-cancer of the oral mucosa. 2nd edition. Berlin: Springer Verlag; 1997.
16. Lingen MW, Pinto A, Mendes RA, et al. Genetics/epigenetics of oral premalignancy: current status and future research. Oral Dis 2011;17(Suppl 1):7–22.

17. Hanahan D, Weinberg RA. Hallmarks of cancer: the next generation. Cell 2011;
    144(5):646–74.
18. Howard JD, Lu B, Chung CH. Therapeutic targets in head and neck squamous
    cell carcinoma: identification, evaluation, and clinical translation. Oral Oncol
    2012;48(1):10–7.
19. Haddad RI, Shin DM. Recent advances in head and neck cancer. N Engl J Med
    2008;359(11):1143–54.
20. Choi S, Myers JN. Molecular pathogenesis of oral squamous cell carcinoma: im-
    plications for therapy. J Dent Res 2008;87(1):14–32.
21. Gasche JA, Goel A. Epigenetic mechanisms in oral carcinogenesis. Future On-
    col 2012;8(11):1407–25.
22. Oliveira LR, Ribeiro-Silva A. Prognostic significance of immunohistochemical
    biomarkers in oral squamous cell carcinoma. Int J Oral Maxillofac Surg 2011;
    40(3):298–307.
23. Shiraki M, Odajima T, Ikeda T, et al. Combined expression of p53, cyclin D1 and
    epidermal growth factor receptor improves estimation of prognosis in curatively
    resected oral cancer. Mod Pathol 2005;18(11):1482–9.
24. Zheng M, Li L, Tang YL, et al. Biomarkers in tongue cancer: understanding the
    molecular basis and their clinical implications. Postgrad Med J 2010;86(1015):292–8.
25. Petti S. Lifestyle risk factors for oral cancer. Oral Oncol 2009;45(4–5):340–50.
26. Saman DM. A review of the epidemiology of oral and pharyngeal carcinoma: up-
    date. Head Neck Oncol 2012;4:1.
27. Sivasithamparam J, Visk CA, Cohen EE, et al. Modifiable risk behaviors in pa-
    tients with head and neck cancer. Cancer 2013;119(13):2419–26.
28. Warnakulasuriya S. Causes of oral cancer–an appraisal of controversies. Br
    Dent J 2009;207(10):471–5.
29. Goldstein BY, Chang SC, Hashibe M, et al. Alcohol consumption and cancers of
    the oral cavity and pharynx from 1988 to 2009: an update. Eur J Cancer Prev
    2010;19(6):431–65.
30. de Visscher JG, van der Waal I. Etiology of cancer of the lip. A review. Int J Oral
    Maxillofac Surg 1998;27(3):199–203.
31. Gillison ML, Broutian T, Pickard RK, et al. Prevalence of oral HPV infection in the
    United States, 2009-2010. JAMA 2012;307(7):693–703.
32. Pickard RK, Xiao W, Broutian TR, et al. The prevalence and incidence of oral hu-
    man papillomavirus infection among young men and women, aged 18-30 years.
    Sex Transm Dis 2012;39(7):559–66.
33. Rautava J, Syrjanen S. Biology of human papillomavirus infections in head and
    neck carcinogenesis. Head Neck Pathol 2012;6(Suppl 1):S3–15.
34. Shaw R, Robinson M. The increasing clinical relevance of human papillomavirus
    type 16 (HPV-16) infection in oropharyngeal cancer. Br J Oral Maxillofac Surg
    2011;49(6):423–9.
35. Tribius S, Hoffmann M. Human papilloma virus infection in head and neck can-
    cer. Dtsch Arztebl Int 2013;110(11):184–90, 90e1.
36. Demarosi F, Lodi G, Carrassi A, et al. Oral malignancies following HSCT: graft
    versus host disease and other risk factors. Oral Oncol 2005;41(9):865–77.
37. Dasanayake AP, Silverman AJ, Warnakulasuriya S. Mate drinking and oral and
    oro-pharyngeal cancer: a systematic review and meta-analysis. Oral Oncol
    2010;46(2):82–6.
38. Conway DI, Petticrew M, Marlborough H, et al. Socioeconomic inequalities and
    oral cancer risk: a systematic review and meta-analysis of case-control studies.
    Int J Cancer 2008;122(12):2811–9.

39. Blot WJ, McLaughlin JK, Winn DM, et al. Smoking and drinking in relation to oral and pharyngeal cancer. Cancer Res 1988;48(11):3282–7.
40. Jeng JH, Chang MC, Hahn LJ. Role of areca nut in betel quid-associated chemical carcinogenesis: current awareness and future perspectives. Oral Oncol 2001;37(6):477–92.
41. Warnakulasuriya S. Living with oral cancer: epidemiology with particular reference to prevalence and life-style changes that influence survival. Oral Oncol 2010;46(6):407–10.
42. Marron M, Boffetta P, Zhang ZF, et al. Cessation of alcohol drinking, tobacco smoking and the reversal of head and neck cancer risk. Int J Epidemiol 2010; 39(1):182–96.
43. Herrero R, Quint W, Hildesheim A, et al. Reduced prevalence of oral human papillomavirus (HPV) 4 years after bivalent HPV vaccination in a randomized clinical trial in Costa Rica. PLoS One 2013;8(7):e68329.
44. Food and Drug Administration. Gardasil [package insert]. Available at: http://www.fda.gov/downloads/BiologicsBloodVaccines/Vaccines/ApprovedProducts/UCM111263.pdf. Accessed February 5, 2014.
45. Food and Drug Administration. Cervarix [package insert and patient information]. Available at: http://www.fda.gov/downloads/BiologicsBloodVaccines/Vaccines/ApprovedProducts/UCM186981.pdf. Accessed February 5, 2014.
46. Diaz ML. Counseling the patient with HPV disease. Obstet Gynecol Clin North Am 2013;40(2):391–402.
47. World Health Organization. International Agency for Research on Cancer. GLOBOCAN 2012: Latest world cancer statistics. 2014. Available at: http://globocan.iarc.fr/Default.aspx. Accessed February 5, 2014.
48. National Cancer Institute. SEER stat fact sheets: oral cavity and pharynx cancer. Available at: http://seer.cancer.gov/statfacts/html/oralcav.html. Accessed February 7, 2014.
49. Marur S, D'Souza G, Westra WH, et al. HPV-associated head and neck cancer: a virus-related cancer epidemic. Lancet Oncol 2010;11(8):781–9.
50. Cleveland JL, Junger ML, Saraiya M, et al. The connection between human papillomavirus and oropharyngeal squamous cell carcinomas in the United States: implications for dentistry. J Am Dent Assoc 2011;142(8):915–24.
51. Huber MA. Adjunctive diagnostic aids in oral cancer screening: an update. Tex Dent J 2012;129(5):471–80.
52. Food and Drug Administration. 510(k) Premarket notification - MicroLux DL, MicroLux BLU, Bio/Screen - K121282. Available at: http://www.accessdata.fda.gov/scripts/cdrh/cfdocs/cfpmn/pmn.cfm?ID=K121282. Accessed February 8, 2014.
53. Food and Drug Administration. 510(k) Premarket notification - OralID - K123169. Available at: http://www.accessdata.fda.gov/scripts/cdrh/cfdocs/cfpmn/pmn.cfm?ID=K123169. Accessed February 8, 2014.
54. Rethman MP, Carpenter W, Cohen EE, et al. Evidence-based clinical recommendations regarding screening for oral squamous cell carcinomas. J Am Dent Assoc 2010;141(5):509–20.
55. Edge SB, Byrd DR, Compton CC, et al. AJCC cancer staging manual. 7th edition. New York: Springer; 2010.
56. Trotta BM, Pease CS, Rasamny JJ, et al. Oral cavity and oropharyngeal squamous cell cancer: key imaging findings for staging and treatment planning. Radiographics 2011;31(2):339–54.
57. Skinner HD, Holsinger FC, Beadle BM. Oropharynx cancer. Curr Probl Cancer 2012;36(6):334–415.

58. Takes RP, Rinaldo A, Silver CE, et al. Future of the TNM classification and staging system in head and neck cancer. Head Neck 2010;32(12):1693–711.
59. Angadi PV, Savitha JK, Rao SS, et al. Oral field cancerization: current evidence and future perspectives. Oral Maxillofac Surg 2012;16(2):171–80.
60. Hanna GJ, Haddad RI, Lorch JH. Induction chemotherapy for locoregionally advanced head and neck cancer: past, present, future? Oncologist 2013; 18(3):288–93.
61. Licitra L, Grandi C, Guzzo M, et al. Primary chemotherapy in resectable oral cavity squamous cell cancer: a randomized controlled trial. J Clin Oncol 2003;21(2):327–33.
62. Duvvuri U, Myers JN. Contemporary management of oropharyngeal cancer: anatomy and physiology of the oropharynx. Curr Probl Surg 2009;46(2):119–84.
63. Furness S, Glenny AM, Worthington HV, et al. Interventions for the treatment of oral cavity and oropharyngeal cancer: chemotherapy. Cochrane Database Syst Rev 2011;(4):CD006386.
64. Haigentz M Jr, Silver CE, Corry J, et al. Current trends in initial management of oropharyngeal cancer: the declining use of open surgery. Eur Arch Otorhinolaryngol 2009;266(12):1845–55.
65. Epstein JB, Thariat J, Bensadoun RJ, et al. Oral complications of cancer and cancer therapy: from cancer treatment to survivorship. CA Cancer J Clin 2012;62(6):400–22.
66. National Cancer Institute. PDQ® oral complications of chemotherapy and head/neck radiation. Bethesda (MD): National Cancer Institute; 2013. Available at: http://cancer.gov/cancertopics/pdq/supportivecare/oralcomplications/Health Professional. Accessed February 5, 2014.
67. Wang X, Hu C, Eisbruch A. Organ-sparing radiation therapy for head and neck cancer. Nat Rev Clin Oncol 2011;8(11):639–48.
68. Lodi G, Porter S. Management of potentially malignant disorders: evidence and critique. J Oral Pathol Med 2008;37(2):63–9.
69. Vladimirov BS, Schiodt M. The effect of quitting smoking on the risk of unfavorable events after surgical treatment of oral potentially malignant lesions. Int J Oral Maxillofac Surg 2009;38(11):1188–93.
70. Dost F, Le Cao K, Ford PJ, et al. Malignant transformation of oral epithelial dysplasia: a real-world evaluation of histopathologic grading. Oral Surg Oral Med Oral Pathol Oral Radiol 2014;117(3):343–52.
71. Holmstrup P, Vedtofte P, Reibel J, et al. Long-term treatment outcome of oral premalignant lesions. Oral Oncol 2006;42(5):461–74.
72. William WN Jr. Oral premalignant lesions: any progress with systemic therapies? Curr Opin Oncol 2012;24(3):205–10.
73. Gonzalez-Moles MA, Scully C, Ruiz-Avila I. Molecular findings in oral premalignant fields: update on their diagnostic and clinical implications. Oral Dis 2012; 18(1):40–7.
74. Gritz ER, Demark-Wahnefried W. Health behaviors influence cancer survival. J Clin Oncol 2009;27(12):1930–2.
75. Fiore MC, Jaén CR, Baker TB, et al. Treating tobacco use and dependence: 2008 update. Clinical practice guideline. Rockville (MD): US Department of Health and Human Services. Public Health Service; 2008. Available at: http://www.ahrq.gov/professionals/clinicians-providers/guidelines-recommendations/tobacco/clinicians/treating_tobacco_use08.pdf. Accessed February 5, 2014.

Oral Mucosal Diseases
Evaluation and Management

Eric T. Stoopler, DMD, FDS RCSEd, FDS RCSEng*, Thomas P. Sollecito, DMD, FDS RCSEd

KEYWORDS

- Oral mucosal disease • Herpes • Candida • Aphthous • Lichen planus • Pemphigus
- Pemphigoid

KEY POINTS

- Oral mucosal diseases are common disorders affecting all segments of the general population.
- These conditions can be of an infectious or noninfectious etiology.
- Several disorders can present with similar features, which makes clinical diagnosis challenging.
- Management protocols vary based on the specific oral mucosal disease.

Oral mucosal diseases represent several common conditions that affect all segments of the general population. Some of these disorders present with signs and symptoms that are pathognomonic for the condition, whereas others present with similar features that can make diagnosis difficult to achieve based on clinical examination only. These disorders may be categorized based on different clinical parameters, such as acute versus chronic conditions, single versus multiple lesions, primary versus recurrent nature, and/or local versus widespread disease.[1] For the purposes of this article, oral mucosal diseases are categorized on the basis of etiology (ie, infectious vs noninfectious) (**Fig. 1**).

INFECTIOUS DISEASES
Candidiasis

The most common oropharyngeal fungal disease(s) are caused by *Candida* species and the most common *Candida* subtype to cause an oropharyngeal infection is *Candida albicans*.[2] *Candida* is an obligate organism located in the human digestive

Department of Oral Medicine, University of Pennsylvania School of Dental Medicine, 240 South 40th Street, Philadelphia, PA 19104, USA
* Corresponding author.
E-mail address: ets@dental.upenn.edu

Med Clin N Am 98 (2014) 1323–1352
http://dx.doi.org/10.1016/j.mcna.2014.08.006
0025-7125/14/$ – see front matter © 2014 Elsevier Inc. All rights reserved.

medical.theclinics.com

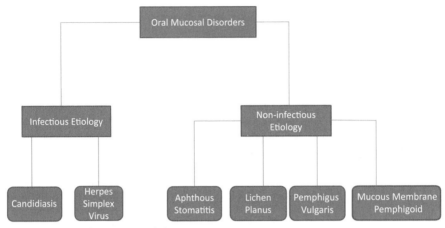

Fig. 1. Etiology of oral mucosal diseases.

and vaginal tracts and up to 60% of immunocompetent individuals may harbor this organism in the oropharynx.[2,3] *Candida* can exist in both the yeast and hyphal phases (dimorphism) and reproduces by multilateral budding. *Candida* is thought to directly invade tissue and cause disease by stimulating a hypersensitive state or by producing toxins.[2] Several factors can alter the oropharyngeal environment to make an individual more susceptible to a *Candida* infection, such as (1) changes to saliva quality and/or quantity, (2) dental prostheses, (3) medications, (4) nutritional deficiencies, and (5) immunosuppressive diseases.[2–4] The most common types of clinical oropharyngeal *Candida* conditions are listed in **Table 1**.

Most infections are diagnosed by the representative clinical features described for each condition. Common adjunctive diagnostic techniques may include exfoliative cytology with potassium hydroxide, Gram stain, or periodic acid-Schiff stain demonstrating hyphae and yeast and/or mucosal biopsy demonstrating budding yeast cells, pseudohyphae, and hyphal structures.[2–5]

Pseudomembranous candidiasis

- Commonly referred to as "thrush" (**Fig. 2**).[2–6]
- Usually presents as white or yellow superficial plaques that can be easily removed with an inflammatory base.
- May present on any mucosal surface.
- Condition may be asymptomatic or associated with burning, stinging, itching, and/or altered taste.

Table 1 Oropharyngeal *Candida* conditions	
Localized to the Oral Cavity	**Candida-Associated Conditions**
Pseudomembranous candidiasis	Angular cheilitis
Erythematous (atrophic) candidiasis	Central papillary atrophy (median rhomboid glossitis)
Chronic hyperplastic candidiasis	

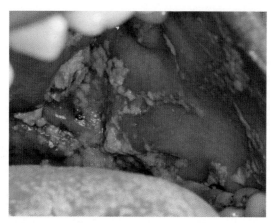

Fig. 2. Pseudomembranous candidiasis on the buccal mucosa.

- Plaques represent accumulation of yeast overgrowth, epithelial cell desquamation, keratin, bacteria, and necrotic tissue.
- Commonly diagnosed in infants, elderly, and patients who are immunosuppressed (disease or medication-induced.)

Erythematous (atrophic) candidiasis

- Commonly appears as red patches (**Fig. 3**).[2–6]
- Most commonly affects the palate and dorsal tongue, but may appear on any mucosal surface.
- Condition may be asymptomatic or associated with burning, stinging, itching, and/or altered taste.
- Most often associated with use of corticosteroids and broad-spectrum antibiotics.
- Denture-associated stomatitis (DAS) is a variant of erythematous candidiasis and affects denture-bearing surfaces.
- DAS is caused by fungal-bacterial contamination of dentures associated with prolonged wearing of denture(s) without removal and/or poor denture hygiene.

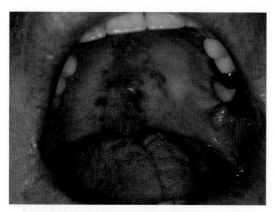

Fig. 3. Erythematous (atrophic) candidiasis on the palate.

Chronic hyperplastic candidiasis

- Commonly appears as a white plaque that cannot be rubbed off (**Fig. 4**).[2–6]
- Affects the buccal mucosa > buccal commissure > palate > tongue, respectively.
- Condition may be asymptomatic or associated with burning, stinging, itching, and/or altered taste.
- Associated with progression to dysplasia (up to 15%) and lesions require long-term monitoring.
- Biopsy is recommended to confirm diagnosis and rule out dysplasia.

Angular cheilitis

- Commonly appears as scaly, fissured, and/or crusted lesions, accompanied by erythema, at the labial commissures (**Fig. 5**).[7–10]
- Condition may be asymptomatic or associated with burning, stinging, or itching.
- Condition is usually representative of a fungal-bacterial infection.
- Typically develops in a chronic, moist environment and is often associated with (1) wrinkling and/or folding of skin, (2) factitial habit, and/or (3) possible vitamin deficiency.

Central papillary atrophy (median rhomboid glossitis)

- Typically appears as an atrophic, erythematous lesion characterized by its geographic shape on the posterior dorsal surface of the tongue (**Fig. 6**).[2,3,11]
- Likely represents a developmental abnormality in the tongue that is superinfected with *Candida*.
- Typically asymptomatic, but can be associated with burning and/or irritation.

Treatment Recommendations

Common antifungal therapies for candida infections localized to the oral cavity include the following[2–7]:

- Clotrimazole troches 10 mg; 1 tablet dissolved on tongue 5× daily × 14 days.
- Nystatin oral suspension 100,000 units/mL; 10-mL swish and expectorate 4× daily × 14 days.
- Fluconazole 100 mg; 2 tablets on day 1, then 100 to 200 mg daily × 7 to 14 days.
- Nystatin–triamcinolone ointment applied 2× daily to affected areas × 14 days (indicated for angular cheilitis).

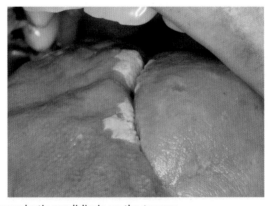

Fig. 4. Chronic hyperplastic candidiasis on the tongue.

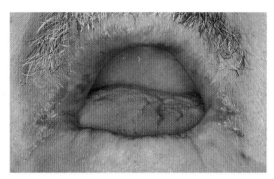

Fig. 5. Angular cheilitis.

If necessary, educate patient on removal of dentures (typically not worn while sleeping) and reinforce importance of denture hygiene. Typically, if the infection has not resolved in 2 weeks, consider referring patient to appropriate health care provider for further evaluation and management.

Herpes Simplex Viral Infections

Herpes simplex viruses (HSV)-1 and -2 are the two most common viral etiologies of oral and perioral infections and are clinically indistinguishable.[12–15] HSV-1 infections typically present after 6 months of age and peak between 2 and 3 years of age, whereas HSV-2 infections typically present after onset of sexual activity.[12–15]

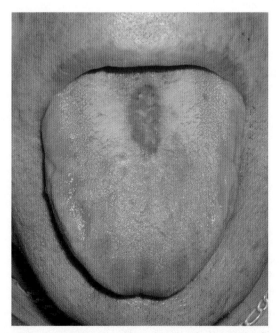

Fig. 6. Central papillary atrophy (median rhomboid glossitis). (*From* Muzyka BC, Epifanio RN. Update on oral fungal infections. Dent Clin North Am 2013;57(4):569; with permission.)

Most HSV infections are subclinical and following resolution of a primary infection, HSV migrates to the trigeminal nerve ganglion, where it can remain latent indefinitely or reactivate to cause clinical infection. HSV infections in immunocompromised patients may have an atypical presentation and can lead to disseminated infection, which can potentially be life-threatening. Most HSV infections are diagnosed by representative clinical features, but adjunctive diagnostic testing may be required to diagnose atypical presentations.[15,16] These tests are briefly described in **Box 1**.

Primary HSV Infections

- Symptomatic clinical infections are typically preceded or accompanied by systemic symptoms that commonly include fever, malaise, gastrointestinal symptoms, headache, and lymphadenopathy, referred to as "prodrome" (**Fig. 7**).[12–15]
- Oral and/or perioral lesions often present within 1 to 2 days after the onset of the prodrome.
- Vesicles and/or ulcers may appear on any mucosal surface, but usually do not affect the gingiva.
- Significant (often generalized) erythema is commonly observed on the gingiva.

Box 1
Adjunctive diagnostic techniques for herpes simplex virus (HSV) infections

Virologic testing

- HSV-infected cells will demonstrate multinucleated giant cells, syncytium, and ballooning degeneration of nuclei.

Cytology smears

- Most commonly used stain is Giemsa
- HSV-infected cells will demonstrate multinucleated giant cells, syncytium, and ballooning degeneration of nuclei.

Direct Fluorescent Assay

- Cellular specimen is incubated with fluorescein isothiocyanate–labeled HSV type–specific monoclonal antibody.
- HSV-infected cells are fluorescent green when examined under a fluorescent microscope.

Polymerase Chain Reaction Test

- Detection of HSV DNA is currently considered the most sensitive testing modality for HSV infection.

Serologic Testing

- Requires sampling of acute and convalescent serum.
- Fourfold or greater antibody rise in convalescent serum is required for the diagnosis of a primary HSV infection.
- Primarily provides retrospective information.

Data from Balasubramaniam R, Kuperstein AS, Stoopler ET. Update on oral herpes virus infections. Dent Clin North Am 2014;58(2):265–80; and Stoopler ET, Pinto A, DeRossi SS, et al. Herpes simplex and varicella-zoster infections: clinical and laboratory diagnosis. Gen Dent 2003;51(3):281–6. [quiz: 287].

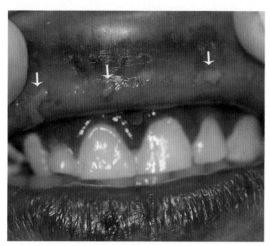

Fig. 7. Primary herpes simplex viral infection (ulcers are noted by *white arrows*). (*From* Balasubramaniam R, Kuperstein AS, Stoopler ET. Update on oral herpes virus infections. Dent Clin North Am 2014;58(2):267; with permission.)

Treatment recommendations

- Most primary HSV infections are self-limiting, only requiring palliative treatment.[13–15,17]
- Antiviral medication may be beneficial if the patient presents within 24 to 48 hours of lesion onset (**Table 2**).

Recurrent HSV Infections

- Reactivation of HSV may be caused by exposure to cold, exposure to sunlight, stress, trauma, or immunosuppression.[13–15,17,18]
- Recurrent herpes labialis (RHL) is the most common form of recurrent HSV infection, typically appearing on the mucocutaneous junction of the lip, and is often referred to as a "cold sore" or "fever blister" (**Fig. 8**).

Treatment recommendations

- Recurrent herpes infections in healthy patients may be treated on a symptomatic basis with topical and/or systemic antiviral medications (**Tables 3 and 4**).[13–15,17,18]

Table 2
Systemic antiviral medications for the treatment of primary herpes simplex virus infection

	Acyclovir		Valacyclovir	Famciclovir
Dose	200 mg[a]	400 mg[b]	1000 mg[a]	250 mg[b]
Frequency	5×/d	3×/d	2×/d	3×/d
Duration	7–10 d	7–10 d	7–10 d	7–10 d

[a] US Food and Drug Administration treatment recommendations for genital herpes.
[b] Recommendations from the Centers for Disease Control and Prevention for genital herpes.
From Stoopler ET, Balasubramaniam R. Topical and systemic therapies for oral and perioral herpes simplex virus infections. J Calif Dent Assoc 2013;41(4):259–62.

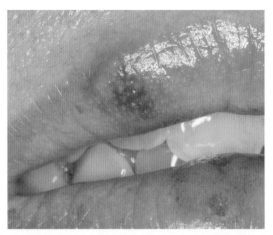

Fig. 8. Recurrent herpes labialis. (*From* Balasubramaniam R, Kuperstein AS, Stoopler ET. Update on oral herpes virus infections. Dent Clin North Am 2014;58(2):268; with permission.)

Table 3
Topical therapies for treatment of oral HSV infections

Category	Agent	Indications	Recommendations
Palliative	Ice, lip balms Over-the-counter topical anesthetic preparations (eg, containing benzocaine)[a]	Primary HSV infections, Recurrent HSL infections, RIH infections	As needed or per manufacturer's instructions.
	Topical lidocaine preparations[b] (Viscous lidocaine 2%, lidocaine gel 2%)	Primary HSV infections, Recurrent HSL infections, RIH infections	Viscous lidocaine 2%: 10 mL swish and spit as needed for pain relief. Lidocaine gel 2%: apply layer to affected area as needed for pain relief.
	Magic Mouthwash[b,c]	Primary infections, RIH infections	10-mL swish and spit as needed for pain relief.
Protective	Sunscreen (SPF 15 or higher)	Recurrent HSL infections	As per manufacturer's instructions.
Antiviral	Acyclovir 5% cream	Recurrent HSL infections	Apply every 2 h from the time of prodrome until lesions are healed.
	Penciclovir 1% cream	Recurrent HSL infections	Apply every 2 h from the time of prodrome until lesions are healed.
	Docosanol 10% cream	Recurrent HSL infections	Apply every 2 h from the time of prodrome until lesions are healed.
	Topical foscarnet, cidofovir, and/or imiquimod	Recalcitrant HSV lesions	Rarely used in healthy individuals; Refer to appropriate health care provider for management with these agents.

Abbreviations: HSL, herpes simplex labialis; HSV, herpes simplex virus; RIH, recurrent intraoral herpes.

[a] US Food and Drug Administration recommends benzocaine products (spray, liquid, gel) should not be used on children younger than 2 years, except under the advice and supervision of a health care professional.

[b] Aspiration of topical lidocaine in the pediatric population has been associated with adverse neurologic and/or cardiovascular side effects.

[c] Various combinations of agents, usually contains topical anesthetic (eg, viscous lidocaine 2%) with coating agents (eg, Maalox) ± diphenhydramine.

From Stoopler ET, Balasubramaniam R. Topical and systemic therapies for oral and perioral herpes simplex virus infections. J Calif Dent Assoc 2013;41(4):259–62.

Table 4 Systemic therapies for treatment of oral HSV infections	
Indication	**Therapy**
Treatment of RHL in the immunocompetent host	• Oral acyclovir 400 mg 3 times a day for 5–7 d • Oral valacyclovir 500 mg–2000 mg twice a day for 1 d • Oral famciclovir 500 mg 2–3 times a day for 3 d
Prophylaxis of RHL in the immunocompetent host[a]	• Oral acyclovir 400 mg 2–3 times a day • Oral valacyclovir 500 mg–2000 mg twice a day
Treatment of recurrent HSV infections in the immunocompromised host	• Oral acyclovir 400 mg 3 times a day for 10 d or longer as necessary • Oral valacyclovir 500–1000 mg twice a day for 10 d or longer as necessary • Oral famciclovir 500 mg twice a day for up to 1 y
Prophylaxis of recurrent HSV infections in the immunocompromised host	• Oral acyclovir 400–800 mg 3 times a day • Oral valacyclovir 500–1000 mg twice a day • Oral famciclovir 500–1000 mg twice a day

Abbreviations: HSV, herpes simplex virus; RHL, recurrent herpes labialis.

[a] Duration of the prophylaxis is based on the extent and frequency of exposure to triggers of RHL episodes, such as sunlight, dental treatment.

Modified from Woo SB, Challacombe SJ. Management of recurrent oral herpes simplex infections. Oral Surg Oral Med Oral Pathol Oral Radiol Endod 2007;103(Suppl 1):S12.e1–18.

- Off-label use of suppressive doses of systemic antivirals to prevent severe, frequent disfiguring recurrences of RHL may be considered in immunocompetent patients.
- Recurrent intraoral herpes can occur on any intraoral mucosal surface and is seen more frequently in immunocompromised patients (**Fig. 9**).
- Recurrent HSV lesions in immunocompromised patients may appear as progressively enlarging ulcers with potential to disseminate and cause generalized infection; therefore, systemic antiviral therapy is typically indicated (see **Table 4**).

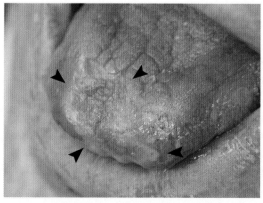

Fig. 9. Recurrent intraoral herpes infection on the tongue (*black arrowheads*) in an immunocompromised patient.

NONINFECTIOUS DISEASES
Recurrent Aphthous Stomatitis

Recurrent aphthous stomatitis (RAS) is a common ulcerative condition affecting the oral mucosa in approximately 20% the general population.[19] The onset of RAS appears to peak in adolescence and teenage years and becomes less frequent with advancing age. Several factors have been attributed to onset of this condition, including genetic predisposition, local trauma, nutritional deficiencies, and underlying systemic diseases (**Box 2**).[19–26]

RAS lesions are usually preceded by prodromal symptoms (burning, tingling) within 48 hours of lesion onset. RAS lesions clinically appear as a symmetric, defined ulcer with a white/gray/yellow pseudomembranous covering surrounded by an erythematous halo, that typically appear on nonkeratinized oral mucosa. RAS is divided into minor, major, and herpetiform variants of the disease based on specific clinical characteristics (**Box 3**, **Figs. 10–12**).[19–26]

Diagnosis of RAS is usually based on the patient's history and clinical examination findings. Advanced diagnostic testing, such as biopsy, is usually not indicated in typical RAS cases, but may be helpful in atypical presentations of the disease. It is important to elicit positive and negative responses to appropriate review of systems questions to determine if RAS may be attributed to an underlying systemic disease, especially for those individuals who present with new onset or worsening of disease

---

Box 2
Etiologic factors commonly associated with recurrent aphthous stomatitis

Hereditary/Genetic Factors

- Genetic predisposition (especially if both parents are RAS positive)
- Human Leukocyte Antigens (HLAs): -A, -B, -DR, -DQ series

Local Factors

- Trauma
- Changes in salivary composition

Nutritional deficiencies

- Iron
- Folate
- Zinc
- B vitamins: -1, -2, -6, -12

Systemic diseases

- Behcet syndrome
- Inflammatory bowel disease (Crohn, ulcerative colitis)
- Celiac disease
- Human Immunodeficiency Virus (HIV)
- Cyclic neutropenia
- MAGIC (mouth and genital ulcers with inflamed cartilage) syndrome
- PFAPA (periodic fever, aphthae, pharyngitis, adenitis [cervical]) syndrome
- Stress

Data from Refs.[19–26]

Box 3
Clinical classification of recurrent aphthous stomatitis (RAS)

Minor RAS (>85% of cases)

- <1 cm in diameter
- Heals within 2 weeks
- Heals without scarring (typically)

Major RAS

- >1 cm in diameter
- Heals greater than 2 weeks
- Heals with scarring (typically)
- May appear asymmetric

Herpetiform RAS (rare)

- Clusters of multiple ulcers throughout the oral mucosa
- May be confused with HSV infection due to clinical appearance

Data from Refs.[19–26]

---

after age 25. Although most RAS cases are idiopathic, if an underlying disease is suspected, the patient should have an appropriate medical workup and/or referral to an appropriate specialist for further evaluation.

RAS therapy is based on the frequency/location/duration of ulcers and associated symptomatology.[20] Topical therapies are directed at palliating symptoms and

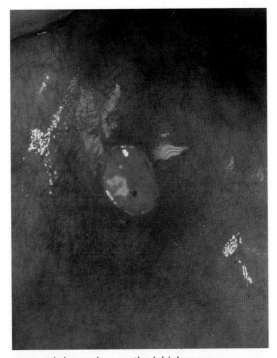

Fig. 10. Minor recurrent aphthous ulcer on the labial mucosa.

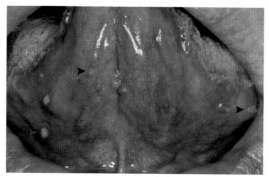

Fig. 11. Minor recurrent aphthous ulcers on the ventral tongue (*red arrowheads,* active lesions; *black arrowheads,* healing lesions).

promoting rapid healing of RAS ulcers, whereas systemic therapies are aimed at preventing recurrences of RAS episodes (**Box 4**).[19–26]

Adverse reactions often are associated with systemic therapies for RAS and discussion regarding the risk/benefit of using these agents, as well as appropriate medical monitoring, must be conducted with the patient before initiation of this type of therapy.

Lichen Planus

Lichen planus (LP) is a mucocutaneous disease frequently affecting the oral cavity. In 40% of the cases, the disease affects both the skin and mucosal tissue. Oral LP (OLP) affects 0.5% to 2.2% of the population and most commonly affects patients in their third to seventh decades. The mean age of diagnosis is 55 years with a female predilection for this disease.[27–29]

OLP lesions can be mildly inflamed with accompanying striae to severely eroded, ulcerated, and painful sores affecting multiple areas of the oral cavity. Significant oral mucosal involvement may impair eating and speaking and impact quality of

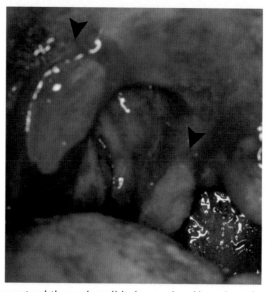

Fig. 12. Major recurrent aphthous ulcers (*black arrowheads*) on the soft palate and uvula.

Box 4
Common therapies for RAS

Topical therapies

- Protective emollients
- Nonsteroidal anti-inflammatory agent
  - Amlexanox 5% paste, apply 4× daily until ulcer(s) resolve
- Corticosteroids
  - Triamcinolone 0.1% paste, apply 2–3× daily until ulcer(s) resolve
  - Fluocinonide 0.05% gel, apply 2–3× daily until ulcer(s) resolve[a]
  - Clobetasol 0.05% gel, apply 2–3× daily until ulcer(s) resolve[a]
  - Betamethasone 0.05% gel, apply 2–3× daily until ulcer(s) resolve[a]
  - Dexamethasone solution 0.5 mg/5 mL, 10-mL swish and spit 2–3× daily until ulcer(s) resolve[a]

Systemic therapies[b]

- Corticosteroids (recommended for management of acute RAS episodes only)
  - Methylprednisolone 4 mg dose pack (24 to 0 mg over 7 days)
- Other (recommended for prevention of RAS episodes)
  - Pentoxifylline 400 mg, 3× daily
  - Colchicine 0.6 mg, 2–3× daily
  - Thalidomide 50 mg, 2× daily (usual effective dose is 100 mg daily)

[a] Generally recommended to coprescribe a prophylactic topical antifungal agent, such as clotrimazole or nystatin, to prevent oral candidiasis.
[b] Use of systemic agents generally requires medical monitoring (serology, frequent physical examinations, etc.).
Data from Refs.[19–26]

---

life.[30] Remission of OLP occurs in fewer than 5% cases. Lichenoid reactions clinically and histopathologically resemble LP but are distinguished from LP when there is an association with a product that subsides when the offending agent is removed.[31,32] LP results from an antigenic challenge from an external source or from keratinocyte autoantigen expression; however, the initiating cause is unclear in most cases. The disorder is a T-cell–mediated process initiated after epithelial antigenic processing by Langerhans cells, similar to a contact allergy reaction. Locally, there is increased expression of cytokines and adhesion molecules. The chronicity of the disease is thought to be related to RANTES, mast cell degranulation, and upregulated release of tumor necrosis factor alpha.[33–37] OLP has been more closely associated with hepatitis C in Japanese, Mediterranean, and the US populations.[38] Rates of malignant transformation of lichen planus to oral squamous cell carcinoma are highly variable based on observational methodology. The estimated rate of malignant transformation to squamous cell carcinoma is approximately 1%.[31,39–41] LP must be clinically differentiated from mucous membrane pemphigoid, pemphigus, paraneoplastic pemphigus, and oral lupus lesion, as these lesions present with similar signs and symptoms. Diagnosis of LP is based on clinical appearance and routine histopathology, whereas direct immunofluorescence (DIF) could differentiate OLP from other chronic oral diseases, such as pemphigoid or pemphigus (**Box 5**).

> **Box 5**
> **Diagnostic testing for lichen planus**
>
> Routine histopathology reveals:
>
> - Hyperkeratosis with thickening of the spinous layer (acanthosis) and saw tooth rete ridges
> - Necrosis of the basal cell layer
> - Dense subepithelial band of chronic inflammatory cells usually T lymphocytes
> - Civatte bodies (necrotic keratinocytes) are often seen
>
> Direct immunofluorescence reveals:
>
> - Fibrinogen deposition in the basement membrane zone
>
> *Data from* Refs.[31,42,43]

Clinical presentation

- OLP can affect all mucosal surfaces and presents as white, lacey lesions: reticular (Wickham striae), atrophic erythematous lesions, bullous lesions, ulcerations, or plaquelike white patches (**Figs. 13–15**).[27,31,43]
- Various presentations often occur in the same patient and within the same lesion
- Often occurs bilaterally
- Atrophic and ulcerative lesions are often painful, and reticular and plaquelike lesions are often asymptomatic
- Can present as desquamative (peeling) gingivitis (**Fig. 16**)
- Cutaneous LP lesions are commonly described as pruritic, polygonal, planar, purple papules, and plaquelike

Treatment

The treatment of OLP involves both topical and systemic immunomodulating medications and palliative strategies to control inflammation/atrophy/ulcer to aid in healing of the mucosa.[31,43] Routine monitoring of OLP is necessary due to the risk of dysplasia and/or malignant transformation (**Box 6**).[44]

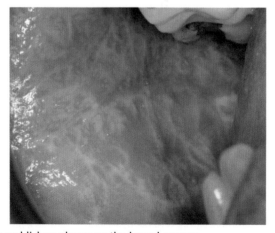

Fig. 13. Reticular oral lichen planus on the buccal mucosa.

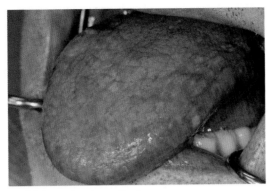

Fig. 14. Plaquelike oral lichen planus on the tongue.

Pemphigus

Pemphigus is an autoimmune mucocutaneous disease resulting in blister (bullae) and ulcer formation. The oral mucosa is often involved before presence of skin lesions. Large areas of oral mucosal involvement impair eating, swallowing, and speaking. Pemphigus should be considered in patients with multiple, chronic (ie, >6 months) ulcers regardless of the presence of skin lesions. Five major categories of pemphigus exist, including pemphigus vulgaris (PV), pemphigus foliaceus (PF), paraneoplastic pemphigus (PNP), drug-induced pemphigus (DIP), and immunoglobulin A pemphigus (IgAP). Although there are various forms of pemphigus, PV and PNP are the more

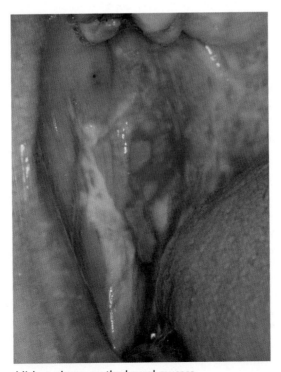

Fig. 15. Erosive oral lichen planus on the buccal mucosa.

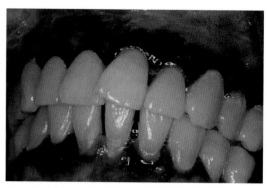

Fig. 16. Desquamative gingivitis in oral lichen planus.

common types affecting the oral cavity.[49] The incidence of pemphigus is estimated to be 0.076 to 5,100,000 person-years with a higher incidence in women (male:female ratio of 1:1.1–2.25).[50] There is significant ethnic clustering, particularly in the Ashkenazi Jewish population, suggesting a probable genetic component.[51]

Box 6
Management of lichen planus

Topical/Intralesional immunomodulating medications

- High-potency corticosteroid gels or rinses applied 2×/d
- Tacrolimus ointment 0.1% applied 2×/d for lesions resistant to steroid therapy
- Intralesional corticosteroid, such as triamcinolone 10 mg/mL, applying 0.1 mL/cm^3
  - Medication considerations
    - Need to consider daily antifungal prophylaxis, such as clotrimazole troches 10 mg 3×/d or nystatin suspension 100,000 units rinses 2×/d
    - Need to consider sugar content of all medications used daily and effect on caries rate. Consider topical fluoride supplements to routine dental care
    - Occlusive trays made by the dentist typically enhances medication placement while preventing salivary washout. Some systemic absorption of medication is possible when using occlusive trays

Systemic medications

- Corticosteroids 0.5 to .75 mg/kg/d (depending on severity and response) used intermittently to control disease or treat recalcitrant lesions
  - Monitor for systemic steroid side effects
- Systemic retinoids have shown to be effective but associated with significant side effects (ie, liver dysfunction, lipidemia)
- Other medications have been used but require further study: (1) oral psoralen with ultraviolet light A (PUVA), (2) levamisole, (3) dapsone, (4) thalidomide
- Biologics, such as tumor necrosis factor–alpha inhibitors, rituximab also have been reported to be effective for oral lichen planus (OLP)
- Low-level laser also has been used for management of OLP

Data from Refs.[45–48]

The etiology and pathogenesis of pemphigus involves autoantibodies that are active against the keratinocytes' cell-to-cell adhesion, resulting in separation or acantholysis.[49,52] The trigger for autoantibody formation and activity is unknown. In PV, IgG is directed against these cellular adhesion molecules known as desmogleins. The two forms of desmoglein (Dsg), Dsg-1 and Dsg-3, are the major cell adhesion molecules of the desmosome. The oral mucosa has a higher concentration of Dsg-3 compared with Dsg-1[53]; therefore, patients with only mucosal disease have autoantibodies against Dsg-3.[53] In PNP, immunoglobulins are focused against Dsg-1 and Dsg-3 and other proteins including desmoplakin 1, 2, plectin, and others.[53] Paraneoplastic pemphigus is commonly associated with underlying lymphoproliferative disorders, such as lymphoma, chronic lymphocytic leukemia, thymoma, and Castleman tumor (**Table 5**).[54]

Pemphigus must be differentiated from other chronic mucocutaneous diseases, such as OLP, mucous membrane pemphigoid, and oral lupus lesions, as they often appear clinically similar. One must also differentiate PV from PNP. The diagnosis of pemphigus is made by routine biopsy of lesional tissue in combination with immunologic testing of the patient's tissue and sera.[49,53] Routine histopathology, together with DIF, indirect immunofluorescence (IIF), and enzyme-linked immunosorbent assays (ELISA) (for known disease-producing antibodies) are often evaluated for an accurate diagnosis and are used for monitoring during management (**Boxes 7 and 8**).

Clinical presentation

- Painful superficial ulcerations of the oral mucosa, often extending to the posterior oropharynx, which can be accompanied by flaccid bullae and superficial ulcerations of the skin (**Figs. 17 and 18**).[49,53,59–61]
- May have esophageal involvement
- Often associated with desquamative (peeling) gingivitis, resulting in chronic bleeding of the gingival tissue (**Fig. 19**)
- Positive Nikolsky sign
  - Formation of a blister with minor inducible trauma or enlargement of a present blister when pressure directed to the fluid-filled tissue
- In PNP, oral lesions might have a clinical appearance similar to OLP (see section on LP), including Wickham striae
- In PNP, the tongue is often involved, associated with ulcers and only partially responsive to medical therapy
- In PNP, blisters and erosions are often seen on palms and soles
- In PNP, bronchial mucosa could be affected leading to bronchiolitis obliterans and ultimately respiratory failure

Treatment

The treatment for pemphigus includes topical and systemic immunomodulating medications and palliative strategies to control blister formation and aid in mucosal healing.[49,53] Some medications will have significant side effects, which can cause both

Table 5		
Primary targets in oral pemphigus vulgaris (PV), skin PV, and paraneoplastic pemphigus (PNP)		
Oral PV	**Skin PV**	**PNP**
Dsg 3	Dsg 1,3	Dsg 1,3 and other proteins including desmoplakin 1, 2, plectin

Box 7
Diagnostic testing for pemphigus

Routine histopathology

- Intraepithelial blister with acantholysis while the basal cell layer will be maintained as a single layer of cells above the basement membrane zone, resulting in a "tombstone appearance" of the basal cells.
- Paraneoplastic pemphigus (PNP) has a variable presentation exhibiting histologic characteristics as seen in lichenoid mucositis and/or erythema multiforme

Direct immunofluorescence (DIF) testing

- The patient's tissue will demonstrate intercellular deposition of IgG and Complement 3 (C3) between epithelial cells leading to a "chicken-wire" appearance under microscopy.
- PNP intercellular staining could be focal and not strong and IgG/C3 staining may involve the basement membrane zone

Indirect immunofluorescence (IIF) testing

- The patient's sera will demonstrate intercellular staining on a substrate
- Sensitivity 75%; specificity 83%
- Positive predictive value 90%
- Correlates with disease activity and possibly useful to follow disease progression and/or response to therapy
- Pemphigus vulgaris (PV) preferred substrate is monkey esophagus
- PNP preferred substrate is rodent bladder

Enzyzme-linked immunosorbent assay (ELISA) testing

- Patient's sera analyzed for titer of Dsg1 and Dsg 3
- Titers correlate well with disease activity
- Comparable to IIF sensitivity but less specific

Data from Refs.[55–58]

Box 8
DIF and IIF testing techniques

DIF Testing Technique

- Tissue transported in Michel solution designed to allow appropriate reaction with immunoreactants
- Perilesional tissue adjacent to newer active area is exposed to fluorescent tagged autoantibodies

IIF Testing Technique

- Dilution of serum incubated with known substrate
- Substrate could include human salt split skin/mucosa, monkey esophagus, or rodent bladder
- A fluorescein-conjugated immunoglobulin antiserum is applied
- The test is reported as a titer

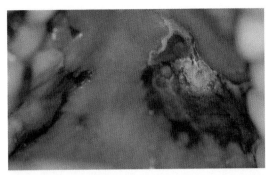

Fig. 17. Pemphigus vulgaris on the palate.

additional oral disease and also affect systemic health. PNP also requires treatment of the underlying neoplasm, with improvement in 75% of patients (**Box 9**).[61]

Mucous Membrane Pemphigoid

Mucous membrane pemphigoid (MMP) is one of several subepithelial blistering disorders (SEBD). MMP results in oral bullae formation, which rupture and result in an ulcer. Large areas of oral mucosal involvement impair eating and speaking. Without appropriate treatment, MMP could result in significant mucosal scarring. Ocular mucosa also may be affected, resulting in blindness from scarring. Pemphigoid should be considered in patients with multiple, chronic (ie, >6 months) oral ulcers, as MMP occurs more commonly in the sixth to eighth decades (although there is a rare childhood form). The true overall incidence of MMP in the population is not clear.[66,67] It has been estimated to be 1.3 to 2.0 per million per year, with a female-to-male ratio of 2:1.[68–70] There is no known racial or geographic predilection.

Genetically, there is thought to be an association between MMP and HLA Class II DQB1*0301.[71,72]

MMP is characterized by the formation of autoantibodies against proteins of the epithelial–connective tissue junction, which is often referred to as the basement membrane zone (BMZ).[66,73] The BMZ proteins targeted by the autoantibodies include bullous pemphigoid antigens 1 and 2 (BPAg1, a 230-kDa protein: BP230, and

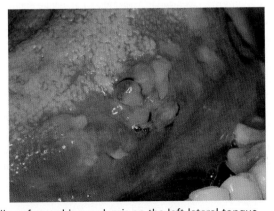

Fig. 18. Small bullae of pemphigus vulgaris on the left lateral tongue.

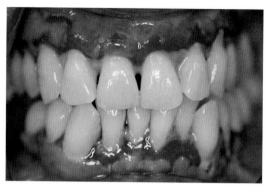

Fig. 19. Desquamative gingivitis in pemphigus vulgaris.

Box 9
Management of pemphigus

Topical/Intralesional immunomodulating medications

- High-potency corticosteroid gels or rinses applied 2×/d
- Tacrolimus ointment 0.1% applied 2×/d
- Intralesional corticosteroid, such as triamcinolone 10 mg/mL applying 0.1 mL/cm³
  - Need to consider daily antifungal prophylaxis, such as clotrimazole troches 10 mg 3×/d or nystatin suspension 100,000-unit rinses 2×/d
  - Need to consider sugar content of all medications used daily and effect on caries rate. May want to consider topical fluoride supplements to routine dental care.

Systemic immunomodulating medications

- Corticosteroids 1 mg/kg/d used over months with gradual taper after clinical remission
  - Monitor systemic steroid side effects
- Rituximab, a monoclonal antibody to CD20 B lymphocytes, is administered for 4 weekly infusions at 375 mg/m² OR 2 infusions of 1000 mg separated by 2 weeks between dosings.
- Other agents could include antimetabolites mycophenolate mofetil, azathioprine, and cyclophosphamide
  - Monitor immunosuppressive medication side effects and management
  - Monitor immunosuppression level
  - Due to immunosuppression monitor for neoplasia
- Intravenous immunoglobulin is sometimes combined with rituximab
- Consider ELISA titer before withdrawal of systemic medications

Palliative strategies

- Topical anesthetic rinses, including viscous lidocaine, magic mouthwash (equal parts viscous lidocaine/Benadryl liquid/topical antacid)
- Frequent gentle dental cleanings will decrease inflammation
- Antimicrobial rinses may aid in healing of immunologic medication responding lesions
- Protective dental trays could alleviate trauma from the dentition

Data from Refs.[62–65]

BPAg2, a 180-kDa protein: BP180).[74,75] BP180 is the most frequently targeted protein in the BMZ in patients with MMP (**Fig. 20, Tables 6 and 7**).

The trigger for autoantibody formation is unknown, but some have reported that it could be related to medications, such as clonidine, methyldopa, and D-penicilli-amine.[76,77] The interaction between the autoantibody and the targeted protein results in an inflammatory process. This inflammatory process is described as a

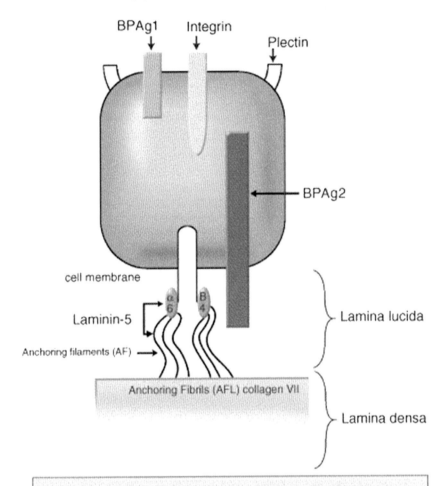

NOTES: 1) Intracellular portion of a hemidesmosome (HDS) includes plectin and BPAg1 (which is a 230-kDa protein plaque).

2) The portion attaching to the BMZ contains BPAg2 (which is a 180-kDa collagen-like transmembrane protein).

3) Anchoring filaments (AF) under HDS contain laminin-5, laminin-6 & uncein.

4) Anchoring fibrils of the BMZ are composed of type VII collagen (200 kDa).

Fig. 20. Hemidesmosome structure. (*From* Sollecito TP, Parisi E. Mucous membrane pemphigoid. Dent Clin North Am 2005;49(1):96, viii; with permission.)

Table 6
Autoantigens identified in MMP

Autoantigens	Location
BPAg2 (BP180)	Hemidesmosome/Lamina lucida (transmembrane)
BPAg1 (BP230)	Hemidesmosome (intracellular)
Integrin subunits α6/β4	Hemidesmosome (transmembrane)
Laminin-5 (laminin-332/epiligrin, α-3, β-3, γ-2 chains)	Lower lamina lucida
Laminin-6	Lower lamina lucida
Type VII collagen	Lamina densa/Sublamina densa

Abbreviations: BP, bullous pemphigoid; MMP, mucous membrane pemphigoid.
From Xu HH, Werth VP, Parisi E, et al. Mucous membrane pemphigoid. Dent Clin North Am 2013;57(4):613; with permission.

complement-mediated process with recruitment of inflammatory cells and mediators that result in separation of the epithelium from the connective tissue by direct cytotoxic action or the effect of lysosomal proteolytic enzymes.[78] Activated fibroblasts induce the clinical features of fibrosis and scarring.[79]

Diagnosis of MMP is made by clinical findings, routine histopathology from lesional tissue, and DIF from perilesional tissue. Occasionally, IIF and ELISA titers are performed to aid in diagnosing MMP when DIF and routine histopathology are equivocal. Because the clinical presentation is similar among chronic oral lesions, one must consider other chronic mucocutaneous diseases, such as OLP, pemphigus, and oral lupus lesions in the differential diagnosis (**Box 10**).[66,80]

DIF and IIF Testing Techniques

For DIF and IIF testing techniques, see **Box 8**.

Clinical presentation

- MMP most commonly affects the oral mucosa (85%), followed by the ocular mucosa (65%), but can affect the nasal mucosa, genital mucosa, esophageal mucosa, and laryngeal mucosa. Skin involvement may be occasionally observed.[67,80]
- Lesions affecting the ocular, esophageal, nasopharyngeal, laryngeal, and genital mucosa are considered high risk due to scarring
- Lesions may heal with scarring
- Ocular scarring might result in blindness from symblepharon formation
- Oral lesions often include desquamative gingivitis (**Fig. 21**)
- Presentation is variable from mild to very severe mucosal lesions with and without scarring (**Fig. 22**)

Treatment

Treatment for MMP includes both topical and systemic immunomodulating medications and palliative strategies to control blister/ulcer/scar formation and aid in healing of the mucosa.[66] Ocular, genital, esophageal, and laryngeal lesions are associated with higher potential for scarring and, therefore, treatment should be focused on prevention of scarring with early intervention and systemic therapy (**Box 11, Fig. 23**).

Table 7
Comparison of MMP with other subepithelial blistering dermatosis

Entity	Clinical Features	DIF	IIF on Salt-Split Substrate	Immunoblotting	Electromicroscope
MMP	Multiple mucosal involvement, scarring, progressive	Linear IgG, IgA, and/or C3 along BMZ	IgG antibodies bind to epidermal or dermal side	BP180, BP230, laminin 5, integrin, type VII collagen	Lamina lucida, sublamina densa
BP	Rare mucosal involvement and scarring	Linear IgG and/or C3 along BMZ	IgG antibodies bind to dermal side	BP180, BP230	Intralamina lucida
EBA	Blisters induced by trauma	Linear IgG along BMZ	IgG antibodies bind to dermal side	Type VII collagen	Sublamina densa
BSLE	Rare scarring, LE symptoms	Linear or granular IgG, IgA and C3 along BMZ	IgG antibodies bind to dermal side	Type VII collagen	Sublamina densa

Abbreviations: BMZ, basement membrane zone; BP, bullous pemphigoid; BSLE, bullous systemic lupus erythematosus; DIF, direct immunofluorescence; EBA, epidermolysis bullosa acquisita; Ig, immunoglobulin; IIF, indirect immunofluorescence; MMP, mucous membrane pemphigoid.
From Xu HH, Werth VP, Parisi E, et al. Mucous membrane pemphigoid. Dent Clin North Am 2013;57(4):619; with permission.

Box 10
Diagnostic testing for pemphigoid

Routine Histopathology

- Oral mucosa reveals a subepithelial split with inflammatory infiltrate of eosinophils, lymphocytes, and neutrophils.

DIF testing

- The patient's tissue will demonstrate a continuous linear deposition of IgG and/or Complement 3 (C3), and occasionally IgA in the BMZ.

IIF testing

- IIF testing of the patient's sera by incubating with various substrates (particularly salt split mucosal tissue) might correlate with disease activity

- IIF may improve sensitivity.

- IIF in combination with other sophisticated immunologic tests might aid in differentiating MMP from other SEBD disorders

ELISA testing

- Patient's sera analyzed for titer of BP-180 and BP-230

- Circulating MMP autoantibodies less common than other SEBDs

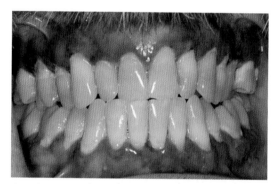

Fig. 21. Desquamative gingivitis in mucous membrane pemphigoid.

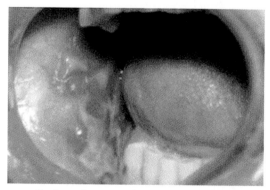

Fig. 22. MMP lesions on the buccal mucosa. (*From* Sollecito TP, Parisi E. Mucous membrane pemphigoid. Dent Clin North Am 2005;49(1):93, viii; with permission.)

Box 11
Management of pemphigoid

Topical/Intralesional Immunomodulating Medications

- High-potency corticosteroid gels or rinses applied 2×/d
- Tacrolimus ointment 0.1% applied 2×/d for lesions resistant to steroid therapy
- Intralesional corticosteroid, such as triamcinolone 10 mg/mL, applying 0.1 mL/cm^3
  - Need to consider daily antifungal prophylaxis, such as clotrimazole troches 10 mg 3×/d or nystatin suspension 100,000-unit rinses 2×/d
  - Need to consider sugar content of all medications used daily and effect on caries rate. Consider topical fluoride supplements to routine dental care
  - Occlusive trays made by the dentist typically enhance medication placement while preventing salivary washout. Some systemic absorption of medication is possible when using occlusive trays.

Systemic Immunomodulating Medications

- Corticosteroids 0.5 to 2.0 mg/kg/d (depending on severity and response) used initially to control disease
  - Monitor for systemic steroid side effects
- Dapsone 50 mg/d, increase 25 mg every 7 days to 100 to 200 mg until desired response and as tolerated
  - Monitor for anemia, hemolysis, and methemoglobinemia (questions for shortness of breath, palpitations, and fatigue, as methemoglobinemia will not be associated with a lower Hg level). Hemoglobin should be evaluated at baseline and after 1 week of therapy and every week after each increase in dose
  - Must screen for glucose-6-phosphate-dehydrogenous (G6PD) deficiency before therapy
  - Dapsone hypersensitivity characterized by fever, lymphadenopathy, hepatitis, and generalized pustules is a serious complication of this medication. Periodic liver function tests are essential
- Minocycline 50–100 mg/d
  - Monitor for side effects, including photosensitivity, hyperpigmentation, nausea, dizziness
- Other agents could include antimetabolites mycophenolate mofetil, azathioprine, and cyclophosphamide
- Biologics, including tumor necrosis factor–alpha inhibitors and rituximab also have been used
- Low-level laser also has been used for management

Palliative Strategies

- Topical anesthetic rinses, including viscous lidocaine, magic mouthwash (equal parts viscous lidocaine/Benadryl liquid/topical antacid)
- Frequent gentle dental cleanings will decrease inflammation
- Antimicrobial rinses may aid in healing of immunologic medication responding to lesions
- Protective dental trays could alleviate trauma from the dentition

Data from Refs.[66,67,81–87]

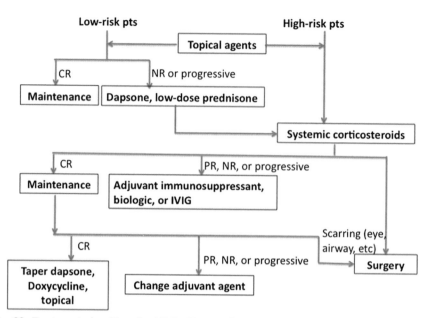

Fig. 23. Treatment algorithm for MMP. CR, complete response; IVIG, intravenous immuno-globulin; NR, no response; PR, partial response; pts, patients. (*From* Xu HH, Werth VP, Parisi E, et al. Mucous membrane pemphigoid. Dent Clin North Am 2013;57(4):625; with permission.)

SUMMARY

Oral mucosal diseases can significantly affect oral function, systemic health, and quality of life for patients. Physicians must have an understanding of the more common oral mucosal diseases observed in clinical practice to appropriately evaluate and manage these conditions.

REFERENCES

1. Sollecito TP, Stoopler ET. Clinical approaches to oral mucosal disorders. Dent Clin North Am 2013;57(4):ix–xi.
2. Muzyka BC, Epifanio RN. Update on oral fungal infections. Dent Clin North Am 2013;57(4):561–81.
3. Farah CS, Lynch N, McCullough MJ. Oral fungal infections: an update for the general practitioner. Aust Dent J 2010;55(Suppl 1):48–54.
4. Laudenbach JM, Epstein JB. Treatment strategies for oropharyngeal candidiasis. Expert Opin Pharmacother 2009;10(9):1413–21.
5. Giannini PJ, Shetty KV. Diagnosis and management of oral candidiasis. Otolaryngol Clin North Am 2011;44(1):231–40, vii.
6. Ship JA, Vissink A, Challacombe SJ. Use of prophylactic antifungals in the immunocompromised host. Oral Surg Oral Med Oral Pathol Oral Radiol Endod 2007;103(Suppl):S6.e1–14.
7. Stoopler ET, Nadeau C, Sollecito TP. How do I manage a patient with angular cheilitis? J Can Dent Assoc 2013;79:d68.
8. Park KK, Brodell RT, Helms SE. Angular cheilitis, part 1: local etiologies. Cutis 2011;87(6):289–95.

9. Park KK, Brodell RT, Helms SE. Angular cheilitis, part 2: nutritional, systemic, and drug-related causes and treatment. Cutis 2011;88(1):27–32.

10. Sharon V, Fazel N. Oral candidiasis and angular cheilitis. Dermatol Ther 2010; 23(3):230–42.

11. Reamy BV, Derby R, Bunt CW. Common tongue conditions in primary care. Am Fam Physician 2010;81(5):627–34.

12. Stoopler ET. Oral herpetic infections (HSV 1-8). Dent Clin North Am 2005;49(1): 15–29, vii.

13. Fatahzadeh M, Schwartz RA. Human herpes simplex virus infections: epidemiology, pathogenesis, symptomatology, diagnosis, and management. J Am Acad Dermatol 2007;57(5):737–63 [quiz: 764–6].

14. Stoopler ET, Balasubramaniam R. Topical and systemic therapies for oral and perioral herpes simplex virus infections. J Calif Dent Assoc 2013;41(4):259–62.

15. Balasubramaniam R, Kuperstein AS, Stoopler ET. Update on oral herpes virus infections. Dent Clin North Am 2014;58(2):265–80.

16. Stoopler ET, Pinto A, DeRossi SS, et al. Herpes simplex and varicella-zoster infections: clinical and laboratory diagnosis. Gen Dent 2003;51(3):281–6 [quiz: 287].

17. Fatahzadeh M, Schwartz RA. Human herpes simplex labialis. Clin Exp Dermatol 2007;32(6):625–30.

18. Woo SB, Challacombe SJ. Management of recurrent oral herpes simplex infections. Oral Surg Oral Med Oral Pathol Oral Radiol Endod 2007;103(Suppl): S12.e1–18.

19. Akintoye SO, Greenberg MS. Recurrent aphthous stomatitis. Dent Clin North Am 2014;58(2):281–97.

20. Stoopler ET, Musbah T. Recurrent aphthous stomatitis. CMAJ 2013;185(5):E240.

21. Scully C. Clinical practice. Aphthous ulceration. N Engl J Med 2006;355(2): 165–72.

22. Chattopadhyay A, Shetty KV. Recurrent aphthous stomatitis. Otolaryngol Clin North Am 2011;44(1):79–88, v.

23. Messadi DV, Younai F. Aphthous ulcers. Dermatol Ther 2010;23(3):281–90.

24. Casiglia JM. Recurrent aphthous stomatitis: etiology, diagnosis, and treatment. Gen Dent 2002;50(2):157–66.

25. Greenberg MS, Pinto A. Etiology and management of recurrent aphthous stomatitis. Curr Infect Dis Rep 2003;5(3):194–8.

26. Baccaglini L, Lalla RV, Bruce AJ, et al. Urban legends: recurrent aphthous stomatitis. Oral Dis 2011;17(8):755–70.

27. Stoopler ET, Sollecito TP, DeRossi SS. Oral lichen planus. Update for the general practitioner. N Y State Dent J 2003;69(6):26–8.

28. Mollaoglu N. Oral lichen planus: a review. Br J Oral Maxillofac Surg 2000;38(4): 370–7.

29. Edwards PC, Kelsch R. Oral lichen planus: clinical presentation and management. J Can Dent Assoc 2002;68(8):494–9.

30. Riordain RN, Meaney S, McCreary C. Impact of chronic oral mucosal disease on daily life: preliminary observations from a qualitative study. Oral Dis 2011;17(3):265–9.

31. De Rossi SS, Ciarrocca K. Oral lichen planus and lichenoid mucositis. Dent Clin North Am 2014;58(2):299–313.

32. Schlosser BJ. Lichen planus and lichenoid reactions of the oral mucosa. Dermatol Ther 2010;23(3):251–67.

33. Thornhill MH, Pemberton MN, Simmons RK, et al. Amalgam-contact hypersensitivity lesions and oral lichen planus. Oral Surg Oral Med Oral Pathol Oral Radiol Endod 2003;95(3):291–9.

34. Sugerman PB, Savage NW, Walsh LJ, et al. The pathogenesis of oral lichen planus. Crit Rev Oral Biol Med 2002;13(4):350–65.
35. Ismail SB, Kumar SK, Zain RB. Oral lichen planus and lichenoid reactions: etiopathogenesis, diagnosis, management and malignant transformation. J Oral Sci 2007;49(2):89–106.
36. Lavanya N, Jayanthi P, Rao UK, et al. Oral lichen planus: an update on pathogenesis and treatment. J Oral Maxillofac Pathol 2011;15(2):127–32.
37. Payeras MR, Cherubini K, Figueiredo MA, et al. Oral lichen planus: focus on etiopathogenesis. Arch Oral Biol 2013;58(9):1057–69.
38. Lodi G, Pellicano R, Carrozzo M. Hepatitis C virus infection and lichen planus: a systematic review with meta-analysis. Oral Dis 2010;16(7):601–12.
39. Lodi G, Scully C, Carrozzo M, et al. Current controversies in oral lichen planus: report of an international consensus meeting. Part 2. Clinical management and malignant transformation. Oral Surg Oral Med Oral Pathol Oral Radiol Endod 2005;100(2):164–78.
40. Epstein JB, Wan LS, Gorsky M, et al. Oral lichen planus: progress in understanding its malignant potential and the implications for clinical management. Oral Surg Oral Med Oral Pathol Oral Radiol Endod 2003;96(1):32–7.
41. Fitzpatrick SG, Hirsch SA, Gordon SC. The malignant transformation of oral lichen planus and oral lichenoid lesions: a systematic review. J Am Dent Assoc 2014;145(1):45–56.
42. Villarroel Dorrego M, Correnti M, Delgado R, et al. Oral lichen planus: immunohistology of mucosal lesions. J Oral Pathol Med 2002;31(7):410–4.
43. Eisen D. The clinical manifestations and treatment of oral lichen planus. Dermatol Clin 2003;21(1):79–89.
44. McCreary CE, McCartan BE. Clinical management of oral lichen planus. Br J Oral Maxillofac Surg 1999;37(5):338–43.
45. Gonzalez-Moles MA, Morales P, Rodriguez-Archilla A. The treatment of oral aphthous ulceration or erosive lichen planus with topical clobetasol propionate in three preparations. A clinical study on 54 patients. J Oral Pathol Med 2002; 31(5):284–5 [author reply: 286–7].
46. Hodgson TA, Sahni N, Kaliakatsou F, et al. Long-term efficacy and safety of topical tacrolimus in the management of ulcerative/erosive oral lichen planus. Eur J Dermatol 2003;13(5):466–70.
47. Zhang J, Zhou G, Du GF, et al. Biologics, an alternative therapeutic approach for oral lichen planus. J Oral Pathol Med 2011;40(7):521–4.
48. Cafaro A, Albanese G, Arduino PG, et al. Effect of low-level laser irradiation on unresponsive oral lichen planus: early preliminary results in 13 patients. Photomed Laser Surg 2010;28(Suppl 2):S99–103.
49. Santoro FA, Stoopler ET, Werth VP. Pemphigus. Dent Clin North Am 2013;57(4): 597–610.
50. Gupta VK, Kelbel TE, Nguyen D, et al. A globally available Internet-based patient survey of pemphigus vulgaris: epidemiology and disease characteristics. Dermatol Clin 2011;29(3):393–404, vii–iii.
51. Sarig O, Bercovici S, Zoller L, et al. Population-specific association between a polymorphic variant in ST18, encoding a pro-apoptotic molecule, and pemphigus vulgaris. J Invest Dermatol 2012;132(7):1798–805.
52. Karpati S, Amagai M, Prussick R, et al. Pemphigus vulgaris antigen, a desmoglein type of cadherin, is localized within keratinocyte desmosomes. J Cell Biol 1993;122(2):409–15.
53. Ettlin DA. Pemphigus. Dent Clin North Am 2005;49(1):107–25, viii–ix.

54. Anhalt GJ. Paraneoplastic pemphigus. J Investig Dermatol Symp Proc 2004; 9(1):29–33.
55. Helou J, Allbritton J, Anhalt GJ. Accuracy of indirect immunofluorescence testing in the diagnosis of paraneoplastic pemphigus. J Am Acad Dermatol 1995;32(3): 441–7.
56. Mutasim DF, Adams BB. Immunofluorescence in dermatology. J Am Acad Dermatol 2001;45(6):803–22 [quiz: 822–4].
57. Avgerinou G, Papafragkaki DK, Nasiopoulou A, et al. Correlation of antibodies against desmogleins 1 and 3 with indirect immunofluorescence and disease status in a Greek population with pemphigus vulgaris. J Eur Acad Dermatol Venereol 2013;27(4):430–5.
58. Zagorodniuk I, Weltfriend S, Shtruminger L, et al. A comparison of anti-desmoglein antibodies and indirect immunofluorescence in the serodiagnosis of pemphigus vulgaris. Int J Dermatol 2005;44(7):541–4.
59. Edgin WA, Pratt TC, Grimwood RE. Pemphigus vulgaris and paraneoplastic pemphigus. Oral Maxillofac Surg Clin North Am 2008;20(4):577–84.
60. Scully C, Mignogna M. Oral mucosal disease: pemphigus. Br J Oral Maxillofac Surg 2008;46(4):272–7.
61. Czernik A, Camilleri M, Pittelkow MR, et al. Paraneoplastic autoimmune multiorgan syndrome: 20 years after. Int J Dermatol 2011;50(8):905–14.
62. Ben Lagha N, Poulesquen V, Roujeau JC, et al. Pemphigus vulgaris: a case-based update. J Can Dent Assoc 2005;71(9):667–72.
63. Hodgson TA, Malik F, Hegarty AM, et al. Topical tacrolimus: a novel therapeutic intervention for recalcitrant labial pemphigus vulgaris. Eur J Dermatol 2003; 13(2):142–4.
64. Lunardon L, Tsai KJ, Propert KJ, et al. Adjuvant rituximab therapy of pemphigus: a single-center experience with 31 patients. Arch Dermatol 2012;148(9):1031–6.
65. Behzad M, Mobs C, Kneisel A, et al. Combined treatment with immunoadsorption and rituximab leads to fast and prolonged clinical remission in difficult-to-treat pemphigus vulgaris. Br J Dermatol 2012;166(4):844–52.
66. Xu HH, Werth VP, Parisi E, et al. Mucous membrane pemphigoid. Dent Clin North Am 2013;57(4):611–30.
67. Sollecito TP, Parisi E. Mucous membrane pemphigoid. Dent Clin North Am 2005; 49(1):91–106, viii.
68. Bernard P, Vaillant L, Labeille B, et al. Incidence and distribution of subepidermal autoimmune bullous skin diseases in three French regions. Bullous Diseases French Study Group. Arch Dermatol 1995;131(1):48–52.
69. Bertram F, Brocker EB, Zillikens D, et al. Prospective analysis of the incidence of autoimmune bullous disorders in Lower Franconia, Germany. J Dtsch Dermatol Ges 2009;7(5):434–40.
70. Woo SB, Greenberg M. Ulcerative, vesicular, and bullous lesions. In: Greenberg M, Glick M, Ship J, editors. Burket's Oral Medicine. 11th Edition. Hamilton (Canada): B.C. Decker Inc; 2008. p. 67.
71. Chan LS, Hammerberg C, Cooper KD. Significantly increased occurrence of HLA-DQB1*0301 allele in patients with ocular cicatricial pemphigoid. J Invest Dermatol 1997;108(2):129–32.
72. Setterfield J, Theron J, Vaughan RW, et al. Mucous membrane pemphigoid: HLA-DQB1*0301 is associated with all clinical sites of involvement and may be linked to antibasement membrane IgG production. Br J Dermatol 2001;145(3):406–14.
73. Chan LS, Yancey KB, Hammerberg C, et al. Immune-mediated subepithelial blistering diseases of mucous membranes. Pure ocular cicatricial pemphigoid

is a unique clinical and immunopathological entity distinct from bullous pemphigoid and other subsets identified by antigenic specificity of autoantibodies. Arch Dermatol 1993;129(4):448–55.

74. Yeh SW, Usman AQ, Ahmed AR. Profile of autoantibody to basement membrane zone proteins in patients with mucous membrane pemphigoid: long-term follow up and influence of therapy. Clin Immunol 2004;112(3):268–72.

75. Carrozzo M, Cozzani E, Broccoletti R, et al. Analysis of antigens targeted by circulating IgG and IgA antibodies in patients with mucous membrane pemphigoid predominantly affecting the oral cavity. J Periodontol 2004;75(10):1302–8.

76. Van Joost T, Van't Veen AJ. Drug-induced cicatricial pemphigoid and acquired epidermolysis bullosa. Clin Dermatol 1993;11(4):521–7.

77. Laskaris G, Satriano RA. Drug-induced blistering oral lesions. Clin Dermatol 1993;11(4):545–50.

78. Eversole LR. Immunopathology of oral mucosal ulcerative, desquamative, and bullous diseases. Selective review of the literature. Oral Surg Oral Med Oral Pathol 1994;77(6):555–71.

79. Bernauer W, Wright P, Dart JK, et al. The conjunctiva in acute and chronic mucous membrane pemphigoid. An immunohistochemical analysis. Ophthalmology 1993;100(3):339–46.

80. Chan LS. Mucous membrane pemphigoid. Clin Dermatol 2001;19(6):703–11.

81. Moghadam-Kia S, Werth VP. Prevention and treatment of systemic glucocorticoid side effects. Int J Dermatol 2010;49(3):239–48.

82. Rogers RS 3rd, Mehregan DA. Dapsone therapy of cicatricial pemphigoid. Semin Dermatol 1988;7(3):201–5.

83. Ciarrocca KN, Greenberg MS. A retrospective study of the management of oral mucous membrane pemphigoid with dapsone. Oral Surg Oral Med Oral Pathol Oral Radiol Endod 1999;88(2):159–63.

84. Poskitt L, Wojnarowska F. Minimizing cicatricial pemphigoid orodynia with minocycline. Br J Dermatol 1995;132(5):784–9.

85. Schulz S, Deuster D, Schmidt E, et al. Therapeutic effect of etanercept in antilaminin 5 (laminin 332) mucous membrane pemphigoid. Int J Dermatol 2011;50(9):1129–31.

86. Shetty S, Ahmed AR. Critical analysis of the use of rituximab in mucous membrane pemphigoid: a review of the literature. J Am Acad Dermatol 2013;68(3):499–506.

87. Cafaro A, Broccoletti R, Arduino PG. Low-level laser therapy for oral mucous membrane pemphigoid. Lasers Med Sci 2012;27(6):1247–50.

Temporomandibular Disorders

Evaluation and Management

Scott S. De Rossi, DMD[a,b,c,]*, Martin S. Greenberg, DDS, FDS RCS[d],
Frederick Liu, DDS, MD[e], Andrew Steinkeler, DMD, MD[e]

KEYWORDS

- Temporomandibular disorders • Orofacial pain • Myalgia • Arthralgia • TMJ surgery

KEY POINTS

- Temporomandibular disorder (TMD) is a multifactorial disease process with various causes, including parafunctional habits (eg, nocturnal bruxing, tooth clenching, lip or cheek biting), emotional distress, acute trauma to the jaw, trauma from hyperextension (eg, dental procedures, oral intubations for general anesthesia, yawning, hyperextension associated with cervical trauma), instability of maxillomandibular relationships, laxity of the joint, and comorbidity of other rheumatic or musculoskeletal disorders.
- Symptoms of TMD include decreased mandibular range of motion, muscle and joint pain, joint crepitus, and functional limitation or deviation of the jaw opening.
- Treatment of patients with TMD initially should be based on the use of conservative, reversible, and evidence-based therapeutic modalities.
- Only after failure of noninvasive options should more invasive and nonreversible treatments be initiated.
- Temporomandibular joint replacement is reserved for severely damaged joints with end-stage disease that has failed all other conservative treatment modalities.

Disclosures: None.
This article includes portions of material previously published in De Rossi SS, Stern I, Sollecito TP. Disorders of the masticatory muscles. Dent Clin North Am 2013;57(3):449–64; and Liu F, Steinkeler A. Epidemiology, diagnosis, and treatment of temporomandibular disorders. Dent Clin North Am 2013;57(3):465–79.
[a] Oral Medicine, Oral Health & Diagnostic Sciences, Georgia Regents University, 1120, 15th Street, Augusta, GA 30912, USA; [b] Dermatology, Georgia Regents University, 1120, 15th Street, Augusta, GA 30912, USA; [c] Otolaryngology/Head & Neck Surgery, Georgia Regents University, 1120, 15th Street, Augusta, GA 30912, USA; [d] Department of Oral Medicine, Hospital Affairs, School of Dental Medicine, University of Pennsylvania, Philadelphia, PA, USA; [e] Department of Oral and Maxillofacial Surgery, School of Dental Medicine, University of Pennsylvania, Philadelphia, PA, USA
* Corresponding author. Oral Medicine, Oral Health & Diagnostic Sciences, Georgia Regents University, 1120, 15th Street, Augusta, GA 30912.
E-mail address: sderossi@gru.edu

Med Clin N Am 98 (2014) 1353–1384
http://dx.doi.org/10.1016/j.mcna.2014.08.009
0025-7125/14/$ – see front matter © 2014 Elsevier Inc. All rights reserved.

medical.theclinics.com

INTRODUCTION

Temporomandibular disorders (TMDs) are a broad group of clinical problems involving the masticatory musculature, the temporomandibular joint (TMJ), surrounding bony and soft tissue components, and combinations of these structures.[1] Symptoms of TMD may include decreased mandibular range of motion, pain in the muscles of mastication, TMJ pain, associated joint noise (clicking, popping, or crepitus) with function, generalized myofascial pain, and a functional limitation (locking) or deviation of jaw opening.[1] TMD is classified as a subtype of secondary headache disorders by the International Headache Society in the International Classification of Headache Disorders. The common perception that all symptoms of the head, face, and jaw without an identifiable cause constitute a TMJ problem is unfounded.

EPIDEMIOLOGY

The prevalence of TMD is thought to be greater than 5% of the population.[2] Lipton and colleagues[3] showed that about 6% to 12% of the population experience clinical symptoms of TMD but only about 5% have significant signs and symptoms warranting treatment. Patients with TMD symptoms present over a broad age range; however, there is a peak occurrence between 20 and 40 years of age.[4] TMD symptoms are more prevalent in women than in men. Contrary to the known increased health risk in postmenopausal women of conditions such as heart disease and stroke, women tend to develop TMD during their premenopausal years.[1,2] The reasons behind the gender disequilibrium in TMD prevalence are not clear, but some clinicians have suggested a hormonal influence.[5–7] Both animal and human studies have suggested that sex hormones may predispose to TMJ dysfunction and cartilaginous breakdown.[5–7] Increased levels of estrogen have been found in patients with TMD.[2] However, no definitive link between these hormones and causation of TMD has been established.

CAUSES

TMD was first described in the 1930s when otolaryngologist JB Costen established the TMJ as a separate source of otalgia (**Box 1**). He assumed that TMJ problems were the result of structural malalignments between the mandible and the cranium and that only dentists could take care of TMJ problems because of the structural corrections that would be required.[2] This relationship between dental occlusion and TMD has been of interest for the past 55 years, often promoting acrimonious and

---

Box 1
Multifactorial causes of TMD

Parafunctional habits (eg, nocturnal bruxing, tooth clenching, lip or cheek biting)

Emotional distress

Acute trauma to the jaw

Trauma from hyperextension (eg, dental procedures, oral intubations for general anesthesia, yawning, hyperextension associated with cervical trauma)

Instability of maxillomandibular relationships

Laxity of the joint

Comorbidity of other rheumatic or musculoskeletal disorders

Poor general health and an unhealthy lifestyle

counterproductive discussions. However, during the past 15 years, a mounting body of evidence has challenged past thinking about the role of dental occlusion in various TMDs. Malocclusions (eg, anterior open bite) may be the result of anatomic changes in the TMJs caused by inflammation and degenerative changes associated with rheumatoid arthritis (RA) as opposed to causing TMD. Recent scientific literature has not supported a relationship between occlusal factors and TMD because occlusal issues fail to meet the Hill criteria of causation for TMD. In addition, the scientific literature has not shown effectiveness of occlusal adjustments such as grinding and/or orthodontic therapy in the treatment of TMD.[2,8,9]

CLASSIFICATION OF TEMPOROMANDIBULAR DISORDERS

In general, TMDs can be divided into articular and nonarticular disorders, and these are synonymous with intracapsular and extracapsular conditions, respectively. Most nonarticular disorders present as myofascial pain focused to the muscles of mastication (**Fig. 1**). Other nonarticular disorders include chronic conditions such as fibromyalgia, muscle strain, and myopathies. Most myofascial pain and dysfunction (MPD) is theorized to arise from clenching, bruxism, or other parafunctional habits. This condition leads to masticatory musculature strain, spasm, pain, and functional limitation.[2] Emotional stress also predisposes to clenching and bruxism, which contributes to myofascial pain.[10] Symptoms include chronic pain in the masticatory muscles, and radiating pain to the ears, neck, and head. The American Academy of Orofacial Pain (AAOP) highlights 3 main diagnostic categories of TMD (**Table 1**).[11]

Articular disorders can be divided into inflammatory and noninflammatory arthropathies. Inflammatory articular disorders include rheumatologic processes such as RA, seronegative spondylopathies such as ankylosing spondylitis, psoriatic arthritis, gout, and infectious arthritis. Noninflammatory articular disk disorders include osteoarthritis, joint damage from prior trauma or surgery, or other cartilage or bone disorders (see **Table 1**). Articular disorders occur mechanistically as a result of an altered balance of anabolic and catabolic cytokines. This cytokine imbalance creates

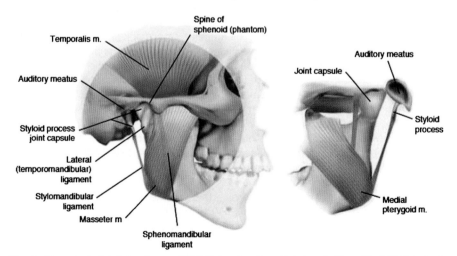

Fig. 1. Musculoskeletal structures of TMJ (lateral and medial views). (*From* Liu F, Steinkeler A. Epidemiology, diagnosis, and treatment of temporomandibular disorders. Dent Clin North Am 2013;57(3):465–79.)

Table 1	
AAOP diagnostic classification of TMDs	
Diagnostic Category	**Diagnoses**
Cranial bones (including the mandible)	Congenital and developmental disorders: aplasia, hypoplasia, hyperplasia, dysplasia (eg, first and second branchial arch anomalies, hemifacial microsomia, Pierre Robin syndrome, Treacher Collins syndrome, condylar hyperplasia, prognathism, fibrous dysplasia)
	Acquired disorders (neoplasia, fracture)
TMJ disorders	Deviation in form
	Disc displacement (with reduction; without reduction)
	Dislocation
	Inflammatory conditions (synovitis, capsulitis)
	Arthritides (osteoarthritis, osteoarthrosis, polyarthritides)
	Ankylosis (fibrous, bony)
	Neoplasia
Masticatory muscle disorders	Myofascial pain
	Myositis spasm
	Protective splinting
	Contracture

Adapted from de Leew R. Orofacial pain: guidelines for assessment, classification, and management. The American Academy of Orofacial Pain. 5th edition. Chicago: Quintessence Publishing; 2013.

an inflammatory milieu that leads to oxidative stress, free radicals, and ultimately joint damage.[12]

Internal derangement equates to changes in the disc-condyle relationship.[11] Disc displacements are categorized as disc displacement with reduction or disc displacement without reduction (**Fig. 2**). The fibrocartilage disc is typically displaced anteromedially but rarely is displaced laterally or posteriorly.[13–15] The anatomy of disc displacement with reduction is an interference between the mandibular condyle and the articular disc during jaw opening or closing. This interference may generate clicking, popping, or crepitus in the joint, which can be associated with discomfort. However, clicking alone is not diagnostic of articular disc displacement. During disc displacement with reduction, the condyle meets the posterior aspect of the disc, which then reduces to its proper position between the condyle and glenoid fossa.[11,15] Articular disc displacement is associated with TMD. One study found MRI evidence of disc displacement in 84% of symptomatic patients with TMD versus 33% of asymptomatic patients.[16] However, MRI findings should not solely dictate treatment, because disc displacement may occur in asymptomatic patients. Disc displacement without reduction results in a closed lock, in which the condylar movement is physically blocked by the anteriorly displaced disc. Acute closed lock is associated with limited mandibular opening and severe pain.[11,15] Common causes of articular and nonarticular TMD are summarized in **Box 2**.

Articular disorders are classified according to the Wilkes Staging Classification for Internal Derangement of the TMJ (stages I–V). The Wilkes classification is based on clinical, radiologic, and anatomic findings (**Box 3**).[17] For research purposes, a more detailed diagnostic classification is used, known as the Research Diagnostic Criteria for Temporomandibular Disorders (RDC/TMD). The RDC/TMD classification system is divided into 3 axes: axis 1 (muscle disorders), axis 2 (disc disorders), and axis 3 (arthralgias).[18,19]

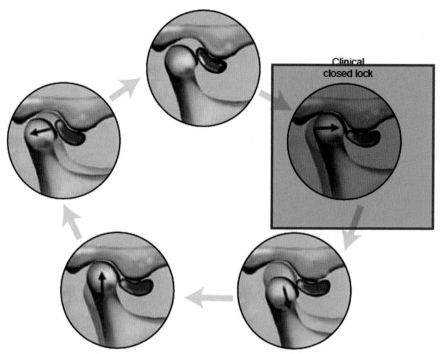

Fig. 2. Motion mechanics seen in TMJ with anteriorly displaced disc and resultant closed lock. (*From* Liu F, Steinkeler A. Epidemiology, diagnosis, and treatment of temporomandibular disorders. Dent Clin North Am 2013;57(3):465–79.)

Box 2
Common causes of articular and nonarticular TMD

Articular disorders

Osteoarthritis

Trauma

Infectious arthritis

Prior surgery (iatrogenic)

Gout/pseudogout (crystal arthropathies)

Psoriatic arthritis

RA/juvenile RA

Ankylosing spondylitis

Nonarticular disorders

Myofascial pain

Acute muscle strain

Muscle spasm

Fibromyalgia

Chronic pain conditions

Myotonic dystrophy

Adapted from Ghali GE, Miloro M, Waite PD, et al, editors. Peterson's principles of oral and maxillofacial surgery. 3rd edition. Shelton (CT): People's Medical Publishing House—USA; 2012.

Box 3
Wilkes staging for internal derangement of the TMJ

I. Early stage

   A. Clinical presentation: no pain or decreased range of motion, possible clicking

   B. Radiographic presentation: disc anteriorly positioned, normal bony contours

   C. Anatomic correlation: anterior displacement, normal anatomic form of bone and disc

II. Early/intermediate stage:

   A. Clinical presentation: episodes of pain, opening clicks, intermittent locking

   B. Radiographic presentation: anterior disc displacement, thickened posterior disc, bony contours normal

   C. Anatomic correlation: early disc deformity, anterior displacement normal bony contours

III. Intermediate stage

   A. Clinical presentation: many painful episodes, intermittent closed locking, multiple functional symptoms, decreased range of motion

   B. Radiographic presentation: anterior disc displacement with disc deformity

   C. Anatomic correlation: marked disc displacement and deformity, normal bony contours

IV. Intermediate/late stage

   A. Clinical presentation: increased pain relative to earlier stages

   B. Radiographic presentation: bony changes such as flattened eminence, condylar deformity, osteosclerotic changes

   C. Anatomic correlation: adhesions of disc, bony changes, evidence of osteoarthritis, osteophytes, no disc perforations

V. Late stage

   A. Clinical presentation: episodic or continuous pain, crepitus, limited range of motion at all times, constant functional difficulties

   B. Radiographic presentation: disc perforations, gross deformities of bony structures and cartilage, progressive arthritic changes

   C. Anatomic correlation: gross hard and soft tissue changes, perforations, adhesions, subcortical cysts

Adapted from Wilkes CH. Internal derangements of the temporomandibular joint: pathological variation. Arch Otolaryngol Head Neck Surg 1989;115:469–77.

DIAGNOSIS OF TEMPOROMANDIBULAR DISORDERS

Diagnosing TMD requires a focused history and physical examination. Pain and limited range of motion are accepted symptoms and signs of TMJ dysfunction warranting treatment. Radiographic studies can also be used as supplemental diagnostic tools. Dental radiographs can be used to rule out dental disorder as a cause of referred pain. Cone beam computed tomography scans and panoramic radiographs provide detailed imaging of the joint's bony structures, but not of the articular disc. MRI is the modality of choice for examining disc position and morphology (gold standard). MRI may also show degenerative bony changes. MRI findings alone should not dictate treatment strategies. Clinicians must combine the patient's clinical presentation, signs, and symptoms along with TMJ imaging when developing a diagnosis and plan of treatment. On MRI, joint effusions are imaging signs of inflammation.[20]

Inflammation indicates a transition from adaptive to pathologic changes within the joint. The MRI diagnosis of anterior disc displacement uses the most superior aspect of the condyle (12 o'clock position) as a reference point.[20] Anterior disc displacement is defined radiographically when the posterior disc tissue is located anterior to the 12 o'clock condylar position. Disc displacement may occur in asymptomatic patients, such that all imaging findings must be placed in clinical context before beginning TMJ treatments.

The algorithm in **Fig. 3** summarizes the Research Diagnostic Criteria Decision Tree for Pain-related TMD/Headache and Joint Disorders.

CLINICAL EVALUATION

The most effective approach for diagnosis of TMDs involves careful review of the chief complaint; the history of present illness (**Table 2**); the dental, medical, and psychosocial behavioral histories (**Box 4**); and a comprehensive head and neck evaluation, including a cranial nerve assessment (**Table 3**).[12] In addition, imaging modalities may be important to rule out other conditions. No single physical finding can be relied on to establish a diagnosis, but a pattern of signs and symptoms may suggest the source of the problem and a diagnosis.[21] However, masticatory muscle tenderness on palpation is the most consistent examination feature present in TMDs.[3,22–26] The clinical features that distinguish patients with TMD from those with non-TMD or masticatory muscle pain most consistently in the literature are restricted passive mouth opening without pain, masticatory muscle tenderness on palpation, limited maximal mouth opening, and an uncorrected deviation on maximum mouth opening and tenderness on muscle or joint palpation.[2,3,22–26]

Objective determination of the presence or absence of parafunctional jaw behavior is challenging.[27] Although the presence of these behaviors may not have proven diagnostic validity, their assessment remains important because it provides potential causative or perpetuating factors and/or effects on the masticatory system. An oral behavior checklist is a useful instrument for determining the presence or awareness of parafunctional behaviors.[28]

Interincisor separation (plus or minus the incisor overlap in centric occlusion) provides the measure of mandibular movement. Maximum interincisal opening (MIO) should be measured using a ruler without pain, as wide as possible with pain, and after opening with clinician assistance. Mouth opening with assistance is accomplished by applying mild pressure against the upper and lower incisors with the thumb and index finger. Passive stretching often allows the clinician to assess and differentiate the limitation of opening caused by a muscle or joint problem by comparing assisted opening with active opening. This comparison provides the examiner with the quality of resistance at the end of the movement. Often, muscle restrictions are associated with a soft end-feel and result in an increase of more than 5 mm more than the active opening (wide opening with pain), whereas joint disorders such as acute nonreducing disc displacements have a hard end-feel and characteristically limit assisted opening to less than 5 mm (normal MIO is ~40 mm; range, 35–55 mm). A simple clinical assessment is to use fingerbreadths, assuming each fingerbreadth to be approximately 15 mm. Measurements of lateral movement are made with the teeth slightly separated, measuring the displacement of the lower midline from the maxillary midline and adding or subtracting the lower-midline displacement at the start of movement. Protrusive movement is measured by adding the horizontal distance between the upper and lower central incisors and adding the distance the lower incisors travel beyond the upper incisors; normal lateral and protrusive movements are ~7 mm.

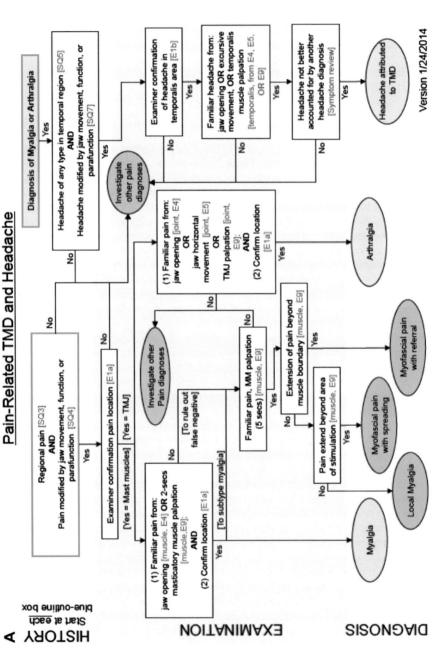

Fig. 3. Research diagnostic criteria decision tree for pain-related TMD/headache (*A*) and joint disorders(*B*). (*From* International RDC-TMD Consortium. Available at: www.rdc-tmdinternational.org. Accessed April 1, 2014.)

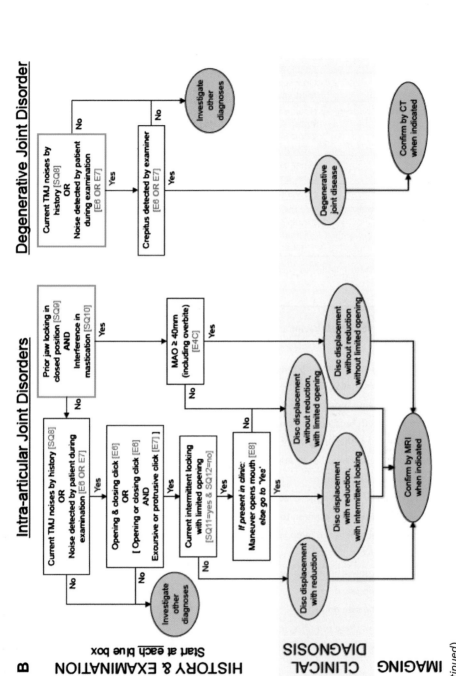

Fig. 3. (*continued*)

Table 2
History of the present illness: pain characteristics

Quality	Common patient descriptors (eg, dull, sharp, tight, aching, tired)
Location	Unilateral vs bilateral Pain confined to a single muscle or referred to a distant area
Intensity	On a scale of 1–10 Mild, moderate, or severe
Onset, duration, pattern	How long has the pain been present? What, if anything, caused the pain? (eg, trauma) What been the course of pain since its onset? (eg, episodic, constant, fluctuating)
Modifiers	What exacerbates or diminishes the pain? Does anything you do or use help or worsen pain?
Chronicity	How long has the pain been present?
Comorbid symptoms and sign	Are there any other conditions or symptoms associated with pain? (eg, depression, acute anxiety, nausea/vomiting, tearing, visual changes, dizziness, numbness/tingling, weakness, generalized pain)

From De Rossi SS, Stern I, Sollecito TP. Disorders of the masticatory muscles. Dent Clin North Am 2013;57(3):449–64.

Box 4
Questions regarding oral behavior and parafunction.

Do you:

Clench or grind your teeth when asleep?

Sleep in a position that puts pressure on your jaw? (eg, side, stomach)

Clench or press teeth together while awake?

Touch or hold teeth together while eating?

Hold, tighten, or tense muscles without clenching or touching teeth together?

Hold out or jut jaw forward or to side?

Press tongue between teeth?

Bite, chew, or play with tongue, cheeks, or lips?

Hold jaw in rigid or tense position to brace or protect jaw?

Bite or hold objects between teeth (eg, pens, pipe, hair, fingernails)?

Use chewing gum?

Play musical instruments that involve mouth or jaw?

Lean with hand on jaw or chin?

Chew food on one side only?

Eat between meals (food requiring lots of chewing)?

Do sustained talking?

Sing?

Yawn excessively?

Hold telephone between head and shoulder?

Adapted from Ohrbach R, Markiewicz M, McCall WD Jr. Oral behaviors checklist: performance validity of targeted behaviors. J Dent Res 2004;83(Spec Issue A):T27–45.

Table 3
Physical examination directed toward mandibular dysfunction

Examination	Observations
Inspection	Facial asymmetry, swelling, and masseter and temporal muscle hypertrophy Opening pattern (corrected and uncorrected deviations, uncoordinated movements, limitations)
Assessment of range of mandibular movement	Maximum opening with comfort, with pain, and with clinician assistance Maximum lateral and protrusive movements
Palpation examination	Masticatory muscles TMJs Neck muscles and accessory muscles of the jaw Parotid and submandibular areas Lymph nodes
Provocation tests	Static pain test (mandibular resistance against pressure) Pain in the joints or muscles with tooth clenching Reproduction of symptoms with chewing (wax, sugarless gum)
Intraoral examination	Signs of parafunction (cheek or lip biting, accentuated linea alba, scalloped tongue borders, occlusal wear, tooth mobility, generalized sensitivity to percussion, thermal testing, multiple fractures of enamel and restorations)

From De Rossi SS, Stern I, Sollecito TP. Disorders of the masticatory muscles. Dent Clin North Am 2013;57(3):449–64; and *Data from* Refs.[2,3,22–26]

The primary finding related to masticatory muscle palpation is pain; however, the methods for palpation are not standardized in clinical practice.[29] The amount of pressure to apply and the exact sites that are most likely associated with TMD are unknown. Some clinicians have recommended attempting to establish a baseline (to serve as a general guide or reference) by squeezing a muscle between the index finger and thumb or by applying pressure in the center of the forehead or thumbnail to gauge what pressure becomes uncomfortable.[18] The RDC/TMD guidelines recommend 0.45 kg (1 lb) of pressure for the joint and 0.9 kg (2 lb) of pressure for the muscles. Palpation should be accompanied by asking the patient about the presence of pain at the palpation site, whether palpation produces pain spread or referral to a distant site, and whether palpation reproduces the pain the patient has been experiencing.[18,30] Reproducing the site and the character of the pain during the examination procedure helps identify the source of the pain. The distant origin of referred pain can also be identified by palpation.[30]

Palpation of the muscles for pain should be done with the muscles in a resting state.[30] There are no standardized methods of assessing the severity of palpable pain, and the patient should be asked to rate the severity by using a scale (eg, a numeric scale from 1 to 10; a visual analog scale; or a ranking such as none, mild, moderate, or severe). The RDC/TMD recommends using the categories of pressure only, mild pain, moderate pain, and severe pain.[18] These ratings may also be useful in assessing treatment progress in addition to asking patients what percent improvement they feel. The lateral pterygoid is in a position that does not allow access for adequate palpation examination even though there are examination protocols and descriptions for palpating this muscle.

Patients with TMDs often have musculoskeletal problems in other regions (eg, neck, back).[31] The upper cervical somatosensory nerves send branches that synapse in the spinal trigeminal nucleus, which is one proposed mechanism to explain referral of pain from the neck to the orofacial region and masticatory muscles.[32–34] The sternocleidomastoid and trapezius muscles are often part of cervical muscle disorders and may refer pain to the face and head. Other cervical muscle groups to include in the palpation examination include the paravertebral (scalene) and suboccipital muscles.

Injections of anesthetics into the TMJ or selected masticatory muscles may help confirm a diagnosis. Elimination of, or a significant decrease in, pain and improved jaw motion should be considered a positive test result. Diagnostic injections may also be helpful in differentiating pain arising from joints or muscle.[2,30] In situations in which a joint procedure is being considered, local anesthetic injection of the joint may confirm the joint as the source of pain. Injecting trigger points or tender areas of muscle should eliminate pain from the site and should also eliminate referred pain associated with the injected trigger point. Interpretation of injections must be in the context of all the diagnostic information because a positive result does not ensure a specific diagnosis. The use of botulin toxin has recently been advocated for trigger point injections and for the management of tension-type headache.[8,30] In several case control studies and randomized trials, descriptive analysis showed that improvements in both objective (range of mandibular movements) and subjective (pain at rest; pain during chewing) clinical outcome variables were higher in Botox-treated groups than in the placebo-treated subjects. Patients treated with Botox had a higher subjective improvement in their perception of treatment efficacy than the placebo subjects. However, Botox does not seem statistically significantly better than saline, local anesthetic, or dry needle.[2,30,35]

MASTICATORY MUSCLE DISORDERS

Mechanisms behind masticatory muscle pain include overuse of a normally perfused muscle or ischemia of a normally working muscle, sympathetic reflexes that produce changes in vascular supply and muscle tone, and changes in psychological and emotional states.[36] Neurons mediating pain from skeletal muscle are subject to strong modulatory influences. Bradykinin, serotonin, substance P, prostaglandins, and neuropeptides sensitize nociceptors and can easily sensitize nociceptive endings. Painful conditions of muscle often result in increased sensitivity of peripheral nociceptors and hyperexcitability in the central nervous system with hyperalgesia.[37]

Muscle disorders can be divided into local and regional disorders, such as myalgia and myofascial pain, associated with TMD; and systemic disorders, such as pain associated with fibromyalgia.[2] The paucity of data on the causes and pathophysiology of muscle pain limits the ability to clearly delineate all groups of muscle disorders. Clinicians often must rely on clinical judgment to establish a diagnosis. Well-designed controlled trials and additional research are necessary for the development of validated diagnostic criteria and treatment protocols.[8,18,38]

Chronic myalgia of the muscle of mastication (MOM) is one aspect of TMD.[2,8] In the past, clinicians and researchers subclassified TMDs into intracapsular disorders and masticatory muscle disorders such as local myalgia, myofascial pain, centrally mediated myalgia, myospasm, myositis, myofibrotic contracture, and masticatory muscle neoplastic disease.[18] Conflicting classification schemes and terminology have led to significant confusion among clinicians and perhaps inaccurate diagnosis and treatment of patients. Many studies continue to group muscle pain and painful TMJ disorders together under the term TMD, although these entities are pathophysiologically and clinically distinct.[8,11,39,40] Although the most common feature of most masticatory muscle disorders is pain, mandibular dysfunction, such as difficulty chewing and mandibular dysfunction, may also occur. Clinicians need to differentiate masticatory muscle disorders from primary TMJ disorders, such as those that involve pain associated with osteoarthritis, disc displacement, or jaw dysfunction (**Table 4**).

The clinical features of masticatory muscle disorders are as follows:

Features of local myalgia
- Sore MOM with pain in cheeks and temples on chewing, wide opening, and often on waking (eg, nocturnal bruxism)
- Bilateral
- Described as stiff, sore, aching, spasm, tightness, or cramping
- Sensation of muscle stiffness, weakness, fatigue
- Possible reduced mandibular range of motion
- Differential diagnosis: myositis, myofascial pain, neoplasm, fibromyalgia

Features of myofascial pain
- Regional dull aching muscle pain
- Trigger points present and pain referral on palpation with/without autonomic symptoms
- Referred pain often felt as headache
- Trigger points can be inactivated with local anesthetic injection
- Sensation of muscle stiffness and/or malocclusion not verified clinically
- Otologic symptoms including tinnitus, vertigo, and pain
- Headache or toothache
- Decreased range of motion
- Hyperalgesia in region of referred pain
- Differential diagnosis: arthralgia, myositis, local myalgia, neoplasia, fibromyalgia

Features of centrally mediated myalgia
- Trigger points and pain referral on palpation
- Sensation of muscle stiffness, weakness, and/or fatigue
- Sensation of malocclusion not verified clinically
- Otologic symptoms including tinnitus, vertigo, and pain
- Decreased range of motion
- Hyperalgesia
- Does not respond to treatment directed at painful muscle tissue
- Differential diagnosis: arthralgia, myositis, myofascial pain, local myalgia, neoplasm, fibromyalgia

Features of myospasm
- Sudden and involuntary muscle contraction
- Acute malocclusion (dependent on muscles involved)
- Decreased range of motion and pain on function and at rest
- Rare disorder in orofacial pain population
- Differential diagnosis: myositis, local myalgia, neoplasm

Features of myositis
- History of trauma to muscle or source of infection
- Often continuous pain affecting the entire muscle
- Pain aggravated by function
- Severe limited range of motion

Table 4
Diagnostic criteria for masticatory muscle disorders

Disorder	Cause	Diagnostic Criteria
Centrally mediated chronic muscle pain	Chronic generalized muscle pain associated with a comorbid disease	History of prolonged and continuous muscle pain Regional dull, aching pain at rest Pain aggravated by function of affected muscles Pain aggravated by palpation
Myalgia (local)	Acute muscle pain Protective muscle splinting Postexercise soreness Muscle fatigue Pain from ischemia	Regional dull, aching pain during function No or minimal pain at rest Local muscle tenderness on palpation Absence of trigger points and pain referral
Myofascial pain	Chronic regional muscle pain	Regional dull, aching pain at rest Pain aggravated by function of affected muscles Provocation of trigger points alters pain complaint and reveals referral pattern >50% reduction of pain with vapocoolant spray or local anesthetic injection to trigger point followed by stretch
Myofibrotic contracture	Painless shortening of muscles	Limited range of motion Firmness on passive stretch (hard stop) Little or no pain unless involved muscle is forced to lengthen
Myositis	Inflammation secondary to direct trauma or infection	Continuous pain localized in muscle area following injury or infection Diffuse tenderness over entire muscle Pain aggravated by function of affected muscles Moderate to severe decreased range of motion caused by pain and swelling
Neoplasia	Benign or malignant	May or may not be painful Anatomic and structural changes Imaging and biopsy needed
Myospasm	Acute involuntary and continuous muscle contraction	Acute onset pain at rest and function Markedly decreased range of motion caused by continuous involuntary muscle contraction Pain aggravated by function of affected muscles Increased electromyogram activity (higher than at rest) Sensation of muscle tightness, cramping, or stiffness

Adapted from de Leew R. Orofacial pain: guidelines for assessment, classification, and management. The American Academy of Orofacial Pain. 5th edition. Chicago: Quintessence Publishing; 2013.

Features of myofibrotic contracture
- Not usually painful
- Often follows long period of limited range of motion or disuse (eg, intermaxillary fixation)
- History of infection or trauma is common
- Differential diagnosis: TMJ ankylosis, coronoid hypertrophy

Features of masticatory muscle neoplasia
- Pain may or may not be present
- Anatomic and structural changes: tumors may be in muscles or masticatory spaces
- Swelling, trismus, paresthesias, and pain referred to teeth
- Positive findings on imaging or biopsy

Some clinicians have stressed classifying myogenic disorders based on an anatomic system, allowing a simpler diagnostic process because the patient evaluation involves careful palpation of the masticatory muscles and joints.[40–42] The clinician needs to determine the causes and pathophysiology that occur with the various masticatory muscle disorders, such as disorders caused by trauma and so forth. A thorough history and clinical examination, an understanding of pain neuroanatomy and neurophysiology, and an in-depth knowledge of muscle pain research are important.[42–44] Various causes of myogenous pain are reviewed in **Table 5**.

Table 5
Causes of myogenous pain

Cause	Criteria
Focal myalgia from direct trauma	History of trauma preceding pain onset Subjective pain in muscles with function Pain reproduced on palpation
Primary myalgia caused by parafunction	No history of trauma Subjective pain in muscle with function Pain reproduced on palpation No trigger points
Secondary myalgia caused by active local disorder or recent medications	History of recent joint, oral soft tissue, or pulpal disease or medication (eg, SSRI) that coincides with muscle pain Subjective pain in muscle with function Pain reproduced on palpation
Myofascial pain	No history of recent trauma Subjective pain in muscles with function Pain reproduced on palpation Trigger points and pain referral
Diffuse chronic muscle pain and fibromyalgia	Subjective pain in multiple sites aggravated by function Widespread pain involving more than 3 body quadrants >3-mo duration Pain on palpation in 11 of 18 body sites

Abbreviation: SSRI, serotonin-selective reuptake inhibitors.
Adapted from Clark GT, Minakuchi H. Oral appliances. In: Laskin DM, Greene CS, Hylander WL, editors. TMDs, an evidence-based approach to diagnosis and treatment. Chicago: Quintessence; 2006. p. 377–90.

A new term, persistent orofacial muscle pain (POMP), was recently introduced to more accurately reflect the interplay between peripheral nociceptive sources in muscles, faulty central nervous system components, and decreased coping ability.[8] POMP likely shares mechanisms with tension-type headache, regional myofascial pain, and fibromyalgia and has genetically influenced traits that determine pain modulation and pharmacogenomics interacting with psychological traits to affect disease onset, clinical progression, and pain experience.[8,9] To date, these factors cannot be identified in individual patients in order to tailor focused, mechanism-based treatment. POMP is consistent with the condition often referred to as centrally mediated myalgia and, as such, treatment needs to be redirected from local and regional therapies to systemic and central ones.

TREATMENT OF MASTICATORY MUSCLE DISORDERS

It is important for the clinician treating patients with TMDs to distinguish clinically significant disorders that require therapy from incidental findings in patients with facial pain from other causes.[2] TMJ abnormalities are often discovered on routine examination and may not require treatment, such as with asymptomatic clicking of the TMJ. The need for treatment is largely based on the level of pain and dysfunction as well as the progression of symptoms. With respect to disorders of MOM, the principles of treatment are based on a generally favorable prognosis and an appreciation of the present lack of clinically controlled trials indicating the superiority, predictability, and safety of treatments.[2,8,18,45] The literature suggests that many treatments have some beneficial effect, although this effect may be nonspecific and not directly related to the particular treatment.[2,8,18]

According to the American Association of Dental Research, it is strongly recommended that, unless there are specific and justifiable indications to the contrary, treatment of patients with TMD, including those with disorders of MOM, initially should be based on the use of conservative, reversible, and evidence-based therapeutic modalities.[45] Studies of the natural history of many TMDs suggest that they tend to improve or resolve over time.[39,41,43] Although no specific therapies have been proved to be uniformly effective, many of the conservative modalities have proved to be at least as effective in providing symptomatic relief as most forms of invasive treatment. Because those modalities do not produce irreversible changes, they present less risk of producing harm. Professional treatment should be augmented with a home care program, in which patients are taught about their disorders and how to manage their symptoms.[45,46]

Treatments that are accessible, not prohibitive because of expense, safe, and reversible should be given priority, such as education, self-care, physical therapy, intraoral appliance therapy, short-term pharmacotherapy, behavioral therapy, and relaxation techniques (**Table 6**). There is evidence to suggest that multimodal therapy and combining treatments produces a better outcome.[47,48] Occlusal therapy continues to be recommended by some clinicians as an initial treatment or as a requirement to prevent recurrent symptoms. However, research does not support occlusal abnormalities as a significant causal factor in TMD including masticatory muscle disorders.[2,49–52]

Avoidance therapy and cognitive awareness play a vital role in patient care but have little scientific evidence to support their use.[2,26,27,43] In general, common sense dictates that, if something hurts, it should be avoided. Four behaviors should be avoided in patients with masticatory muscle pain:

1. Avoidance of clenching by reproducing a rest position in which the patient's lips are closed but the teeth are slightly separated

Table 6
Initial treatment of masticatory muscle disorders

Treatment Component	Description
Education	Explanation of the diagnosis and treatment Reassurance about the generally good prognosis for recovery and natural course Explanation of patient's and doctor's roles in therapy Information to enable patient to perform self-care
Self-care	Eliminate oral habits (eg, tooth clenching, chewing gum) Provide information on jaw care associated with daily activities
Physical therapy	Education regarding biomechanics of jaw, neck, and head posture Passive modalities (heat and cold therapy, ultrasonography, laser, and TENS) Range-of-motion exercises (active and passive) Posture therapy Passive stretching, general exercise, and conditioning program
Intraoral appliance therapy	Cover all the teeth on the arch on which the appliance is seated Adjust to achieve simultaneous contact against opposing teeth Adjust to a stable comfortable mandibular posture Avoid changing mandibular position Avoid long-term continuous use
Pharmacotherapy	NSAIDs, acetaminophen, muscle relaxants, antianxiety agents, tricyclic antidepressants
Behavioral/relaxation techniques	Relaxation therapy Hypnosis Biofeedback Cognitive-behavior therapy

Abbreviations: NSAIDs, nonsteroidal antiinflammatory drugs; TENS, transcutaneous electrical nerve stimulation.

From De Rossi SS, Stern I, Sollecito TP. Disorders of the masticatory muscles. Dent Clin North Am 2013;57(3):449–64; and *Data from* Refs.[2,43,51,52]

2. Avoidance of poor head and neck posture
3. Avoidance of testing the jaw or jaw joint clicking
4. Avoidance of other habits such as nail biting, lip biting, and gum chewing (**Box 5**).

Many patients report benefit from heat or ice packs applied to painful MOM. The local application of heat can increase circulation and relax muscles, whereas ice may serve as an anesthetic for painful muscles. In addition, stretch therapy must be part of a self-care program. Stretches should be done multiple times daily to maximize effectiveness. The most effective stretching exercise is passive stretching, which is summarized in **Box 6**.

Physiotherapy helps to relieve musculoskeletal pain and restore normal function by altering sensory input; reducing inflammation; decreasing, coordinating, and strengthening muscle activity; and promoting the rehabilitation of tissues.[11] A licensed professional therapist is recommended for treatment. Despite the absence of well-controlled clinical trials, physiotherapy is a well-recognized, effective, and conservative therapy for many disorders of the MOM.

Physical therapy techniques:
- Posture training
- Exercises
- Mobilization

Box 5
Patients instructions for self-care

Be aware of habits or patterns of jaw use.

- Avoid tooth contact except during chewing and swallowing.
- Notice any contact the teeth make.
- Notice any clenching, grinding, gritting, or tapping of teeth or any tensing or rigid holding of the jaw muscles.
- Check for tooth clenching while driving, studying, doing computer work, reading, or engaging in athletic activities, and also when at work or in social situations and when experiencing overwork, fatigue, or stress.
- Position the jaw to avoid tooth contacts.
- Place the tip of the tongue behind the top teeth and keep the teeth slightly apart; maintain this position when the jaw is not being used for functions such as speaking and chewing.

Modify your diet.

- Choose softer foods and only those foods that can be chewed without pain.
- Cut foods into smaller pieces; avoid foods that require wide mouth opening and biting off with the front teeth or foods that are chewy and sticky and that require excessive mouth movements.
- Do not chew gum.

Do not test the jaw.

Do not open wide or move the jaw around excessively to assess pain or motion.

Avoid habitually maneuvering the jaw into positions to assess its comfort or range.

Avoid habitually clicking the jaw if a click is present.

Avoid certain postures.

- Do not lean on or cup the chin when performing desk work or at the dining table.
- Do not sleep on the stomach or in postures that place stress on the jaw.

Avoid elective dental treatment while symptoms of pain and limited opening are present.

During yawning, support the jaw by providing mild pressure underneath the chin with the thumb and index finger or with the back of the hand.

Apply moist hot compresses to the sides of the face and to the temple areas for 10–20 minutes twice daily.

From De Rossi SS, Stern I, Sollecito TP. Disorders of the masticatory muscles. Dent Clin North Am 2013;57(3):449–64.

Physical agents and modalities

- Electrotherapy and transcutaneous electrical nerve stimulations (TENS)
- Ultrasonography
- Iontophoresis
- Vapocoolant spray
- Trigger point injections with local anesthetic or botulin toxin
- Acupuncture
- Laser treatment

SPLINT THERAPY

Splints, orthotics, orthopedic appliances, bite guards, nightguards, or bruxing guards are used in TMD treatment and often for disorders of masticatory muscles (**Box 7**).[2]

Box 6
Patient exercise instructions

Certain exercises can help to relieve the pain that that comes from tired, cramped muscles. They can also help if you have difficulty opening your mouth. The exercises described here work by helping to relax tense muscles and are referred to as passive stretching. The more often you do these exercises, the more you will relax the muscles that are painfully tense.

Do these exercises 2 times daily:

1. Ice down both sides of face for 5 to 10 minutes before beginning (ice cubes in sandwich bags or packs of frozen vegetables work well for this).

2. Place thumb of one hand on the edge of the upper front teeth and the index and middle fingers of the other hand on the edge of the lower front teeth, with the thumb under the chin.

3. The starting position for the stretches is with the thumb of one hand and index finger of the other hand just touching.

4. Gently pull open the lower jaw, using the hand only, until you feel a passive stretch, not pain. Hold for 10 seconds, then allow the lower jaw to close until the thumb and index finger are once again contacting; it is crucial when doing these exercises not to use the jaw muscles to open and close, but rather manual manipulation only (ie, the fingers do all the work).

5. Repeat the above stretching action 10 times, performing 2 to 3 sets per day, 1 in the morning and 1 or 2 in the evening.

6. When finished with the exercises, moist heat can be applied to both sides of the face for 5 to 10 minutes (heating a wet washcloth in the microwave for about 1 minute works well for this).

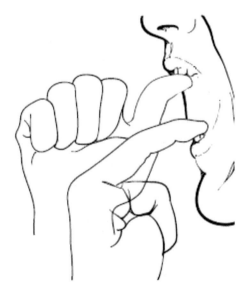

Demonstration of a passive stretch using the fingers.

From De Rossi SS, Stern I, Sollecito TP. Disorders of the masticatory muscles. Dent Clin North Am 2013;57(3):449–64.

Box 7
Splint therapy

- The appliance most commonly used is described as a stabilization appliance or muscle relaxation splint.
- These splints are designed to cover a full arch and are adjusted to avoid altering jaw position or placing orthodontic forces on the teeth.
  - Should be adjusted to provide bilateral even contact with the opposing teeth on closure and in a comfortable mandibular posture
  - Should be reexamined periodically and readjusted as necessary to accommodate changes in mandibular posture or muscle function that may affect the opposing tooth contacts on the appliance
- At the beginning of appliance therapy, a combination of appliance use during sleep and for periods during the waking hours is appropriate.
  - Factors such as tooth clenching when driving or exercising or pain symptoms that tend to increase as the day progresses may be better managed by increasing splint use during these times
- To avoid the possibility of occlusal change, appliances should not be worn continuously (ie, 24 hours per day) for prolonged periods.
- Full-coverage appliance therapy during sleep is a common practice to reduce the effects of bruxism and is not usually associated with occlusal change.

From De Rossi SS, Stern I, Sollecito TP. Disorders of the masticatory muscles. Dent Clin North Am 2013;57(3):449–64.

Their use is considered to be a reversible part of initial therapy. Several studies on splint therapy have shown a treatment effect, although researchers disagree as to the reason for the effect.[11,41] In a review of the literature on splint therapy, Clark and colleagues[26] found that patients reported a 70% to 90% improvement with splint therapy.[43] A recent review of the research on splint therapy suggests that using a splint as part of therapy for masticatory myalgia, arthralgia, or both may be supported by the literature in case control studies.[51] In contrast, there is insufficient evidence in reviewing randomized controlled trials published to support the use of stabilization splint therapy rather than other active interventions in treatment of myofascial pain (MFP). It seems better than no treatment, but only as effective as other active interventions for MFP.[51–53] A systematic review and meta-analysis by Ebrahim and colleagues[48] of 11 eligible studies of 1567 patients showed promising results for pain reduction, very low evidence for effect on quality of life, and high research bias.

PHARMACOLOGIC THERAPY

Both clinical and controlled experimental studies suggest that medications may promote patient comfort and rehabilitation when used as part of comprehensive treatment. Although there is a tendency for clinicians to rely on favorite agents, no single medication has proved to effective for the entire spectrum of TMDs.[2,8,26,43,47] With respect to pain associated with disorders of the MOM, analgesics, nonsteroidal anti-inflammatory agents, corticosteroids, benzodiazepines, muscle relaxants, and low-dose antidepressants have shown efficacy.[31,43,47] Many of the medications used for fibromyalgia can be used for patients with masticatory muscle disorders (**Table 7**).[31] These medications are versatile and effective at treating the multiple symptoms associated with chronic muscle pain.

Table 7
Medications used for fibromyalgia that may be beneficial for masticatory muscle pain

Medication Class	Effect
TCAs	Moderately helpful for pain Strong side effects (xerostomia, fatigue)
SSRIs	Less strong side effects than TCAs More effective for anxiety/depression than pain
Muscle relaxants	Moderately helpful for local muscle pain Strong side effects (xerostomia, sedation)
Serotonin-norepinephrine reuptake inhibitors	Moderately helpful for fibromyalgia-related pain
Low-potency opioids	Moderately helpful for fibromyalgia-related pain
NSAIDs	Helpful for acute inflammatory pain but not chronic muscle pain or fibromyalgia-related pain

Abbreviation: TCAs, tricyclic antidepressants.
From De Rossi SS, Stern I, Sollecito TP. Disorders of the masticatory muscles. Dent Clin North Am 2013;57(3):449–64.

TREATMENT OF INTRACAPSULAR DISORDERS

The treatment of TMJ osteoarthrosis and internal derangement can be divided into 3 broad categories: noninvasive, minimally invasive, and invasive management. The management plan can vary depending on the specific diagnosis and severity of TMJ disorder, but the underlying principles of treatment apply universally.[2]

1. Multidisciplinary approach involving multiple specialties, including general dentistry, oral medicine, orofacial pain, orthodontics, oral surgery, physical therapy, and psychiatry, may be necessary to address the problem fully from all aspects.
2. Progression of treatment only after failure of more conservative modalities. The least invasive and most reversible treatments should be tried first. Only after a failure to alter the disease process and clinical symptoms should more invasive and often nonreversible treatments be initiated.

Goals of treatment:
1. Decreasing joint pain
2. Increasing joint function and opening
3. Preventing further joint damage
4. Improving overall quality of life and reducing disease-related morbidities

NONINVASIVE TREATMENT OPTIONS
Occlusal or Stabilization Splints

Various types of splints have been used by physicians since the eighteenth century for the treatment of TMJ disorders.[54] Today the use of splints has become one of the most common in-office initial treatments for TMD-associated pain. Since their inception, splints have been thought to work by unloading the condyle and protecting the TMJ and articular disc from degeneration and excessive articular strain.[54] Although there are varying designs, they all function similarly to disengage the condylar head from the fossa and articular disc.

A recent meta-analysis of randomized controlled trials evaluating intraoral orthopedic appliances for TMDs showed that hard stabilization appliances have good evidence of modest efficacy in the treatment of TMJ disorder pain compared with nonoccluding appliances and no treatment.[52] Other types of appliances, including soft stabilization appliances, anterior positioning appliances, and anterior bite appliances, have some evidence of efficacy in reducing TMD pain.[52,55] However, a Cochrane Database review of stabilization splint therapy for TMJ pain revealed that there is insufficient evidence either for or against the use of stabilization splint therapy.[52] Further randomized controlled studies with larger sample sizes and longer duration of follow-up are needed to study the effectiveness of splint therapy for TMD pain (**Table 8**).

Pharmacotherapy

Pharmacologic therapy in conjunction with other treatment modalities often plays an important role in the management of articular disc and TMJ disorders. Pharmacotherapy has 2 main goals[56]:

1. Treatment of the underlying disease process
2. Alleviation of disease-associated symptoms such as pain and swelling

There are various classes of medications that function to target each of the two treatment goals. Often, it is necessary to use a combination of medications to treat both the pain and the inflammatory disease process depending on the severity of disease. However, care must be taken to avoid the prolonged use of certain medications, particularly analgesics, to prevent drug tolerance and dependency. The health provider's ultimate goal should be symptomatic relief for a period of time in the hopes that this will break the disease cycle and lead to permanent improvement.

Despite the frequent use of pharmacologic agents, numerous review articles have shown insufficient evidence to support or not support the effectiveness of pharmacologic interventions for pain in patients with TMJ disorders.[57,58] There is an obvious need for further randomized control trials to study the effectiveness of pharmacologic interventions to treat pain associated with TMD. The medication classes are often similar for intracapsular and myogenic disorders (**Table 9**).

Physical Therapy

Physical therapy is commonly used in the outpatient setting to relieve musculoskeletal pain, reduce inflammation, and restore oral motor function. Physical therapy plays an adjunctive role in virtually all TMJ disorder treatment regimens. Various physical therapy modalities are available to the outpatient health provider. Although the evidence is weak, there are numerous systematic review articles that support the efficacy of exercise therapy, thermal therapy, and acupuncture to reduce symptoms such as pain, swelling, and TMJ hypomobility (**Table 10**).[59–61]

Table 8 Major types of occlusal splints used in TMD therapy	
Splint Type	**Design**
Stabilization splint	Hard acrylic with full coverage of maxillary and mandibular dentition in centric occlusion
Repositioning splint	Hard acrylic with full coverage of maxillary or mandibular dentition with inclines to guide mandible to a more anterior position
Soft splint	Similar to hard stabilization splints but made from a less expensive pliable material

From Liu F, Steinkeler A. Epidemiology, diagnosis, and treatment of temporomandibular disorders. Dent Clin North Am 2013;57(3):465–79.

Table 9
Types of medication used in TMD treatment

Class	Examples	Function
NSAIDs	Ibuprofen, naproxen, diclofenac, aspirin, etodolac, and others	Reduce inflammation and pain
Opioids	Codeine, oxycodone, morphine, hydromorphone, meperidine	Reduce pain
Corticosteroids	Prednisone, dexamethasone, hydrocortisone	Reduce inflammation and pain
Muscle relaxants	Cyclobenzaprine, carisoprodol, baclofen, and others	Reduce muscle spasm
Antidepressants	Amitriptyline, trazodone, fluoxetine, sertraline	Reduce muscle tension
Anxiolytics	Alprazolam, lorazepam, oxazepam, diazepam, buspirone	Reduce tension and muscle spasm

From Liu F, Steinkeler A. Epidemiology, diagnosis, and treatment of temporomandibular disorders. Dent Clin North Am 2013;57(3):465–79; and *Data from* List T, Axelsson S, Leijon G. Pharmacologic interventions in the treatment of temporomandibular disorders, atypical facial pain, and burning mouth syndrome. A qualitative systematic review. J Orofac Pain 2003;17(4):301–10.

MINIMALLY INVASIVE TREATMENT OPTIONS
Intra-articular Injections

Different therapeutic solutions can be injected directly into the TMJ space and allow the targeted treatment of inflammation and joint degeneration (see **Table 9**). The TMJ has 2 unconnected cavities, superior and inferior, partitioned by the articular disc. The superior space injection is the commonly used technique. However, a recent review article showed that an inferior space injection, or simultaneous injections of the upper and lower spaces, seemed to be more effective, with increasing mouth opening and decreasing TMJ-associated pain (**Table 11**).[62]

Arthrocentesis/Arthroscopy

Arthrocentesis and arthroscopy are safe and quick minimally invasive procedures that are used in patients who are resistant to more conservative treatment modalities.

Table 10
Description of treatment modalities for articular disk and TMJ osteoarthrosis

Modality	Description
Exercise therapy	Techniques include manual therapy, postural exercises, muscle stretching, and strengthening exercises. Passive and active stretching of muscles or range-of-motion exercise are performed to increase oral opening and decrease pain
Thermal therapy	Involves the superficial application of a dry or moist heat/cold pad directly to the affected area typically in 20-min intervals. Used in conjunction with exercise therapy in the treatment of inflammation and TMJ hypomobility
Acupuncture	Thought to stimulate the production of endorphins, serotonin, and acetylcholine within the central nervous system, or may relieve pain by acting as a noxious stimulus. Treatments involve placement of needles in the face and hands, and are typically given weekly for a total of 6 wk[61]

Table 11
Types of intra-articular injections used in treatment of TMJ and articular disk disorders

	Hyaluronic Acid	Corticosteroids
Benefits	Sodium hyaluronate is a natural component of TMJ synovial fluid, and lubricates and maintains the normal internal environment of the joints[63]	Reduction of inflammatory factors and reducing the activity of the immune system
Adverse effects	Mild pain and swelling at injection site, mostly transient	Infection and destruction of articular cartilage. Long-term repeat injections should be avoided[64]
Efficacy	Improved long-term clinical signs of TMD and overall improvement of symptoms compared with placebo. No difference in radiological progression of disease[63]	Same short-term and long-term improvements in symptoms, clinical signs, and overall condition compared with hyaluronic acid[63]

Often they are combined with immediate postoperative intra-articular injections and the use of occlusal splints, pharmacotherapy, and physical therapy during the recovery period (**Tables 12** and **13**).[65–67]

INVASIVE TREATMENT OPTIONS

It is strongly recommended that, unless there are specific and justifiable indications to the contrary, treatment of patients with TMD initially should be based on the use of conservative, reversible, and evidence-based therapeutic modalities. Studies of the natural history of many TMDs suggest that they tend to improve or resolve over

Table 12
Arthrocentesis for TMD treatment

	Arthrocentesis[65–67]
Description	Saline lavage of the superior joint space, hydraulic pressure and manipulation to release adhesions, and elimination of intra-articular inflammatory mediators (see **Fig. 3**). Less invasive than arthroscopy and can be done in outpatient setting with local anesthesia and intravenous sedation
Indication	Limited opening with anteriorly displaced articular disc without reduction Chronic pain with good range of movement and displaced articular disc with reduction Painful degenerative osteoarthritis
Contraindications	TMJ with bony or fibrous ankylosis Extracapsular source of pain Patients who have not undergone noninvasive treatment modalities
Efficacy	Recent studies report 83.5% treatment success rate in patients with internal derangement and osteoarthritis, defined as an improvement in maximum jaw opening and a reduction in pain level and mandibular dysfunction

From Liu F, Steinkeler A. Epidemiology, diagnosis, and treatment of temporomandibular disorders. Dent Clin North Am 2013;57(3):465–79.

Table 13 Arthroscopy for TMD treatment	
	Arthroscopy[68]
Description	Involves insertion of an arthroscope and inspection of the TMJ under fluid distention under general anesthesia. Allows irrigation of joint space, lysis of these adhesions, and mobilization of the joint under direct visualization (**Fig. 4**)
Indication	Limited opening and pain secondary to internal derangement TMJ hypomobility secondary to fibrosis or adhesions Degenerative osteoarthritis
Contraindications	TMJ with severe bony or fibrous ankylosis Extracapsular source of pain Patients who have not undergone noninvasive treatment modalities Practitioner with lack of open joint surgery experience
Efficacy	A large multicenter study reports >90% success rate as defined as improved mobility, pain, and function.[40] Arthroscopy led to greater improvement in opening after 12 mo than arthrocentesis; however, there was no difference in pain[39]

From Liu F, Steinkeler A. Epidemiology, diagnosis, and treatment of temporomandibular disorders. Dent Clin North Am 2013;57(3):465–79.

time. Although no specific therapies have been proved to be uniformly effective, many of the conservative modalities have proved to be at least as effective in providing symptomatic relief as most forms of invasive treatment.[45] However, surgical interventions are occasionally necessary to restore function and reduce pain.

Arthroplasty

TMJ arthroplasty involves the reshaping of the articular surface to remove osteophytes, erosions, and irregularities found in osteoarthritis refractory to other treatment modalities.[64] These patients frequently also present with articular disc degeneration or displacement, which can be repositioned, repaired, or removed. All such procedures should be performed by an experienced oral and maxillofacial surgeon under general anesthesia, and done using an open surgical approach through a periauricular skin incision (**Fig. 5**). Complications are rare but can include wound infection, facial nerve injury, permanent occlusal changes, relapsing joint pain, and life-threatening vascular injuries. As with all TMJ-related surgeries, early postoperative physical therapy and range-of-motion exercises are vital to achieving long-term functional improvements.

- Disc repositioning: reposition of the disc back to its normal anatomic position in patients with internal derangement. This procedure is most effective in discs that are normal appearing (white, firm, shiny) with minimal displacement.
- Disc repair: small disc perforations can be repaired with a tension-free primary closure.
- Discectomy alone: removal of the articular disc is indicated in patients with severe disc perforation, complete loss of disc elasticity, and who are persistently symptomatic even after disc repositioning.[41] Although studies have shown there is generally an improvement in pain and maximal mouth opening following the surgical removal of the disc, patients also showed signs of fibrous adhesions, narrowing of joint space, and osteophyte formation on MRI.[69–71]
- Discectomy with graft replacement: the placement of a graft is thought to protect the joint from further degeneration and prevent the formation of fibrous

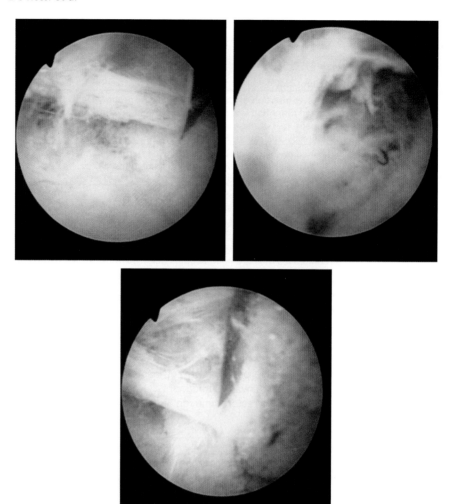

Fig. 4. Arthroscopic views of TMJ space showing evidence of multiple disk adhesions. (*From* Liu F, Steinkeler A. Epidemiology, diagnosis, and treatment of temporomandibular disorders. Dent Clin North Am 2013;57(3):465–79.)

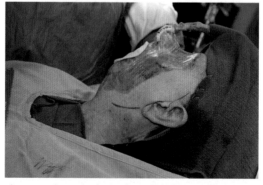

Fig. 5. Open surgical approach made through outlined periauricular and endaural skin incision. (*From* Liu F, Steinkeler A. Epidemiology, diagnosis, and treatment of temporomandibular disorders. Dent Clin North Am 2013;57(3):465–79.)

Box 8
Criteria for successful TMJ disc surgery

1. Mild, brief pain of no concern to the patient

2. Vertical range of motion greater than 35 mm and lateral range of motion greater than 6 mm

3. Ability to tolerate a regular diet

4. Stabilization of any degenerative radiological changes

5. Absence of symptoms for at least 2 years

6. Absence of significant surgical complications

From Liu F, Steinkeler A. Epidemiology, diagnosis, and treatment of temporomandibular disorders. Dent Clin North Am 2013;57(3):465–79; and *Data from* Holmlund AB. Surgery for TMJ internal derangement. Evaluation of treatment and criteria for success. Int J Oral Maxillofac Surg 1993;22:75–7.

---

adhesions. The use of autogenous sources, such as temporalis flaps, auricular cartilage, and dermal grafts, results in superior clinical outcomes compared with alloplastic grafts.[72] Studies have shown that autogenous graft does not prevent remodeling of the joint but may help to reduce the onset of crepitus resulting from discectomy alone.[72] However, it was shown that discectomy with dermis graft replacement does result in a statistically significant improvement in pain, chewing, and general health (**Box 8**).

Total Joint Replacement

TMJ replacement is intended primarily to restore form and function and any pain relief gained is only a secondary benefit.[72] The need for TMJ replacement typically indicates severely damaged joints with end-stage disease that has failed all other

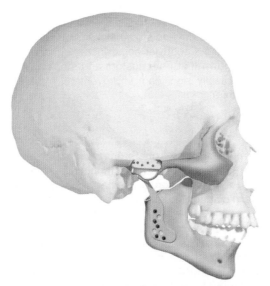

Fig. 6. Total joint replacement consisting of a fossa and condylar component held in place by screw fixation. (*From* Liu F, Steinkeler A. Epidemiology, diagnosis, and treatment of temporomandibular disorders. Dent Clin North Am 2013;57(3):465–79.)

Box 9
Indications and relative contraindications for TMJ alloplastic replacement

Indications[72]

1. Ankylosis or reankylosis with severe anatomic abnormalities

2. Failure of autogenous grafts in patients who underwent multiple operations

3. Destruction of autogenous graft tissue by pathosis

4. Severe inflammatory joint disease that results in anatomic mutilation of the total joint components and functional disability

5. Failure of Proplast-Teflon implant

6. Failure of Vitek-Kent total or partial joints

Relative contraindications

1. Pediatric patients with immature facial skeleton

2. Patient with unrealistic expectations or lack of understanding of procedure

3. Uncontrolled systemic disease

4. Allergy to implant material

5. Active infection at implantation site

From Liu F, Steinkeler A. Epidemiology, diagnosis, and treatment of temporomandibular disorders. Dent Clin North Am 2013;57(3):465–79.

---

more conservative treatment modalities. Autogenous costochondral bone grafts have frequently been used in TMJ reconstruction because of their gross anatomic similarity to the mandibular condyle, ease of adaptation to the recipient site, and their growth potential in juveniles.[73] However, because of potential harvest site morbidity and failure during the transplantation process or from functional loading, the use of alloplastic materials has become increasingly popular in the adult population. At present, various custom and stock titanium joint designs are available that consists of both a fossa and a condylar component held in place by screw fixation (**Fig. 6**). Studies have shown that both custom and stock alloplastic TMJ replacements resulted in statistically significant improvement in pain level, jaw function, and incisal opening (**Box 9**).[74,75]

SUMMARY

TMDs remain a common cause of visits to primary care physicians, internists, pediatricians, and emergency departments. Although the exact cause and fundamental pathogenesis of these disorders remains poorly understood, significant advances in the clinical diagnosis, radiographic imaging, and classification of these disorders have improved long-term management. It is clear that there are several types of disorders of the masticatory muscles and the TMJ as well as associated structures and each may have a complex cause, clinical course, and response to therapy. Host susceptibility plays a role at several stages of these disorders, including pain modulation and response to therapy. Future research in the area of genetics, pain, and arthritides offers greater possibility in defining this heterogeneous group of disorders and providing more focused and effective treatment strategies.

REFERENCES

1. Wadhwa S, Kapila S. TMJ disorders: future innovations in diagnostics and therapeutics. J Dent Educ 2008;72(8):930–47.
2. Scrivani SJ, Keith DA, Kaban LB. Temporomandibular disorders. N Engl J Med 2008;359:2693–705.
3. Lipton JA, Ship JA, Larach-Robinson D. Estimated prevalence and distribution of reported orofacial pain in the United States. J Am Dent Assoc 1993;124: 115–21.
4. Manfredini D, Guarda-Nardini L, Winocur E, et al. Research diagnostic criteria for temporomandibular disorders: a systematic review of axis I epidemiologic findings. Oral Surg Oral Med Oral Pathol Oral Radiol Endod 2011;112: 453–62.
5. Abubaker AO, Raslan WF, Sotereanos GC. Estrogen and progesterone receptors in temporomandibular joint discs of symptomatic and asymptomatic persons: a preliminary study. J Oral Maxillofac Surg 1993;51:1096–100.
6. Milam SB, Aufdemorte TB, Sheridan PJ, et al. Sexual dimorphism in the distribution of estrogen receptors in the temporomandibular joint complex of the baboon. Oral Surg Oral Med Oral Pathol 1987;64:527–32.
7. Aufdemorte TB, Van Sickels JE, Dolwick MF, et al. Estrogen receptors in the temporomandibular joint of the baboon (*Papio cynocephalus*): an autoradiographic study. Oral Surg Oral Med Oral Pathol 1986;61:307–14.
8. Benoliel R, Svensson P, Heir GM, et al. Persistent orofacial muscle pain. Oral Dis 2011;17(Suppl 1):23–41.
9. Benoliel R, Sharav Y. Chronic orofacial pain. Curr Pain Headache Rep 2010;14: 33–40.
10. Rasmussen O. Description of population and progress of symptoms in a longitudinal study of temporomandibular joint arthropathy. Scand J Dent Res 1981; 89:196–203.
11. de Leew R. Orofacial pain: guidelines for assessment, classification, and management. The American Academy of Orofacial Pain. 5th edition. Chicago: Quintessence Publishing; 2013.
12. Ghali GE, Miloro M, Waite PD, et al, editors. Peterson's principles of oral and maxillofacial surgery. 3rd edition. Shelton (CT): Peoples Medical Publishing House; 2012.
13. Blankestijn J, Boering G. Posterior dislocation of the temporomandibular disc. Int J Oral Surg 1985;14:437–43.
14. Liedberg J, Westesson P, Kurita K. Side-ways and rotational displacement of the temporomandibular joint disk: diagnosis by arthrography and correlation to cryosectional morphology. Oral Surg Oral Med Oral Pathol 1990;69:757–63.
15. Sanders B. Management of internal derangements of the temporomandibular joint. Semin Orthod 1995;1(4):244–57.
16. Tallents RH, Katzberg RW, Murphy W, et al. Magnetic resonance imaging findings in asymptomatic volunteers and symptomatic patients with temporomandibular disorders. J Prosthet Dent 1996;75:529.
17. Wilkes C. Internal derangement of the temporomandibular joint. In: Clark G, Sanders B, Bertolami C, editors. Advances in diagnostic and surgical arthroscopy of the temporomandibular joint. Philadelphia: Sanders; 1993.
18. Dworkin SF, Leresche L. Research diagnostic criteria for temporomandibular disorders: review, criteria, examinations and specifications, critique. J Craniomandib Disord 1992;6:301–55.

19. Michelotti A, Iodice G, Vollaro S, et al. Evaluation of the short-term effectiveness of education versus and occlusal splint for the treatment of myofascial pain of the jaw muscles. J Am Dent Assoc 2012;145:47–53.

20. Shaefer J, Riley C, Caruso P, et al. Analysis of criteria for MRI diagnosis of TMJ disc displacement and arthralgia. Int J Dent 2012;2012:283163.

21. Mohl ND. The anecdotal tradition and the need for evidence-based care for temporomandibular disorders. J Orofac Pain 1999;13:227–31.

22. Schiffman E, Fricton JR, Haley D, et al. The prevalence and treatment needs of subjects with temporomandibular disorders. J Am Dent Assoc 1989;120:295–301.

23. Kurita K, Westesson PL, Yuasa H, et al. Natural course of untreated symptomatic temporomandibular joint disc displacement without reduction. J Dent Res 1998;77:361–5.

24. Milam SB. TMJ osteoarthritis. In: Laskin DM, Greene CS, Hylander WL, editors. TMDs, an evidence-based approach to diagnosis and treatment. Chicago: Quintessence; 2006. p. 105–23.

25. Rammelsberg P, Leresche L, Dworkin S, et al. Longitudinal outcome of temporomandibular disorders: a 5-year epidemiologic study of muscle disorders defined by Research Diagnostic Criteria for Temporomandibular Disorders. J Orofac Pain 2003;17:9–20.

26. Clark GT, Seligman DA, Solberg WK, et al. Guidelines for the examination and diagnosis of temporomandibular disorders. J Craniomandib Disord 1989;3: 7–14.

27. Dworkin SF. Psychological and psychosocial assessment. In: Laskin DM, Greene CS, Hylander WL, editors. TMDs, an evidence-based approach to diagnosis and treatment. Chicago: Quintessence; 2006. p. 203–17.

28. Markiewicz M, Ohrbach R, McCall WD Jr. Oral behaviors checklist: reliability of performance in targeted waking-state behaviors. J Orofac Pain 2006;20(4):306–16.

29. National Institutes of Health Technology Assessment Conference on Management of Temporomandibular Disorders. Oral Surg Oral Med Oral Pathol Oral Radiol Endod 1997;83:49–183.

30. Simons DG. Neurophysiologic basis of pain caused by trigger points. APS J 1994;3:17–9.

31. Clauw DJ. Fibromyalgia: an overview. Am J Med 2009;122:S3–13.

32. Diatchenko L, Slade GD, Nackley AG, et al. Genetic basis for individual variations in pain perception and the development of a chronic pain condition. Hum Mol Genet 2005;14:135–43.

33. Fillingim RD. Sex differences in analgesic responses: evidence from experimental pain models. Eur J Anaesthesiol Suppl 2002;26:16–24.

34. Raphael KG, Marbach JJ, Galagher RM. Somatosensory amplification and affective inhibition are elevated in myofascial face pain. Pain Med 2000;1:247–53.

35. Myburgh C, Larsen AH, Hartvifgsen J. A systematic, critical review of manual palpation for identifying myofascial trigger points: evidence and clinical significance. Arch Phys Med Rehabil 2008;89:1169–76.

36. Nijs J, Daenen L, Cras P, et al. Nociception affects motor output: a review on sensory-motor interaction with focus on clinical implications. Clin J Pain 2012; 28(2):175–81.

37. Staud R. Is it all central sensitization? Role of peripheral tissue nociception in chronic musculoskeletal pain. Curr Rheumatol Rep 2010;12(6):448–54.

38. Look JO, John MT, Tai F, et al. The research diagnostic criteria for temporomandibular disorders II: reliability of Axis I diagnoses and selected clinical measures. J Orofac Pain 2010;24:25–34.

39. Dworkin S, Huggins K, LeResche L, et al. Epidemiology of signs and symptoms in temporomandibular disorders: clinical signs in cases and controls. J Am Dent Assoc 1990;120:273–81.

40. Anderson GC, Gonzalez YM, Ohrbach R, et al. The research diagnostic criteria for temporomandibular disorders. VI: future directions. J Orofac Pain 2010;24:19–88.

41. Lobbezo F, Drangsholt M, Peck C, et al. Topical review: new insights into the pathology and diagnosis of the temporomandibular joint. J Orofac Pain 2004;18: 181–91.

42. Sessle BJ. The neural basis of temporomandibular joint and masticatory muscle pain. J Orofac Pain 1999;13:238–45.

43. Clark GT, Minakuchi H. Oral appliances. In: Laskin DM, Greene CS, Hylander WL, editors. TMDs, an evidence-based approach to diagnosis and treatment. Chicago: Quintessence; 2006. p. 377–90.

44. Lund JP. Muscular pain and dysfunction. In: Laskin DM, Greene CS, Hylander WL, editors. Temporomandibular disorders, an evidence-based approach to diagnosis and treatment. Chicago: Quintessence; 2006. p. 99.

45. Greene CS. Managing the care of patients with temporomandibular disorders: a new guideline for care. J Am Dent Assoc 2010;141(9):1086–8.

46. Glaros AG, Burton E. Parafunctional clenching, pain, and effort in temporomandibular disorders. J Behav Med 2004;27:91–100.

47. Galdon MJ, Dura E, Andreu Y, et al. Multidimensional approach to the differences between muscular and articular temporomandibular patients: coping, distress, and pain characteristics. Oral Surg Oral Med Oral Pathol 2006;102:40–6.

48. Ebrahim S, Montoya L, Busse JW, et al. The effectiveness of splint therapy in patients with temporomandibular disorders. J Am Dent Assoc 2012;143:847–57.

49. Henrikson T, Nilner M. Temporomandibular disorders, occlusion and orthodontic treatment. J Orthod 2003;30:129–37.

50. Poggio CE, Schmitz JH, Worthington HV, et al. Interventions for myogenous temporomandibular disorder (TMD) patients. The Cochrane Library 2010;(11).

51. Kreiner M, Betancor E, Clark GT. Occlusal stabilization appliances. Evidence of their efficacy. J Am Dent Assoc 2001;132:770–7.

52. Fricton J, Look JO, Wright E, et al. Systematic review and meta-analysis of randomized controlled trials evaluating intraoral orthopedic appliances for temporomandibular disorders. J Orofac Pain 2010;24(3):237–54.

53. Truelove E, Huggins KH, Mancl L, et al. The efficacy of traditional, low-cost and nonsplint therapies for temporomandibular disorders: a randomized clinical trial. J Am Dent Assoc 2006;137:1099–107.

54. Klasser GD, Greene CS. Oral appliances in the management of temporomandibular disorders. Oral Surg Oral Med Oral Pathol Oral Radiol Endod 2009; 107(2):212–23.

55. Al-Ani MZ, Davies SJ, Gray RJ, et al. Stabilisation splint therapy for temporomandibular pain dysfunction syndrome. Cochrane Database Syst Rev 2004;(1):CD002778.

56. Dionne RA. Pharmacologic treatments for temporomandibular disorders. Oral Surg Oral Med Oral Pathol Oral Radiol Endod 1997;83(1):134–42.

57. Mujakperuo HR, Watson M, Morrison R, et al. Pharmacological interventions for pain in patients with temporomandibular disorders. Cochrane Database Syst Rev 2010;(10):CD004715.

58. List T, Axelsson S, Leijon G. Pharmacologic interventions in the treatment of temporomandibular disorders, atypical facial pain, and burning mouth syndrome. A qualitative systematic review. J Orofac Pain 2003;17(4):301–10.

59. McNeely ML, Armijo Olivo S, Magee DJ. A systematic review of the effectiveness of physical therapy interventions for temporomandibular disorders. Phys Ther 2006;86(5):710–25.
60. Cho SH, Whang WW. Acupuncture for temporomandibular disorders: a systematic review. J Orofac Pain 2010;24(2):152–62.
61. Rosted P. Practical recommendations for the use of acupuncture in the treatment of temporomandibular disorders based on the outcome of published controlled studies. Oral Dis 2001;7(2):109–15.
62. Li C, Zhang Y, Lv J, et al. Inferior or double joint spaces injection versus superior joint space injection for temporomandibular disorders: a systematic review and meta-analysis. J Oral Maxillofac Surg 2012;70(1):37–44.
63. Shi Z, Guo C, Awad M. Hyaluronate for temporomandibular joint disorders [review]. Cochrane Database Syst Rev 2003;(1):CD002970.
64. Tanaka E, Detamore MS, Mercuri LG. Degenerative disorders of the temporomandibular joint: etiology, diagnosis, and treatment. J Dent Res 2008;87:296.
65. Guo C, Shi Z, Revington P. Arthrocentesis and lavage for treating temporomandibular joint disorders. Cochrane Database Syst Rev 2009;(4):CD004973.
66. Nitzan DW. Arthrocentesis for management of severe closed lock of the temporomandibular joint. Oral Maxillofac Surg Clin North Am 1994;6:245–57.
67. Monje-Gil F, Nitzan D, González-Garcia R. Temporomandibular joint arthrocentesis. Review of the literature. Med Oral Patol Oral Cir Bucal 2012;17(4):e575–81.
68. Rigon M, Pereira LM, Bortoluzzi MC, et al. Arthroscopy for temporomandibular disorders. Cochrane Database Syst Rev 2011;(5):CD006385.
69. McCain JP, Sanders B, Koslin MG, et al. Temporomandibular joint arthroscopy: a 6-year multicenter retrospective study of 4,831 joints. J Oral Maxillofac Surg 1992;50(9):926–30.
70. Hansson LG, Eriksson L, Westesson PL. Magnetic-resonance evaluation after temporomandibular-joint discectomy. Oral Surg Oral Med Oral Pathol 1992;74:801–10.
71. Miloro M, Henriksen B. Discectomy as the primary surgical option for internal derangement of the temporomandibular joint. J Oral Maxillofac Surg 2010;68:782–9.
72. Dimitroulis G. A critical review of interpositional grafts following temporomandibular joint discectomy with an overview of the dermis-fat graft. Int J Oral Maxillofac Surg 2011;40:561–8.
73. MacIntosh RB. The use of autogenous tissue in temporomandibular joint reconstruction. J Oral Maxillofac Surg 2000;58:63–9.
74. Wolford LM, Pitta MC, Reiche-Fischel O, et al. TMJ Concepts/Techmedica custom-made TMJ total joint prosthesis: 5-year follow-up study. Int J Oral Maxillofac Surg 2003;32(3):268–74.
75. Giannakopoulos HE, Sinn DP, Quinn PD. Biomet microfixation temporomandibular joint replacement system: a 3-year follow-up study of patients treated during 1995 to 2005. J Oral Maxillofac Surg 2012;70(4):787–94.

Orofacial Pain Syndromes
Evaluation and Management

Ramesh Balasubramaniam, BDSc, MS[a],*, Gary D. Klasser, DMD[b]

KEYWORDS

- Orofacial pain • Neuropathic pain • Neurovascular pain • Vascular pain • Diagnosis
- Management

KEY POINTS

- Recognition and understanding of orofacial pain conditions by primary care physicians is important, as patients often present with complaints associated with these disorders.
- An accurate history and examination enable clinicians to render a correct diagnosis and formulate an appropriate course of therapy, which may include a referral to an orofacial pain expert. Neuropathic orofacial pain may be episodic or continuous.
- Neurovascular pain and vascular pain can manifest in the orofacial region.

INTRODUCTION

It is important to recognize and understand various orofacial pain syndromes, as the first health practitioner visited by patients is often the primary care physician. Therefore, having knowledge in the evaluation and management of orofacial pain syndromes is beneficial. Unfortunately, these conditions may be rather complex and this often leads to misdiagnosis and/or incomplete diagnosis, resulting in misdirected and/or incomplete treatment, despite well-intentioned efforts.

In this article, the evaluation and management of various neuropathic, neurovascular, and vascular pains are discussed.

NEUROPATHIC PAIN

Neuropathic pain (NP) is currently defined by the International Association for the Study of Pain (IASP)[1] as "pain caused by a lesion or disease of the somatosensory nervous

Disclosure Statement: The authors do not have any relationship with a commercial company that has a direct financial interest in the subject matter or materials discussed in the article or with a company making a competing product.
[a] School of Dentistry, University of Western Australia, Perth, Australia; [b] School of Dentistry, Louisiana State University, New Orleans, LA, USA
* Corresponding author. Perth Oral Medicine & Dental Sleep Centre, Unit 6, 24 McCourt Street, West Leederville, Western Australia 6007, Australia.
E-mail address: ramesh.balasubramaniam@uwa.edu.au

system."[1] In spite of this definition, clinically in many cases, there may be no demonstrable lesion or disease. Costigan and colleagues[2] designate NP as "dysfunctional pain." Dysfunctional pain is considered a malfunction (which can be considered a disease unto itself) of the somatosensory nervous system, involving both spontaneous and stimulus-dependent pain (evoked by both low-intensity and high-intensity stimuli), but without known structural nervous system lesions or active peripheral inflammation.

Classification of NP based on a temporal component may be divided into episodic and continuous. Episodic NP is characterized by sudden episodes of electriclike, severe, shooting pain that lasts only a few seconds to several minutes and is referred to as neuralgia.[3] Often there exists a perioral and/or intraoral trigger zone whereby nontraumatic stimuli, such as light touch, provoke severe paroxysmal pain.[3] Continuous NPs are pain disorders originating in neural structures and present as constant, ongoing, and unremitting pain. Patients usually experience varying and fluctuating intensities of pain, often without total remission.

Episodic

Trigeminal neuralgia

Trigeminal neuralgia[4] (TN) is mainly a unilateral painful (moderate to severe) disorder characterized by brief, electric-shocklike pains, which are abrupt in onset and termination, and limited to the distribution of one or more divisions of the trigeminal nerve (usually the maxillary [V2] and mandibular [V3] divisions are affected). Often there are pain-free (refractory) periods between attacks. The International Classification of Headache Disorders-3 (ICHD-3) suggests 3 main variants (**Table 1**) and presents diagnostic criteria for each one, including its many subvariants.[5] The prevalence of TN in the general population is between 0.01% and 0.3%.[6] The gender ratio of women to men is approximately 2:1. Disease onset usually occurs after the age of 40 years with peak age of onset between the ages of 50 and 60 years.

Evaluation involves a thorough history and comprehensive examination (applicable for all neuropathic disorders), which includes a cranial nerve examination, mainly to rule out other possible causes for symptom presentation. Magnetic resonance imaging (MRI) of the brain and associated structures is the most useful imaging technique to determine the presence of other conditions that may mimic the symptoms of TN.

Medical management typically consists of the following[7,8]:

- First-line therapy: carbamazepine (200–1200 mg/d) or oxcarbazepine (600–1800 mg/d).
- Second-line therapy: combination of first-line therapy with lamotrigine (400 mg/d) or a switch to lamotrigine or baclofen (40–80 mg/d).
- Third-line therapy: phenytoin, gabapentin, pregabalin, valproate, tizanidine, and tocainide.

If a medical approach is unsuccessful or results in marked deterioration in activities of daily living due to medication side effects, surgical procedures (not without serious adverse effects) should be considered.

- Peripheral surgical procedures: cryotherapy, neurectomy or alcohol injection, microvascular decompression (nondestructive surgical technique) of the nerve/vessel contact or percutaneous ablative techniques (radiofrequency thermocoagulation, balloon compression, and glycerol rhizotomy) of the Gasserian ganglion.
- Stereotactic radiosurgery: gamma knife surgery (a focused beam of radiation aimed at the trigeminal root in the posterior fossa)[9]

Features	Classical TN	Classical TN with Concomitant Persistent Facial Pain	Symptomatic TN
Previously used term	Tic douloureux	Atypical TN; TN type 2	—
Description	TN developing without apparent cause other than neurovascular compression (usually located at the trigeminal root entry to the brainstem and most frequently by the superior cerebellar artery)	TN with persistent background facial pain	TN attributed to a structural lesion other than vascular compression such as multiple sclerosis
Note	Imaging (preferably MRI) is recommended to exclude secondary causes and, in most patients, to demonstrate neurovascular compression of the trigeminal nerve	Neurovascular compression on MRI is less likely to be demonstrated. Responds poorly to conservative treatment and to neurosurgical interventions. Less likely to be triggered by innocuous stimuli.	—

Table 1
Description of TN variants

Abbreviations: MRI, magnetic resonance imaging; TN, trigeminal neuralgia.
 Data from Headache Classification Committee of the International Headache Society (IHS). The International Classification of Headache Disorders, 3rd edition (beta version). Cephalalgia 2013;33(9):629–808; with permission.

The American Academy of Neurology and the European Federation of Neurological Societies have published guidelines regarding TN management (medical and surgical).[10]

Other neuralgias

Glossopharyngeal neuralgia (GPN), known as vagoglossopharyngeal neuralgia, is typically a unilateral painful (mild to moderate) disorder characterized by brief, electric-shocklike pains, is abrupt in onset and termination, and is localized to the ear, the base of the tongue, posterior aspects of the throat (especially the tonsillar fossa), or beneath the angle of the jaw (distributions of the auricular and pharyngeal branches of the vagus nerve and branches of the glossopharyngeal nerve). Bilaterality of presentation may occur in up to 25% of patients.[11] GPN is commonly provoked by swallowing, talking, coughing, and/or yawning; has similar characteristics as TN; and may coexist with TN in 10% to 12% of patients with GPN.[12,13] Other common triggers of attack are sneezing, clearing the throat, touching the gums or oral mucosa, blowing the nose, or rubbing the ear.[11] Cardiac dysrhythmias and syncope may occur due to stimulation of the vagus nerve. GPN incidence in the general population has been reported to be 0.2 per 100,000 persons per year.[11,12] As observed in TN, a significant association between symptoms of GPN and multiple sclerosis has been reported.[13] Computed tomography or MRI may reveal lesions, as well as neurovascular compression.

Management is similar to that of TN:

- First-line therapy: carbamazepine (200–1200 mg/d) or oxcarbazepine (600–1800 mg/d).[14]
- Second-line therapy: local anesthetic to the tonsil and pharyngeal wall can prevent attacks for a few hours.[12]

If medical treatment is unsuccessful, surgical procedures include microvascular decompression, intracranial sectioning of the glossopharyngeal nerve and the upper rootlets of the vagus nerve, or gamma-knife surgery. The major complications include dysphagia, hoarseness, and facial paresis.[4,15–17]

Occipital neuralgia (ON) is a unilateral or bilateral paroxysmal, shooting or stabbing severe pain in the posterior part of the scalp, in the distribution of the greater, lesser, or third occipital nerves. It is important to distinguish ON from occipital pain referred from the atlantoaxial or upper zygapophyseal joints or from tender trigger points in neck muscles or their insertions.[18,19] Imaging studies are necessary to exclude underlying pathologic conditions.

Management with injection of local anesthetics and corticosteroids may provide temporary and even long-lasting pain relief.[20]

Continuous

Peripheral painful trigeminal traumatic neuropathy

Peripheral painful trigeminal traumatic neuropathy (PPTTN), also known as anesthesia dolorosa, is a unilateral (bilateral in 10% of cases) facial or oral pain (moderate to severe intensity and usually burning and/or stabbing) following trauma (within 3–6 months of the event) to the trigeminal nerve.[5,21] Often, there is clinical evidence of either positive (hyperalgesia, allodynia) and/or negative (hypoesthesia, hypoalgesia) signs of trigeminal nerve dysfunction.[21] The traumatic event may be mechanical, chemical, thermal, or caused by radiation.[5] In orofacial pain clinics, reported onset most often has a clear association with craniofacial or oral trauma,[22,23] but pain may begin after minor dental trauma, such as root canal therapy.[24,25] The duration of the pain ranges widely from paroxysmal to constant (most cases), and may be mixed.[5,21] It has been reported that after considerable injury to trigeminal nerve branches, chronic pain develops in approximately 3% to 5% of patients,[22,26] as compared to approximately 5% to 17% in other body regions.[27,28] Diagnostic testing may involve quantitative sensory testing or advanced neurophysiological testing; however, this is not always possible to do intraorally.[21]

Management consists of antidepressants and anticonvulsants to modulate pain.[21] Microsurgical repair has shown to be effective in only 1 of 7 patients.[29] Dorsal root entry zone lesioning (DREZ) has shown some promise,[30,31] as has sensory thalamic neurostimulation.[32] It has been reported that most cases that have undergone peripheral surgical procedures, such as exploratory procedures or apicoectomies, have resulted in pain escalation.[33]

Persistent idiopathic facial pain

Persistent idiopathic facial pain (PIFP), previously termed atypical facial pain, is persistent facial and/or oral pain (mild to severe; superficial or deep), with varying presentations but recurring daily for more than 2 hours per day over more than 3 months, in the absence of clinical neurologic deficit.[5,34,35] However, sensory deficits have been reported in up to 60% of cases.[36,37] PIPF has been characterized as being poorly localized, not following the distribution of a peripheral nerve, while having a dull, aching, or nagging quality (may have sharp exacerbations); is aggravated by stress; and, with time, may spread to a wider area of the craniocervical region.[5] PIPF may originate from a minor operation or injury to the orofacial region but persists after healing of the initial noxious event or presents without any demonstrable local cause.[38] Patients experiencing PIPF often report multiple ineffective dental interventions in the area of complaint.[39,40]

Before definitive diagnosis, all other local or systemic causes must be excluded. Imaging studies of the brain and skull base may be necessary in ruling out underlying pathology. Psychophysical or neurophysiological tests may demonstrate sensory abnormalities; however, this may not be clinically practical.[41]

The Canadian Pain Society, the Neuropathic Pain Special Interest Group of the IASP, and the European Federation of Neurological Societies Task Force developed guidelines regarding the pharmacologic management of neuropathic pain.[42–44] Medications commonly used for neuropathic pain management are tricyclic antidepressants (amitriptyline, desipramine, nortriptyline), anticonvulsants (gabapentin, pregabalin), serotonin noradrenaline reuptake inhibitors (venlafaxine, duloxetine, milnacipran), topical lidocaine, and analgesics (opioids, tramadol). Surgical procedures have been trialed; however, these techniques are not currently approved by the Food and Drug Administration (FDA) for chronic pain.[45–48]

Neuritis

Peripheral neuritis Currently, peripheral neuritis is used to describe localized nerve pathologies secondary to inflammation. Inflammation may affect the nerve either by direct effects of mediator secretion, mainly cytokines or secondary to pressure induced by the accompanying edema.[49,50] Temporary perineural inflammation in the orofacial region is most likely due to dental and other invasive procedures, but this is usually asymptomatic. However, misplaced dental implants or periapical inflammation close to a nerve trunk can produce chronic symptoms. Other conditions, such as temporomandibular joint pathologies,[51] paranasal sinusitis,[52] or early malignancies[53] can induce symptomatic perineural inflammation, pain, and other aberrant sensations.

Early administration of anti-inflammatory medication (corticosteroids or nonsteroidal anti-inflammatory drugs) can be beneficial.[54]

Herpes zoster/postherpetic neuralgia Acute herpes zoster (HZ) or shingles is a reactivation of latent varicella-zoster virus (VZV) infection that may occur decades after the primary infection. HZ is a disease of the dorsal root and cranial nerve ganglion and therefore induces a dermatomal vesicular eruption. HZ affects trigeminal nerves in approximately 10% to 15% of all cases. The ophthalmic branch is affected in more than 80% of the trigeminal cases, particularly in elderly men, and may cause sight-threatening keratitis.[5] The vesicles and pain are dermatomal and unilateral and will appear intraorally when the maxillary or mandibular branches of the trigeminal nerve are affected. The incidence of HZ is higher among people aged 60 to 70 (6–7 cases per 1000 person-years) and older than 80 years (>10 cases per 1000 person-years).[55] HZ typically begins with prodromal symptoms, such as malaise, headache, photophobia, abnormal skin sensations, and occasionally fever. These symptoms may occur 1 to 5 days before the appearance of the rash.[56] Diagnosis may be obtained by analyzing fluid from vesicles with the use of polymerase chain reaction testing, viral culture, or direct immunofluorescence antigen staining.[57]

Management for HZ should be directed at controlling pain, accelerating healing, and reducing the risk of complications, such as dissemination, postherpetic neuralgia (PHN), and local secondary infection.[58]

- Antivirals (acyclovir, valacyclovir, famciclovir) initiated less than 72 hours from onset of rash, particularly in patients older than 50 years, decrease rash duration, pain severity, and the incidence of PHN.[59,60]
- Nonopioid analgesics: acetaminophen or nonsteroidal anti-inflammatory drugs used to control fever and mild to moderate pain.
- Opioids: used for severe pain.
- Corticosteroids added to antivirals: decreases the pain of HZ[61]; however, a systematic review found no significant difference between corticosteroids and placebo in preventing PHN 6 months after onset of the rash.[62]
- Adjunctive therapies: antidepressants (amitriptyline, desipramine, venlafaxine, bupropion) or gabapentinoids (gabapentin, pregabalin) provide analgesia, shorten illness duration, and reduce the risk of PHN.[63,64]

PHN, a neuropathic pain syndrome due to replication of the varicella-zoster virus in the basal ganglia causing nerve injury and manifesting as pain in the affected dermatome, is the most common complication of HZ. It occurs in approximately 30% of patients older than 80 years and in approximately 20% of patients 60 to 65 years old; it is rare in patients younger than 50 years.[65] Postherpetic pain may include allodynia, hyperpathia, and dysesthesia.[66] Women are at greater risk of PHN with additional risk factors, including older age, moderate to severe rash, moderate to severe acute pain during the rash, ophthalmic involvement, and history of prodromal pain.[66,67] PHN may persist from 30 days to more than 6 months after the lesions have healed, and most cases resolve spontaneously.[65]

Management of established PHN should be immediate, as it improves prognosis, with ophthalmic PHN having the worst prognosis.[68] Management options include antidepressants, gabapentinoids, opioids, and topical lidocaine patches.[69] Invasive modalities include epidural and intrathecal steroids and a variety of neurosurgical techniques.[70]

HZ and PHN are relatively preventable conditions. The Shingles Prevention Study found the HZ vaccine to be 51.3% effective in preventing HZ and 66.5% effective in preventing PHN (when defined as pain rated as at least a 3 of 10 on a severity scale that persisted for at least 90 days after rash onset).[71] Vaccination also has been shown to reduce the incidence of PHN by 39% among patients who develop HZ.[72] Currently, the Centers for Disease Control and Prevention recommends that patients aged 60 years and older should be vaccinated regardless of their prior exposure to VZV.[72] However, the vaccine is approved for patients as young as 50 years of age as well.

Burning mouth syndrome

Burning mouth syndrome (BMS), also known as stomatodynia, glossodynia, oral dysesthesia, or stomatopyrosis, is a poorly understood pain condition that is most probably neuropathic. BMS is most common in postmenopausal women with reported prevalence rates in the general population varying from 0.7% to 15%,[73,74] with individuals younger than 30 years rarely affected.[75] For clinical utility, BMS may be classified into "primary BMS" or essential/idiopathic BMS for which a neuropathological cause is likely; and "secondary BMS" resulting from local or systemic pathologic conditions.[76] By definition, primary BMS cannot be attributed to any systemic or local cause and therefore is essentially a diagnosis by exclusion (**Table 2**).[77,78] The condition is characterized by a burning (mild to severe) sensation in the mucosa devoid of clinical findings and without abnormalities in laboratory testing or imaging, often accompanied by dysgeusia and xerostomia. Burning pain commonly presents with a bilateral symmetric distribution, most frequently involving the anterior two-thirds of the tongue,

Table 2
Factors needed to be ruled out before a diagnosis of burning mouth syndrome

Local	Systemic
Poorly fitting dental prostheses/mechanical irritations	Nutritional deficiencies (iron, B complex vitamins, zinc)
Dental anomalies	Endocrine disorders (diabetes, thyroid disorders, hormone deficiencies, menopause)
Parafunctional habits (clenching, bruxism, tongue posturing)	Anemia
Allergic contact stomatitis (dental restorations, denture materials, oral care products, foods, preservatives, additives, flavorings)	Gastrointestinal disorders (esophageal reflux)
Oral/perioral infections (bacteria, fungal, viral)	Medication (angiotensin-converting enzyme inhibitors, antihyperglycemics, chemotherapeutic agents)
Hyposalivation (radiation therapy, salivary gland disorders, medications)	Connective tissue/autoimmune diseases
Xerostomia	Neuropathy/neuralgia
Oral mucosal lesions (lichen planus, benign migratory glossitis)	
Tongue alterations (scalloped and/or fissured tongue)	
Chemical irritants	
Taste alteration/dysfunction	
Neurologic alterations	
Myofascial pain	

the dorsum and lateral borders of the tongue, the anterior hard palate, and the mucosa of the lower lip, and often presenting in multiple sites.[79,80] BMS is typically of spontaneous onset and lasts from months to several years,[78,81] with spontaneous remission reported in 3% of patients approximately 5 years after onset.[82] Minimal symptoms are reported by most patients on awakening, with gradual increase in intensity of symptoms as the day progresses, climaxing in the evening. Most patients report an intensification of the burning sensation while experiencing personal stressors and fatigue, with aggravation on eating acidic/hot/spicy foods. However, in about half the patients, oral intake/stimulation and distraction reduce or alleviate the symptoms.[83] A possible association with anxiety, depression, and personality disorders is described in the literature, particularly in postmenopausal women,[75,76] but it is unclear if pain initiated the psychological disorder or vice versa.[84–86]

Management approaches include 3 strategies, which may be used singularly or in combination.

- Behavioral strategies: cognitive behavioral approaches and/or group psychotherapy.
- Topical medications: anxiolytics (clonazepam), atypical analgesics (capsaicin), antimicrobials (lysozyme-lactoperoxidase), artificial sweeteners (sucralose), and low-level laser therapy.
- Systemic medications: antidepressants (amitriptyline, trazodone, paroxetine, milnacipran), anxiolytics (clonazepam, diazepam, chlordiazepoxide), anticonvulsants (gabapentin, topiramate), antioxidants (alpha lipoic acid), atypical

analgesics/antipsychotics (capsaicin, olanzapine), histamine receptor antagonists (lafutidine, which is not FDA approved for use in the United States), monoamine oxidase inhibitors (moclobemide, which is not FDA approved for use in the United States), salivary stimulants (pilocarpine), dopamine agonists (pramipexole), and herbal supplements (hypericum perforatum or St. John's wort).

Recently, a randomized controlled trial indicated that systemic use of clonazepam should be considered as first-line treatment.[87]

NEUROVASCULAR PAIN

Primary headache disorders are often associated with orofacial pain.[88–91] These include migraine, tension-type headache, and trigeminal autonomic cephalalgias (TACs). The reader is encouraged to review the ICHD-3 for an extensive overview of all the headache disorders.[5]

Migraine

The 2 most common types of migraine are migraine without aura (80% of cases) and migraine with aura (20% of cases).[92] Fifteen percent of migraineurs will report daily or chronic (near daily) headache.[93] Migraine affects 6% of men and 18% of women in the adult population.[94,95] Its prevalence peaks between the ages of 35 and 45.[96] Migraine is associated with significant burden and decreased quality of life.[95,97]

Clinical features
Patients with migraine often report a trigger(s) for their migraine. Potential triggers include stress; altered sleep patterns; certain foods, such as cheese and chocolate; alcohol (wine); bright or flashing lights; menstruation; or changes in barometric pressure.[98,99] The clinical presentation of migraine may occur in phases.

- Phase 1 (prodrome): occurs hours or days before the headache onset. Associated with cravings, lethargy, tiredness, stiff neck, and difficulty concentrating.[100]
- Phase 2 (aura): occurs in patients with migraine with aura. Auras may be visual, such as scotomas or fortification spectrum; sensory, such as numbness, and pins and needles; or motor, such as dysarthria.[101] The aura develops within 5 to 20 minutes after the trigger and may last up to 60 minutes.
- Phase 3 (headache): headache is typically a unilateral pain localized around the ocular, temporal, and frontal regions. Occipital and neck area also may be involved.[102–104] Patients report throbbing or pulsating pain at moderate to severe intensity.[93,101,102,105] Aggravation of the pain with physical activities and sudden head movements is often reported.[101,102] Duration of the headache is usually between 4 and 72 hours, although it can last longer.[105] Most patients report fewer than 1 headache monthly, although some patients may suffer up to 4 migraines a month.[94,105] Migraine also may be chronic, whereby the headache may occur more than 15 days per month.[5] Many migraine sufferers report nausea (80%), vomiting (50%), and photophobia and/or phonophobia (>50%).[102,103]
- Phase 4 (postdrome): feeling of being washed out, irritable, depressed, and tired. Migraine is associated with anxiety, depression, allergies, stroke, and other pain conditions.[106–109]

Facial migraine
There are reports in the literature of patients who present with lower facial pain associated with nausea, photophobia, or phonophobia and autonomic symptoms consistent with migraine or TACs except it is a headache of the lower face.[110–113] Benoliel

and colleagues[114] proposed the term "neurovascular orofacial pain" along with criteria for its diagnosis (**Table 3**).

Management

Management for migraine is divided into 3 categories: behavioral interventions, preventive medications, and abortive medications. Behavioral changes may be adopted by the patient to prevent an attack. Patient education, information regarding sleep hygiene, diet, and stress may be used to prevent a migraine. In some cases, patients may have regular migraine and will need to use a preventive medication (**Table 4**). In the event of a migraine episode, an abortive medication may be used (**Table 5**).

Tension-type Headache

Tension-type headaches (TTH) are a common headache with a 1-year prevalence of greater than 80%.[115,116] The age of onset is 20 to 30 years, with peak prevalence in the third and fifth decades.[117] The ICHD-3 classifies TTH into infrequent (<12 episodes/year) or frequent (>12 and <180 headache days per year), episodic, chronic, or probable. The headache may be associated with or without pericranial tenderness.[5] The clinical features of episodic and chronic TTH are summarized in **Table 6**.

Episodic TTH may be precipitated by stress, fatigue, lack of sleep, disturbed meals, menstruation, and alcohol.[118,119] Patients with chronic TTH usually report a long

Table 3
Proposed criteria for neurovascular orofacial pain

Diagnostic Criteria	Notes
A At least 5 attacks of facial pain fulfilling criteria B–E	
B Severe, unilateral oral and/or perioral	May refer to orbital and/or temporal regions. Side shift may occur; rarely are bilateral cases reported.
C At least 1 of the following characteristics: 1. Toothache with no local pathology 2. Throbbing 3. Awakens from sleep	Frequently painful vital teeth will be hypersensitive to cold stimuli. Some of the teeth in the painful region may have undergone root canal therapy with no long-lasting pain relief.
D Episodic attacks lasting 60 min to >24 h	Chronic unremitting cases that may result in subclassification into episodic and chronic forms have been observed.
E Accompanied by at least 1 of the following: 1. Ipsilateral lacrimation and/or conjunctival injection 2. Ipsilateral rhinorrhea and/or nasal congestion 3. Ipsilateral cheek swelling 4. Photophobia and/or phonophobia 5. Nausea and/or vomiting	
F Not attributed to another disorder	Dental pathology may be very difficult to differentiate and needs careful assessment.

Data from Benoliel R, Birman N, Eliav E, et al. The International Classification of Headache Disorders: accurate diagnosis of orofacial pain? Cephalalgia 2008;28(7):752–62; with permission.

Table 4
Preventive medications for migraine

Class/Drug	Recommended Dose
Antiepileptic	
Divalproex sodium	750–1500 mg BID
Topiramate	100 mg hs or 50 mg BID
Gabapentin	1200–1500 mg TID
Antidepressant	
TCA: Amitriptyline	20–40 mg nocte
SSRI: Venlafaxine extended release	150 mg once daily
Antihypertensive: Beta-blockers	
Propranolol	80–160 mg BID
Nadolol	80–160 mg once daily
Metoprolol	100–200 mg BID
Antihypertensive: Calcium Channel Blockers	
Flunarizine	10 mg hs

Abbreviations: BID, twice daily; hs, hora somni; SSRI, Selective serotonin reuptake inhibitor; TCA, Tricyclic antidepressant; TID, 3 times daily.

Adapted from Pringsheim T, Davenport W, Mackie G, et al. Canadian Headache Society guideline for migraine prophylaxis. Can J Neurol Sci 2012;39(2 Suppl 2):S1–59.

history of episodic headaches that evolved into the chronic form, which is associated with depression, anxiety, and lack of sleep.[120] Management for TTH is summarized in **Table 7**.

Trigeminal Autonomic Cephalalgias

A collective group of headaches, trigeminal autonomic cephalalgias (TACs), are characterized by head and facial pain with accompanying autonomic features. The ICHD-3 classifies TACs as follows[5]: cluster headache (CH), episodic or chronic; paroxysmal hemicranias,[121] episodic or chronic; short-lasting unilateral neuralgiform headache attacks; and hemicrania continua (HC).

Cluster headache

CH affects 120 to 300 individuals per 100,000 in the general population.[122–124] It is a severe unilateral, short-lasting pain overlying the orbital, supraorbital, or temporal sites accompanied by ipsilateral autonomic features, such as conjunctival injections,

Table 5
Abortive medications for migraine

Clinical Phenotype	Strategy	Medications
Mild – moderate pain	1.a. Acetaminophen 1.b. NSAID	Acetaminophen ± metoclopramide Ibuprofen, diclofenac potassium, naproxen sodium, ASA, all ± metoclopramide
Moderate – severe pain/ NSAID failure	2.a. NSAID with triptan rescue	NSAID ± metoclopramide + a triptan later for rescue if necessary

Abbreviations: ASA, acetylsalicylic acid; NSAID, nonsteroidal anti-inflammatory drugs.

Adapted from Worthington I, Pringsheim T, Gawel MJ, et al. Canadian Headache Society Guideline: acute drug therapy for migraine headache. Can J Neurol Sci 2013;40(5 Suppl 3):S1–80.

Table 6
Clinical presentation of episodic and chronic tension-type headache

Subgroup	Episodic	Chronic
Frequency	May be infrequent (<12 episodes/y) or frequent (>12 and <180 headache days per year)	Chronic (>15 episodes per month)
Location	Bilateral frontotemporal region	Bilateral frontotemporal region
Quality	Pressing or tightening	Pressing or tightening
Intensity	Mild to moderate intensity with or without pericranial tenderness	Mild to moderate intensity with or without pericranial tenderness
Duration	Lasting 30 min to 7 d	Lasting hours to days, or unremitting
Associated features	Does not worsen with routine physical activity. Not associated with nausea, but photophobia or phonophobia may be present	Does not worsen with routine physical activity. May be associated with photophobia, phonophobia, or mild nausea

Data from Headache Classification Committee of the International Headache Society (IHS). The International Classification of Headache Disorders, 3rd edition (beta version). Cephalalgia 2013;33(9):629–808; with permission.

lacrimation, nasal congestion, rhinorrhea, forehead and facial sweating, miosis, and ptosis.[123,125,126] Occasionally, the pain may radiate to involve the maxilla, nostril, gingiva, palate, mandible, teeth, and neck.[127–129] The pain is so severe that patients may be restless, pace, and bang their head.[126,130,131] The autonomic features typically cease after an attack, which may last between 15 minutes and 3 hours.[132] The features of CH are reviewed in **Table 8**. Chronic CH affects 10% of patients.[5,133] An MRI of the brain and skull base is necessary to exclude central pathology.[134]

Management for CH may include avoiding triggers, such as nitrates, alcohol, and smoking, and treating obstructive sleep apnea.[135,136] There are also abortive and preventive interventions for CH (**Table 9**).

Paroxysmal hemicrania
PH affects 1 individual per 50,000 in the general population.[137] It is a severe, short-lasting, strictly unilateral pain localized to the orbital, supraorbital, frontal, temporal, and occipital sites associated with ipsilateral autonomic features, such as lacrimation,

Table 7
Management for tension-type headache (TTH)

Pharmacologic	Abortive (for episodic TTH)	Preventive (for chronic TTH)
	Ibuprofen	Amitriptyline
	Naproxen	Nortriptyline
	Acetaminophen	Botulinum toxin
Nonpharmacologic	**Behavioral therapies**	**Physical therapies**
	Relaxation	Physiotherapy
	Biofeedback training	Massage
	Cognitive behavioral therapy	Accupuncture
		Chiropractic manipulations
		Oral appliances

Date from Refs.[160–169]

Table 8
Clinical features of trigeminal autonomic cephalalgias

Features	Cluster Headache	Paroxysmal Hemicrania	Short-Lasting Unilateral Neuralgiform Headache Attacks	Hemicrania Continua
Sex, male:female	5:1	1:2	2:1	1:2
Age, y	20–40	30	40–70	30
Pain				
Type	Boring	Boring	Electriclike	Throbbing or sharp
Severity	Very severe	Very severe	Severe	Varying severity
Location	Orbital	Orbital	Orbital	Temporal/frontal
Duration	15–180 min	2–30 min	15–240 s	Continuous
Frequency	1–8/d	2–40/d	3–200/d	Constant
Autonomic	Yes	Yes	Yes	Yes
Trigger	Alcohol, nitrates	Mechanical	Cutaneous	

Adapted from Balasubramaniam R, Klasser GD, Delcanho R. Trigeminal autonomic cephalalgias: a review and implications for dentistry. J Am Dent Assoc 2008;139(12):1616–24; and *Data from* Charlson RW, Robbins MS. Hemicrania continua. Curr Neurol Neurosci Rep 2014;14(3):436.

conjunctival injection, nasal congestion, rhinorrhea, ptosis, and facial flushing.[5,138,139] It may confuse the clinician, as the pain can present in the facial structures.[110,140,141] It is an excruciating pain of boring or stabbing quality and patients may be agitated, restless, or aggressive.[5,138,139] The pain may occur spontaneously or be triggered by glyceryl trinitrate, alcohol, or manipulation of the head and neck.[142,143] The clinical presentation of PH is summarized in **Table 8**. There is a chronic and episodic form of the pain with the latter having bouts of pain ranging from 2 weeks to 4.5 months with periods of remission between 1 and 36 months.[5,139,142,144]

Table 9
Management of cluster headache

Intervention	Dose	Route of Administration
Abortive		
100% oxygen	7–12 L/min for 15–30 min	Inhalation with non-rebreathing mask
Sumatriptan	6 mg	Subcutaneous injection
Sumatriptan	20 mg	Nasal spray
Zolmitriptan	1 mg	Nasal spray
Preventive		
Verapamil	360–720 mg/d	Oral
Lithium	300–1200 mg/d	Oral
Prednisone	60–80 mg/d, taper across 1 to 4 wk	Oral

Adapted from Balasubramaniam R, Klasser GD, Delcanho R. Trigeminal autonomic cephalalgias: a review and implications for dentistry. J Am Dent Assoc 2008;139(12):1616–24.

Management for PH is indomethacin and resolution of the pain within 24 hours is considered pathognomonic. The recommended dose for indomethacin is 75 to 150 mg 3 times daily.[5,138,139,145]

Short-lasting unilateral neuralgiform headache attacks

The prevalence of this extremely rare headache is 6.6 individuals per 100,000 in the general population.[146] There are 2 forms of headache attacks: (1) short-lasting unilateral neuralgiform headache attacks with conjunctival injections and tearing (SUNCT), when no other autonomic features are apparent; (2) Short-lasting unilateral neuralgiform headache attacks with cranial autonomic symptoms (SUNA), when not limited to conjunctival injections and tearing.[5] This is a moderate or severe unilateral head pain localized to the orbital, supraorbital, temporal, and frontal areas.[147,148] The pain occurs at least once and up to 200 times a day. Common autonomic features are conjunctival injections and tearing and occur 1 to 2 seconds after the attack that last between 2 and 600 seconds.[5,137,147] Attacks may occur spontaneously or with innocuous stimulation similar to TN. Unlike TN there are no refractory periods between attacks (see **Table 8**).[147]

First-line therapy for SUNCT is lamotrigine 100–300 mg per day or intravenous lidocaine 1.5 to 3.5 mg/kg per hour. Failing a therapeutic response, gabapentin 800 to 2700 mg per day or topiramate 50 to 300 mg per day may be used.[145,149]

Hemicrania continua

Hemicrania continua (HC) affects approximately 900 individuals per 100,000 in the general population.[150] HC is a continuous unilateral headache localized to the temporal and frontal areas and, to a lesser extent, the orbital and retroorbital of varying intensity without side change.[5,151–154] Cases of bilateral pain are rare.[155] It is associated with mild autonomic features, namely lacrimation, conjunctival injection, nasal symptoms, and ptosis or miosis.[155] Typically, the quality of pain is described as throbbing, stabbing, or sharp. Similar to PH, HC responds to indomethacin.[5,156]

VASCULAR HEADACHE
Giant Cell Arteritis

Giant cell arteritis, also known as temporal arteritis, is the result of granulomatous inflammation of the temporal artery, typically occurring in individuals older than 50 years. Patients may complain of a swollen, tender temporal artery, headache, hip and shoulder pain, fatigue, and malaise. Jaw claudication, aching, and cramping of the masseter and temporal muscles are common complaints and easily confused with temporomandibular disorders.[157] A delayed diagnosis may result in blindness due to anterior ischemic optic neuropathy.[158]

Investigation typically reveals an elevated erythrocyte sedimentation rate of greater than 50 mm per hour. The diagnosis may be confirmed by temporal artery biopsy. Prompt treatment with corticosteroids is necessary to avoid blindness.[159]

SUMMARY

Patients will often visit their primary medical practitioner with orofacial pain complaints. Hence, it is important to recognize and have an understanding of these conditions to properly evaluate and potentially manage these disorders. If the practitioner is uncertain or uncomfortable with these conditions, then patient referral to a knowledgeable health care practitioner should be considered for further evaluation and management.

REFERENCES

1. International Association for the Study of Pain Committee on Taxonomy. 2011. Available at: http://www.iasppain.org/AM/Template.cfm?Section=Pain_Definitions&Template=/CM/HTMLDisplay.cfm&ContentID=1728-Neuropathicpain. Accessed February 15, 2014.
2. Costigan M, Scholz J, Woolf CJ. Neuropathic pain: a maladaptive response of the nervous system to damage. Annu Rev Neurosci 2009;32:1–32.
3. Scrivani SJ, Mathews ES, Maciewicz RJ. Trigeminal neuralgia. Oral Surg Oral Med Oral Pathol Oral Radiol Endod 2005;100(5):527–38.
4. Kandan SR, Khan S, Jeyaretna DS, et al. Neuralgia of the glossopharyngeal and vagal nerves: long-term outcome following surgical treatment and literature review. Br J Neurosurg 2010;24(4):441–6.
5. Headache Classification Committee of the International Headache Society (IHS). The International Classification of Headache Disorders, 3rd edition (beta version). Cephalalgia 2013;33(9):629–808.
6. Mueller D, Obermann M, Yoon MS, et al. Prevalence of trigeminal neuralgia and persistent idiopathic facial pain: a population-based study. Cephalalgia 2011; 31(15):1542–8.
7. Gronseth G, Cruccu G, Alksne J, et al. Practice parameter: the diagnostic evaluation and treatment of trigeminal neuralgia (an evidence-based review): report of the Quality Standards Subcommittee of the American Academy of Neurology and the European Federation of Neurological Societies. Neurology 2008;71(15): 1183–90.
8. Zhang J, Yang M, Zhou M, et al. Non-antiepileptic drugs for trigeminal neuralgia. Cochrane Database Syst Rev 2013;(12):CD004029.
9. Chan MD, Shaw EG, Tatter SB. Radiosurgical management of trigeminal neuralgia. Neurosurg Clin N Am 2013;24(4):613–21.
10. Cruccu G, Gronseth G, Alksne J, et al. AAN-EFNS guidelines on trigeminal neuralgia management. Eur J Neurol 2008;15(10):1013–28.
11. Katusic S, Williams DB, Beard CM, et al. Incidence and clinical features of glossopharyngeal neuralgia, Rochester, Minnesota, 1945-1984. Neuroepidemiology 1991;10(5–6):266–75.
12. Rushton JG, Stevens JC, Miller RH. Glossopharyngeal (vagoglossopharyngeal) neuralgia: a study of 217 cases. Arch Neurol 1981;38(4):201–5.
13. Minagar A, Sheremata WA. Glossopharyngeal neuralgia and MS. Neurology 2000;54(6):1368–70.
14. Rozen TD. Trigeminal neuralgia and glossopharyngeal neuralgia. Neurol Clin 2004;22(1):185–206.
15. Patel A, Kassam A, Horowitz M, et al. Microvascular decompression in the management of glossopharyngeal neuralgia: analysis of 217 cases. Neurosurgery 2002;50(4):705–10 [discussion: 710–11].
16. Kondo A. Follow-up results of using microvascular decompression for treatment of glossopharyngeal neuralgia. J Neurosurg 1998;88(2):221–5.
17. Stieber VW, Bourland JD, Ellis TL. Glossopharyngeal neuralgia treated with gamma knife surgery: treatment outcome and failure analysis. Case report. J Neurosurg 2005;102(Suppl):155–7.
18. Goadsby PJ, Bartsch T. On the functional neuroanatomy of neck pain. Cephalalgia 2008;28(Suppl 1):1–7.
19. Bogduk N. The anatomy and pathophysiology of neck pain. Phys Med Rehabil Clin N Am 2011;22(3):367–82, vii.

20. Vanelderen P, Lataster A, Levy R, et al. 8. Occipital neuralgia. Pain Pract 2010; 10(2):137–44.
21. Benoliel R, Zadik Y, Eliav E, et al. Peripheral painful traumatic trigeminal neuropathy: clinical features in 91 cases and proposal of novel diagnostic criteria. J Orofac Pain 2012;26(1):49–58.
22. Benoliel R, Birenboim R, Regev E, et al. Neurosensory changes in the infraorbital nerve following zygomatic fractures. Oral Surg Oral Med Oral Pathol Oral Radiol Endod 2005;99(6):657–65.
23. Benoliel R, Eliav E, Elishoov H, et al. Diagnosis and treatment of persistent pain after trauma to the head and neck. J Oral Maxillofac Surg 1994;52(11):1138–47 [discussion: 1147–8].
24. Polycarpou N, Ng YL, Canavan D, et al. Prevalence of persistent pain after endodontic treatment and factors affecting its occurrence in cases with complete radiographic healing. Int Endod J 2005;38(3):169–78.
25. Klasser GD, Kugelmann AM, Villines D, et al. The prevalence of persistent pain after nonsurgical root canal treatment. Quintessence Int 2011;42(3):259–69.
26. Jaaskelainen SK, Teerijoki-Oksa T, Virtanen A, et al. Sensory regeneration following intraoperatively verified trigeminal nerve injury. Neurology 2004; 62(11):1951–7.
27. Beniczky S, Tajti J, Timea Varga E, et al. Evidence-based pharmacological treatment of neuropathic pain syndromes. J Neural Transm 2005;112(6):735–49.
28. Macrae WA. Chronic pain after surgery. Br J Anaesth 2001;87(1):88–98.
29. Gregg JM. Studies of traumatic neuralgia in the maxillofacial region: symptom complexes and response to microsurgery. J Oral Maxillofac Surg 1990;48(2): 135–40 [discussion: 141].
30. Nashold BS Jr, el-Naggar A, Mawaffak Abdulhak M, et al. Trigeminal nucleus caudalis dorsal root entry zone: a new surgical approach. Stereotact Funct Neurosurg 1992;59(1–4):45–51.
31. Kanpolat Y, Savas A, Ugur HC, et al. The trigeminal tract and nucleus procedures in treatment of atypical facial pain. Surg Neurol 2005;64(Suppl 2): S96–100 [discussion: S100–1].
32. Siegfried J. Sensory thalamic neurostimulation for chronic pain. Pacing Clin Electrophysiol 1987;10(1 Pt 2):209–12.
33. Benoliel R, Kahn J, Eliav E. Peripheral painful traumatic trigeminal neuropathies. Oral Dis 2012;18(4):317–32.
34. Aggarwal VR, McBeth J, Lunt M, et al. Development and validation of classification criteria for idiopathic orofacial pain for use in population-based studies. J Orofac Pain 2007;21(3):203–15.
35. Agostoni E, Frigerio R, Santoro P. Atypical facial pain: clinical considerations and differential diagnosis. Neurol Sci 2005;26(Suppl 2):s71–4.
36. Jaaskelainen SK, Forssell H, Tenovuo O. Electrophysiological testing of the trigeminofacial system: aid in the diagnosis of atypical facial pain. Pain 1999; 80(1–2):191–200.
37. Pfaffenrath V, Rath M, Pollmann W, et al. Atypical facial pain–application of the IHS criteria in a clinical sample. Cephalalgia 1993;13(Suppl 12):84–8.
38. Sardella A, Demarosi F, Barbieri C, et al. An up-to-date view on persistent idiopathic facial pain. Minerva Stomatol 2009;58(6):289–99.
39. Truelove E. Management issues of neuropathic trigeminal pain from a dental perspective. J Orofac Pain 2004;18(4):374–80.
40. Marbach JJ. Orofacial phantom pain: theory and phenomenology. J Am Dent Assoc 1996;127(2):221–9.

41. Forssell H, Tenovuo O, Silvoniemi P, et al. Differences and similarities between atypical facial pain and trigeminal neuropathic pain. Neurology 2007;69(14):1451–9.

42. Attal N, Cruccu G, Baron R, et al. EFNS guidelines on the pharmacological treatment of neuropathic pain: 2010 revision. Eur J Neurol 2010;17(9):1113.e88.

43. Dworkin RH, O'Connor AB, Audette J, et al. Recommendations for the pharmacological management of neuropathic pain: an overview and literature update. Mayo Clin Proc 2010;85(Suppl 3):S3–14.

44. Moulin DE, Clark AJ, Gilron I, et al. Pharmacological management of chronic neuropathic pain—consensus statement and guidelines from the Canadian Pain Society. Pain Res Manag 2007;12(1):13–21.

45. Rasche D, Ruppolt M, Stippich C, et al. Motor cortex stimulation for long-term relief of chronic neuropathic pain: a 10 year experience. Pain 2006;121(1–2):43–52.

46. Raslan AM, Nasseri M, Bahgat D, et al. Motor cortex stimulation for trigeminal neuropathic or deafferentation pain: an institutional case series experience. Stereotact Funct Neurosurg 2011;89(2):83–8.

47. Franzini A, Messina G, Cordella R, et al. Deep brain stimulation of the posteromedial hypothalamus: indications, long-term results, and neurophysiological considerations. Neurosurg Focus 2010;29(2):E13.

48. Moore NZ, Lempka SF, Machado A. Central neuromodulation for refractory pain. Neurosurg Clin N Am 2014;25(1):77–83.

49. Zelenka M, Schafers M, Sommer C. Intraneural injection of interleukin-1beta and tumor necrosis factor-alpha into rat sciatic nerve at physiological doses induces signs of neuropathic pain. Pain 2005;116(3):257–63.

50. Eliav E, Gracely RH, Nahlieli O, et al. Quantitative sensory testing in trigeminal nerve damage assessment. J Orofac Pain 2004;18(4):339–44.

51. Eliav E, Teich S, Nitzan D, et al. Facial arthralgia and myalgia: can they be differentiated by trigeminal sensory assessment? Pain 2003;104(3):481–90.

52. Benoliel R, Biron A, Quek SY, et al. Trigeminal neurosensory changes following acute and chronic paranasal sinusitis. Quintessence Int 2006;37(6):437–43.

53. Eliav E, Teich S, Benoliel R, et al. Large myelinated nerve fiber hypersensitivity in oral malignancy. Oral Surg Oral Med Oral Pathol Oral Radiol Endod 2002;94(1):45–50.

54. Benoliel R, Eliav E. Neuropathic orofacial pain. Oral Maxillofac Surg Clin North Am 2008;20(2):237–54, vii.

55. Donahue JG, Choo PW, Manson JE, et al. The incidence of herpes zoster. Arch Intern Med 1995;155(15):1605–9.

56. Gnann JW Jr, Whitley RJ. Clinical practice. Herpes zoster. N Engl J Med 2002;347(5):340–6.

57. Sauerbrei A, Eichhorn U, Schacke M, et al. Laboratory diagnosis of herpes zoster. J Clin Virol 1999;14(1):31–6.

58. Volpi A, Gross G, Hercogova J, et al. Current management of herpes zoster: the European view. Am J Clin Dermatol 2005;6(5):317–25.

59. Dworkin RH, Nagasako EM, Johnson RW, et al. Acute pain in herpes zoster: the famciclovir database project. Pain 2001;94(1):113–9.

60. Schmader K. Herpes zoster in older adults. Clin Infect Dis 2001;32(10):1481–6.

61. Wareham DW, Breuer J. Herpes zoster. BMJ 2007;334(7605):1211–5.

62. Chen N, Yang M, He L, et al. Corticosteroids for preventing postherpetic neuralgia. Cochrane Database Syst Rev 2010;(12):CD005582.

63. Dworkin RH, Johnson RW, Breuer J, et al. Recommendations for the management of herpes zoster. Clin Infect Dis 2007;44(Suppl 1):S1–26.

64. Bowsher D. The effects of pre-emptive treatment of postherpetic neuralgia with amitriptyline: a randomized, double-blind, placebo-controlled trial. J Pain Symptom Manage 1997;13(6):327–31.
65. Fashner J, Bell AL. Herpes zoster and postherpetic neuralgia: prevention and management. Am Fam Physician 2011;83(12):1432–7.
66. High KP. Preventing herpes zoster and postherpetic neuralgia through vaccination. J Fam Pract 2007;56(10 Suppl A):51A–7A [quiz: 58A].
67. Lang PO, Hasso Y, Michel JP. Stop shingles in its tracks. J Fam Pract 2009; 58(10):531–4.
68. Bowsher D. Postherpetic neuralgia and its treatment: a retrospective survey of 191 patients. J Pain Symptom Manage 1996;12(5):290–9.
69. Dubinsky RM, Kabbani H, El-Chami Z, et al, Quality Standards Subcommittee of the American Academy of Neurology. Practice parameter: treatment of postherpetic neuralgia: an evidence-based report of the Quality Standards Subcommittee of the American Academy of Neurology. Neurology 2004;63(6):959–65.
70. Watson CP, Oaklander AL. Postherpetic neuralgia. Pain Pract 2002;2(4): 295–307.
71. Oxman MN, Levin MJ, Johnson GR, et al. A vaccine to prevent herpes zoster and postherpetic neuralgia in older adults. N Engl J Med 2005;352(22): 2271–84.
72. Harpaz R, Ortega-Sanchez IR, Seward JF, Advisory Committee on Immunization Practices (ACIP) Centers for Disease Control and Prevention (CDC). Prevention of herpes zoster: recommendations of the Advisory Committee on Immunization Practices (ACIP). MMWR Recomm Rep 2008;57(RR-5):1–30 [quiz: CE2–4].
73. Lipton JA, Ship JA, Larach-Robinson D. Estimated prevalence and distribution of reported orofacial pain in the United States. J Am Dent Assoc 1993;124(10): 115–21.
74. Tammiala-Salonen T, Hiidenkari T, Parvinen T. Burning mouth in a Finnish adult population. Community Dent Oral Epidemiol 1993;21(2):67–71.
75. Bergdahl M, Bergdahl J. Burning mouth syndrome: prevalence and associated factors. J Oral Pathol Med 1999;28(8):350–4.
76. Scala A, Checchi L, Montevecchi M, et al. Update on burning mouth syndrome: overview and patient management. Crit Rev Oral Biol Med 2003;14(4):275–91.
77. Woda A, Pionchon P. A unified concept of idiopathic orofacial pain: clinical features. J Orofac Pain 1999;13(3):172–84 [discussion: 185–95].
78. Rhodus NL, Carlson CR, Miller CS. Burning mouth (syndrome) disorder. Quintessence Int 2003;34(8):587–93.
79. Grushka M. Clinical features of burning mouth syndrome. Oral Surg Oral Med Oral Pathol 1987;63(1):30–6.
80. van der Ploeg HM, van der Wal N, Eijkman MA, et al. Psychological aspects of patients with burning mouth syndrome. Oral Surg Oral Med Oral Pathol 1987; 63(6):664–8.
81. Zakrzewska JM, Forssell H, Glenny AM. Interventions for the treatment of burning mouth syndrome. Cochrane Database Syst Rev 2005;(1):CD002779.
82. Sardella A, Lodi G, Demarosi F, et al. Burning mouth syndrome: a retrospective study investigating spontaneous remission and response to treatments. Oral Dis 2006;12(2):152–5.
83. Suarez P, Clark GT. Burning mouth syndrome: an update on diagnosis and treatment methods. J Calif Dent Assoc 2006;34(8):611–22.
84. Al Quran FA. Psychological profile in burning mouth syndrome. Oral Surg Oral Med Oral Pathol Oral Radiol Endod 2004;97(3):339–44.

85. Maina G, Albert U, Gandolfo S, et al. Personality disorders in patients with burning mouth syndrome. J Pers Disord 2005;19(1):84–93.

86. Schiavone V, Adamo D, Ventrella G, et al. Anxiety, depression, and pain in burning mouth syndrome: first chicken or egg? Headache 2012;52(6):1019–25.

87. Heckmann SM, Kirchner E, Grushka M, et al. A double-blind study on clonazepam in patients with burning mouth syndrome. Laryngoscope 2012;122(4): 813–6.

88. Franco AL, Goncalves DA, Castanharo SM, et al. Migraine is the most prevalent primary headache in individuals with temporomandibular disorders. J Orofac Pain 2010;24(3):287–92.

89. Goncalves DA, Camparis CM, Speciali JG, et al. Temporomandibular disorders are differentially associated with headache diagnoses: a controlled study. Clin J Pain 2011;27(7):611–5.

90. Goncalves DA, Speciali JG, Jales LC, et al. Temporomandibular symptoms, migraine, and chronic daily headaches in the population. Neurology 2009;73(8): 645–6.

91. Goncalves DA, Bigal ME, Jales LC, et al. Headache and symptoms of temporomandibular disorder: an epidemiological study. Headache 2010;50(2):231–41.

92. Russell MB, Rasmussen BK, Fenger K, et al. Migraine without aura and migraine with aura are distinct clinical entities: a study of four hundred and eighty-four male and female migraineurs from the general population. Cephalalgia 1996; 16(4):239–45.

93. Stewart WF, Lipton RB, Kolodner K. Migraine disability assessment (MIDAS) score: relation to headache frequency, pain intensity, and headache symptoms. Headache 2003;43(3):258–65.

94. Rasmussen BK, Jensen R, Schroll M, et al. Epidemiology of headache in a general population–a prevalence study. J Clin Epidemiol 1991;44(11):1147–57.

95. Lipton RB, Stewart WF, Diamond S, et al. Prevalence and burden of migraine in the United States: data from the American Migraine Study II. Headache 2001; 41(7):646–57.

96. Bigal ME, Liberman JN, Lipton RB. Age-dependent prevalence and clinical features of migraine. Neurology 2006;67(2):246–51.

97. Cavallini A, Micieli G, Bussone G, et al. Headache and quality of life. Headache 1995;35(1):29–35.

98. Rasmussen BK. Migraine and tension-type headache in a general population: precipitating factors, female hormones, sleep pattern and relation to lifestyle. Pain 1993;53(1):65–72.

99. Chabriat H, Danchot J, Michel P, et al. Precipitating factors of headache. A prospective study in a national control-matched survey in migraineurs and nonmigraineurs. Headache 1999;39(5):335–8.

100. Kelman L. The premonitory symptoms (prodrome): a tertiary care study of 893 migraineurs. Headache 2004;44(9):865–72.

101. Russell MB, Olesen J. A nosographic analysis of the migraine aura in a general population. Brain 1996;119(Pt 2):355–61.

102. Rasmussen BK, Jensen R, Olesen J. A population-based analysis of the diagnostic criteria of the International Headache Society. Cephalalgia 1991;11(3): 129–34.

103. Rasmussen BK, Olesen J. Symptomatic and nonsymptomatic headaches in a general population. Neurology 1992;42(6):1225–31.

104. Kelman L. Migraine pain location: a tertiary care study of 1283 migraineurs. Headache 2005;45(8):1038–47.

105. Steiner TJ, Scher AI, Stewart WF, et al. The prevalence and disability burden of adult migraine in England and their relationships to age, gender and ethnicity. Cephalalgia 2003;23(7):519–27.
106. Scher AI, Bigal ME, Lipton RB. Comorbidity of migraine. Curr Opin Neurol 2005; 18(3):305–10.
107. Sacco S, Ornello R, Ripa P, et al. Migraine and hemorrhagic stroke: a meta-analysis. Stroke 2013;44(11):3032–8.
108. Marcus DA, Bhowmick A. Fibromyalgia comorbidity in a community sample of adults with migraine. Clin Rheumatol 2013;32(10):1553–6.
109. Ligthart L, Gerrits MM, Boomsma DI, et al. Anxiety and depression are associated with migraine and pain in general: an investigation of the interrelationships. J Pain 2013;14(4):363–70.
110. Benoliel R, Elishoov H, Sharav Y. Orofacial pain with vascular-type features. Oral Surg Oral Med Oral Pathol Oral Radiol Endod 1997;84(5):506–12.
111. Daudia AT, Jones NS. Facial migraine in a rhinological setting. Clin Otolaryngol Allied Sci 2002;27(6):521–5.
112. Penarrocha M, Bandres A, Penarrocha M, et al. Lower-half facial migraine: a report of 11 cases. J Oral Maxillofac Surg 2004;62(12):1453–6.
113. Czerninsky R, Benoliel R, Sharav Y. Odontalgia in vascular orofacial pain. J Orofac Pain 1999;13(3):196–200.
114. Benoliel R, Birman N, Eliav E, et al. The international classification of headache disorders: accurate diagnosis of orofacial pain? Cephalalgia 2008;28(7): 752–62.
115. Rasmussen BK. Epidemiology of headache. Cephalalgia 1995;15(1):45–68.
116. Lyngberg AC, Rasmussen BK, Jorgensen T, et al. Incidence of primary headache: a Danish epidemiologic follow-up study. Am J Epidemiol 2005;161(11):1066–73.
117. Lyngberg AC, Rasmussen BK, Jorgensen T, et al. Has the prevalence of migraine and tension-type headache changed over a 12-year period? A Danish population survey. Eur J Epidemiol 2005;20(3):243–9.
118. Spierings EL, Ranke AH, Honkoop PC. Precipitating and aggravating factors of migraine versus tension-type headache. Headache 2001;41(6):554–8.
119. Karli N, Zarifoglu M, Calisir N, et al. Comparison of pre-headache phases and trigger factors of migraine and episodic tension-type headache: do they share similar clinical pathophysiology? Cephalalgia 2005;25(6):444–51.
120. de Filippis S, Salvatori E, Coloprisco G, et al. Headache and mood disorders. J Headache Pain 2005;6(4):250–3.
121. Pringsheim T, Davenport W, Mackie G, et al. Canadian Headache Society guideline for migraine prophylaxis. Can J Neurol Sci 2012;39(2 Suppl 2):S1–59.
122. Katsarava Z, Obermann M, Yoon MS, et al. Prevalence of cluster headache in a population-based sample in Germany. Cephalalgia 2007;27(9):1014–9.
123. Sjaastad O, Bakketeig LS. Cluster headache prevalence. Vaga study of headache epidemiology. Cephalalgia 2003;23(7):528–33.
124. Ekbom K, Svensson DA, Pedersen NL, et al. Lifetime prevalence and concordance risk of cluster headache in the Swedish twin population. Neurology 2006;67(5):798–803.
125. Ekbom K. Patterns of cluster headache with a note on the relations to angina pectoris and peptic ulcer. Acta Neurol Scand 1970;46(2):225–37.
126. Campbell JK. Diagnosis and treatment of cluster headache. J Pain Symptom Manage 1993;8(3):155–64.
127. Brooke RI. Periodic migrainous neuralgia: a cause of dental pain. Oral Surg Oral Med Oral Pathol 1978;46(4):511–6.

128. Gross SG. Dental presentations of cluster headaches. Curr Pain Headache Rep 2006;10(2):126–9.
129. Alonso AA, Nixdorf DR. Case series of four different headache types presenting as tooth pain. J Endod 2006;32(11):1110–3.
130. Blau JN. Behaviour during a cluster headache. Lancet 1993;342(8873):723–5.
131. Bahra A, May A, Goadsby PJ. Cluster headache: a prospective clinical study with diagnostic implications. Neurology 2002;58(3):354–61.
132. Lance JW, Anthony M. Migrainous neuralgia or cluster headache? J Neurol Sci 1971;13(4):401–14.
133. Ekbom K, Svensson DA, Traff H, et al. Age at onset and sex ratio in cluster headache: observations over three decades. Cephalalgia 2002;22(2):94–100.
134. Purdy RA, Kirby S. Headaches and brain tumors. Neurol Clin 2004;22(1):39–53.
135. Schurks M, Kurth T, de Jesus J, et al. Cluster headache: clinical presentation, lifestyle features, and medical treatment. Headache 2006;46(8):1246–54.
136. Chervin RD, Zallek SN, Lin X, et al. Timing patterns of cluster headaches and association with symptoms of obstructive sleep apnea. Sleep Res Online 2000;3(3):107–12.
137. Lance JW, Goadsby PJ. Mechanism management headache. 7th edition. Philadelphia: Elsevier, Butterworth Heinemann; 2005.
138. Cittadini E, Matharu MS, Goadsby PJ. Paroxysmal hemicrania: a prospective clinical study of 31 cases. Brain 2008;131(Pt 4):1142–55.
139. Goadsby PJ, Lipton RB. A review of paroxysmal hemicranias, SUNCT syndrome and other short-lasting headaches with autonomic feature, including new cases. Brain 1997;120(Pt 1):193–209.
140. Benoliel R, Sharav Y. Paroxysmal hemicrania. Case studies and review of the literature. Oral Surg Oral Med Oral Pathol Oral Radiol Endod 1998;85(3):285–92.
141. Moncada E, Graff-Radford SB. Benign indomethacin-responsive headaches presenting in the orofacial region: eight case reports. J Orofac Pain 1995;9(3):276–84.
142. Antonaci F, Sjaastad O. Chronic paroxysmal hemicrania (CPH): a review of the clinical manifestations. Headache 1989;29(10):648–56.
143. Giffin NJ. Paroxysmal hemicrania triggered by GTN. Cephalalgia 2007;27(8):953–4.
144. Boes CJ, Swanson JW. Paroxysmal hemicrania, SUNCT, and hemicrania continua. Semin Neurol 2006;26(2):260–70.
145. Pareja JA, Alvarez M. The usual treatment of trigeminal autonomic cephalalgias. Headache 2013;53(9):1401–14.
146. Williams MH, Broadley SA. SUNCT and SUNA: clinical features and medical treatment. J Clin Neurosci 2008;15(5):526–34.
147. Matharu MS, Cohen AS, Boes CJ, et al. Short-lasting unilateral neuralgiform headache with conjunctival injection and tearing syndrome: a review. Curr Pain Headache Rep 2003;7(4):308–18.
148. Pareja JA, Sjaastad O. SUNCT syndrome. A clinical review. Headache 1997;37(4):195–202.
149. Balasubramaniam R, Klasser GD, Delcanho R. Trigeminal autonomic cephalalgias: a review and implications for dentistry. J Am Dent Assoc 2008;139(12):1616–24.
150. Sjaastad O, Bakketeig LS. The rare, unilateral headaches. Vaga study of headache epidemiology. J Headache Pain 2007;8(1):19–27.
151. Cittadini E, Goadsby PJ. Hemicrania continua: a clinical study of 39 patients with diagnostic implications. Brain 2010;133(Pt 7):1973–86.

152. Moura LM, Bezerra JM, Fleming NR. Treatment of hemicrania continua: case series and literature review. Rev Bras Anestesiol 2012;62(2):173–87.
153. Prakash S, Golwala P. A proposal for revision of hemicrania continua diagnostic criteria based on critical analysis of 62 patients. Cephalalgia 2012;32(11): 860–8.
154. Sjaastad O, Spierings EL. "Hemicrania continua": another headache absolutely responsive to indomethacin. Cephalalgia 1984;4(1):65–70.
155. Goadsby PJ, Cittadini E, Burns B, et al. Trigeminal autonomic cephalalgias: diagnostic and therapeutic developments. Curr Opin Neurol 2008;21(3):323–30.
156. Antonaci F, Pareja JA, Caminero AB, et al. Chronic paroxysmal hemicrania and hemicrania continua. Parenteral indomethacin: the 'indotest.'. Headache 1998; 38(2):122–8.
157. Wall M, Corbett JJ. Arteritis. In: Olesen J, Goadsby PJ, Ramadan NM, et al, editors. Headaches. Philadelphia: Lippincott Williams & Wilkins; 2006. p. 901–10.
158. Gayral L, Neuwirth E. Oto-neuroophthalmologic manifestations of cervical origin; posterior cervical sympathetic syndrome of Barre-Lieou. N Y State J Med 1954; 54(13):1920–6.
159. Wight S, Osborne N, Breen AC. Incidence of ponticulus posterior of the atlas in migraine and cervicogenic headache. J Manipulative Physiol Ther 1999;22(1): 15–20.
160. Steiner TJ, Lange R, Voelker M. Aspirin in episodic tension-type headache: placebo-controlled dose-ranging comparison with paracetamol. Cephalalgia 2003;23(1):59–66.
161. Brennum J, Kjeldsen M, Olesen J. The 5-HT1-like agonist sumatriptan has a significant effect in chronic tension-type headache. Cephalalgia 1992;12(6):375–9.
162. Cady RK, Gutterman D, Saiers JA, et al. Responsiveness of non-IHS migraine and tension-type headache to sumatriptan. Cephalalgia 1997;17(5):588–90.
163. Tomkins GE, Jackson JL, O'Malley PG, et al. Treatment of chronic headache with antidepressants: a meta-analysis. Am J Med 2001;111(1):54–63.
164. Stillman MJ. Pharmacotherapy of tension-type headaches. Curr Pain Headache Rep 2002;6(5):408–13.
165. Holroyd KA. Behavioral and psychologic aspects of the pathophysiology and management of tension-type headache. Curr Pain Headache Rep 2002;6(5): 401–7.
166. Bogaards MC, ter Kuile MM. Treatment of recurrent tension headache: a meta-analytic review. Clin J Pain 1994;10(3):174–90.
167. Holroyd KA, O'Donnell FJ, Stensland M, et al. Management of chronic tension-type headache with tricyclic antidepressant medication, stress management therapy, and their combination: a randomized controlled trial. JAMA 2001; 285(17):2208–15.
168. Fernandez-de-Las-Penas C, Alonso-Blanco C, Cuadrado ML, et al. Are manual therapies effective in reducing pain from tension-type headache? A systematic review. Clin J Pain 2006;22(3):278–85.
169. Magnusson T, Carlsson GE. A 21/2-year follow-up of changes in headache and mandibular dysfunction after stomatognathic treatment. J Prosthet Dent 1983; 49(3):398–402.

Salivary Gland Disorders

Louis Mandel, DDS

KEYWORDS

• Salivary gland disease • Secretory dysfunction • Diagnosis

KEY POINTS

- Patients with salivary gland disease present with unique objective and/or subjective signs.
- An accurate diagnosis for these patients requires a range of techniques that includes the organized integration of information derived from their history, clinical examination, imaging, serology, and histopathology.
- This article highlights the signs and symptoms of the salivary gland disorders seen in the Salivary Gland Center, and emphasizes the methodology used to achieve a definitive diagnosis and therapy.

INTRODUCTION

Patients with salivary gland disease (SGD) present with unique objective and/or subjective signs. An accurate diagnosis for these patients requires a range of techniques that includes the organized integration of information derived from their history, clinical examination, imaging, serology, and histopathology. This article highlights the signs and symptoms of the salivary gland disorders seen in the Salivary Gland Center (SGC), and emphasizes the methodology used to achieve a definitive diagnosis and therapy.

SIALADENOSIS

Sialadenosis, or sialosis, is characterized by an asymptomatic bilateral enlargement of the salivary glands, usually the parotids and rarely the submandibulars, with no detectable underlying gland abnormality. The swellings are persistent, do not fluctuate in size, are usually symmetric, and when palpated are normal in tone and painless.

Sialadenosis occurs most commonly in relation to alcoholism, but can develop in diabetes mellitus (**Fig. 1**A), malnutrition, and even idiopathically.[1] It has been reported that the common denominator uniting these disparate systemic conditions is an autonomic neuropathy manifesting itself as a demyelinating polyneuropathy.[2,3] The neuropathy results in excessive salivary acinar protein synthesis and/or a failure of its adequate secretion. The resulting intracytoplasmic engorgement of the acinar cell

Department of Oral and Maxillofacial Surgery, Salivary Gland Center, Columbia University College of Dental Medicine, 630 West 168th Street, New York, NY 10032, USA
E-mail address: LM7@Columbia.edu

Med Clin N Am 98 (2014) 1407–1449
http://dx.doi.org/10.1016/j.mcna.2014.08.008
0025-7125/14/$ – see front matter © 2014 Elsevier Inc. All rights reserved.

medical.theclinics.com

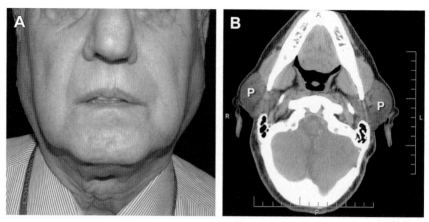

Fig. 1. (*A*) Bilateral parotid sialadenosis (diabetes mellitus). (*B*) Computed tomography (CT) scan (axial view) of the same diabetic patient. Note increased density of enlarged parotid glands (P).

by zymogen granules causes cell enlargement, which in turn leads to the visible clinical parotid hypertrophy.[4,5] The cellular hypertrophy may be facilitated by defective myoepithelial cells that fail to mechanically support the secreting acini.[6] Recently it has been suggested that aquaporin water channels, combined with a disturbance in body water, may play a role in the pathophysiologic events that initiate sialadenosis.[7,8]

Diagnosis is best achieved by integrating the patient's medical history, the clinical signs and symptoms of the glandular swelling, and information derived from available investigative procedures. A computed tomography (CT) scan of the parotid glands will clearly reveal their bilateral enlargements and their increased density (see **Fig. 1**B). The acinar cell hypertrophy seen in sialadenosis displaces the adipose cells and causes the observed increased gland density. Conversely, the CT scan may reveal a significant lucent parotid enlargement, which probably represents a marked fatty infiltration that reflects an end stage of sialadenosis.[9] Sialographic imaging of the duct system will reveal normal duct distribution and caliber. However, because of the glandular hypertrophy, the ducts will be widely dispersed. Fine-needle aspiration biopsy can be performed to histologically substantiate acinar cell hypertrophy.[1]

No effective therapy has been reported for elimination of the glandular swelling. Treatment is best directed toward care of the underlying medical condition. Some diminution in gland size will occur, but the long-term prognosis varies.

BULIMIA NERVOSA

Bulimia nervosa (BN), induced vomiting after an episode of binge eating, characteristically starts in a young woman whose self-image is that she is obese. Dieting may not be entirely successful, and because it is accompanied by periods of hunger, an eating binge occurs, which is then countered by self-induced purging. Before long the individual resorts to bingeing and vomiting not only when hungry but also when depressed, tense, or anxious.[10] The emetic episodes may be practiced for many years and as frequently as 20 times a day. Inevitably, systemic and local complications develop, including parotid swellings, dental damage, sialometaplasia necrotica, and electrolyte depletion.[11,12]

The frequent and continued emetic episodes often lead to bilateral, occasionally unilateral, parotid swellings whose signs and symptoms are similar to those seen in sialadenosis (**Fig. 2**A). The parotid enlargements are usually painless, persistent, do

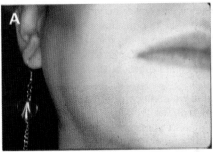 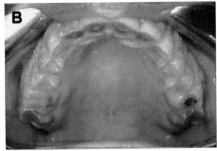

Fig. 2. (A) Bulimic patient with parotid swelling. Opposite parotid was also enlarged. (B) The same bulimic patient. Note extensive loss of palatal and occlusal enamel.

not fluctuate in size, and are normal in tone. Diagnosis is often impeded because patients are secretive about their purging episodes.

The pathophysiology of the parotid hypertrophy (PH) in BN is probably identical to that seen in sialadenosis. Accumulation of intracellular zymogen granules, resulting from a dysregulation of the acinar cell's sympathetic nerve supply, leads to the enlargement of individual parenchymal cells,[12] with confirmation obtained by electron microscopy and fine-needle aspiration biopsy.[2] CT contrast enhancement may be noted, and reflects the augmented vascularity associated with an active bulimic. Intraorally, dental defects are present along the palatal/lingual dental surfaces (see **Fig. 2**B). The constant projection of gastric acid from repeated vomiting against these surfaces results in corrosive demineralization of tooth enamel, with varying degrees of dentin exposure. Because vomiting is initiated by placing fingers into the mouth, a callused knuckle may develop from repetitive rubbing against the incisal edges of the maxillary anterior teeth. In addition, an unusual ulcerative lesion, sialometaplasia necrotica, may occur in the palate of BN patients for unknown reasons.[13]

The serum electrolyte study can be an important tool in diagnosing BN.[11] The multiple emetic episodes often result in hypokalemia and hypochloremia. Their alterations depend on many factors but include duration and frequency of vomiting, use of adjunctive agents, and nutritional replacement. The electrolyte depletions may require hospitalization for cardiac dysrhythmias.

In addition to restoring any abnormal electrolyte levels, the need to stop purging is apparent. Because of the underlying emotional problems, treatment includes psychiatric care supplemented with group, family, and behavioral therapies. As a rule, discontinuation of the vomiting will result in normal serum electrolyte levels and a gradual decrease of parotid gland swelling. Dental care is indicated for dental damage caused by the emetic effect on teeth.

ANOREXIA

Anorexia, a form of self-starvation, is frequently observed in bulimic patients. Extreme diet restriction, usually combined with emetic episodes, is used to attain the goal of thinness. Such practices lead to the signs and symptoms associated with bulimia.

PNEUMOPAROTID

Pneumoparotid, the retrograde forcing of air through the parotid orifice and into the salivary ducts, has been observed to cause unilateral or bilateral parotid swellings.[14,15]

It can occur in wind-instrument players, glass blowers, or any individual who increases intraoral pressure by forcefully blowing up the cheeks consciously or as a neurotic habit (**Fig. 3**A).[14,15] The anatomic design of the parotid duct orifice, as it exits on the intraoral buccal papillary fold, discourages such air reflux. Nevertheless, significant increases in intraoral pressure distort the musculature around the orifice and favor the entrance of air into the duct.

The extraoral parotid swelling is painless, and when palpated a crackling sensation, reflecting tissue emphysema, will be appreciated. The tell-tale sign of frothy, bubbly saliva exiting from Stensen orifice, when the gland is manually pressured, confirms the diagnosis (see **Fig. 3**B). This unique feature represents the mixture of air and saliva within the limited confines of the duct lumen.[14] Infection may become a consequence of continued forced reflux.

A CT scan will show evidence of a dilated Stensen duct caused by the contained air.[16] Similar duct changes will be noted in the gland proper. Sialography will confirm the dilation of the major duct and its tributaries.

Spontaneous regression of the pneumoparotid swelling can be expected within a few days. Because infection is a possibility, therapy requires cessation of the autoinsufflation. An unintentional habit often is involved, and a conscious effort to stop may be difficult. Psychiatric care may be indicated.

ANESTHESIA MUMPS

Anesthesia mumps is seen in association with general anesthesia during the intra-anesthetic or postanesthetic periods. Straining, coughing, and sneezing of the patient, during a difficult anesthetic procedure or postanesthetic period, serve to increase positive pressure in the oral cavity. Simultaneously adjunctive agents, such as succinyl-choline, cause a loss of muscle tone around the Stensen orifice and facilitate retrograde passage of air into the parotid duct. Bilateral or unilateral parotid swelling will usually be noted in the recovery room, often during extubation. The swellings are transient in nature, and subsidence within 1 to 5 days can be expected.[17]

ACUTE PAROTITIS

Acute parotitis (AP) is a bacterial suppurative process characterized by the sudden onset of a painful unilateral, occasionally bilateral, parotid swelling with the submandibular salivary gland infrequently involved. The infection is initiated by an ascending ductal infection and dehydration in those patients who are debilitated, immunocompromised, or systemically ill. It also may develop in those patients recovering from

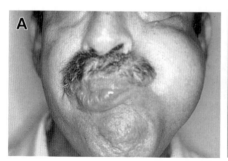 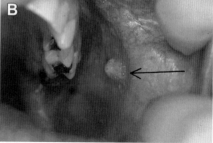

Fig. 3. (*A*) Pneumoparotid patient with habit of constantly blowing cheek out. (*B*) Aerated saliva exiting from Stensen duct in the same patient (*arrow*).

abdominal surgery who have had inadequate fluid replacement (**Fig. 4**A), and in the newborn via either a retrograde ductal or hematogenous route.[18] AP can lead to fatal consequences in a compromised patient.

Dehydration is the primary cause of AP and is brought about by factors that include sweating, emesis, blood loss, diarrhea, and insufficient fluid replacement. Hyposalivation develops, which may be accentuated by systemic medications with antisialogogic side effects.[19] Failure to eat with the loss of mastication's stimulatory effect on saliva and poor oral hygiene also favor the onset of AP. The ensuing loss of the lavaging and antibacterial actions of saliva allow for a significant increase in the oral bacteria, and in turn take part in encouraging the development of the ascending ductal infection that implicates the gland proper.

The most frequent organism involved is *Staphylococcus aureus*, although anaerobic and mixed infections have been recognized.[20] With bacterial localization in the gland parenchyma, swelling and pain develop. Extraoral palpation reveals a swelling that is firm, painful, warm, and erythematous. Intraorally the parotid orifice is red and prominent, and a free flow of pus is evident when the gland is manually pressured (see **Fig. 4**B). Trismus, fever, leukocytosis, and toxicity often accompany AP.

Diagnosis is based on the presence of dehydration, hyposalivation, and the classic local and systemic symptoms associated with an acute suppurative process that involves the parotid gland of a systemically compromised patient. Imaging (CT, magnetic resonance imaging [MRI]) of the involved parotid shows a localized abscess with peripheral enhancement from the vascular inflammatory infiltrate. Gland density increases in tandem with the extent of the inflammatory infiltrate.

Preventive treatment begins with improved fluid and electrolyte control to avoid dehydration. Prophylactic and therapeutic use of appropriate antibiotics is indicated. Rehydration and systemic supportive measures are mandatory. Because the parotid duct acts as an adequate draining mechanism, a conservative approach, minus surgical intervention, is an option. If the patient does not respond to this therapy, surgical incision and drainage are required.

CHRONIC PAROTITIS

Chronic parotitis (CP) is distinguished by a long history of unilateral moderately painful intermittent swellings interspersed with periods of asymptomatic remission. The waxing and waning continue with the extent of gland destruction, increasing with each flare-up. Usually a patient is observed with a swollen, tender parotid gland

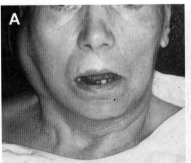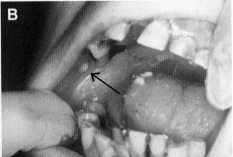

Fig. 4. (*A*) Acute right parotitis following abdominal surgery. (*B*) Acute parotitis (same patient). Note pus exiting from Stensen duct (*arrow*) in extremely dry mouth.

triggered by eating. Signs and symptoms of CP vary from a mild to a severe intractable form. The swellings may persist for hours, days, or weeks, but the repetitive nature eventually causes concern. The etiologic course of CP probably begins with decreased salivary production or impedance of its delivery.[21,22] The resulting failure of sufficient ductal lavage by saliva favors a low-grade ascending duct infection from the oral cavity. The intraluminal bacterial activity leads to inflammation, formation of mucous plugs, and stricturing. Occasionally a plug becomes lodged within the strictured duct's lumen, obstructs flow, and causes gland swelling during meals when increased saliva is produced. The swelling will subside as saliva seeps past the block or when the plug is flushed out by the salivary flow. However, a prolonged exacerbation can develop as a result of infection, obstruction, and stasis, and mimic the manifestations of AP. With the descending spiral that results from repeated bouts of glandular swelling, some patients develop severely compromised glands, which act as a substrate for further acute exacerbations.

During an episodic flare-up, the parotid swelling is indurated, tender, and may involve either a segment or the entire portion of the gland. Cervical lymphadenopathy is usually not present, and fever and malaise may be absent. Intraorally, a flow of saliva mixed with pus may be seen exiting from the Stensen orifice when the parotid is pressured extraorally. With remission, normal salivary quality and quantity will be observed.

Imaging is an indispensable modality in diagnosis. Sialography will depict the duct system clearly and a "sausage-like" pattern will be seen (**Fig. 5**). This duct appearance reflects the duct wall dilatation and stricturing that results from the effects of chronic bacterial infection. The damming effect of the stricture causes a reservoir effect with salivary retention and duct dilatation. The Stensen duct is primarily involved, but the gland's secondary ducts also demonstrate changes that are in direct proportion to CP's duration and severity.[21,23]

In contrast to sialography's depiction of the duct system, the CT scan serves to provide data concerning the parotid's parenchyma. An increased density and enhancement are apparent, which result from fibrosis and the infiltration of inflammatory agents into the normal moderately lucent parotid.

A conservative approach can be used when managing the parotid swelling. Antibiotics, ductal irrigations, probing to break up blockages, glandular massage, and sialogogic agents to increase salivary flow all have therapeutic value. However, sialendoscopy is now becoming the standard of care because it can be used for diagnosis and therapy.[24] The instrumentation is designed to visualize the major duct and to therapeutically irrigate and simultaneously balloon existing duct strictures. Retrograde

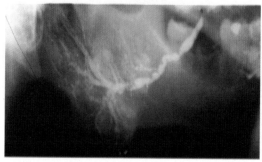

Fig. 5. Chronic parotitis shown by parotid sialogram. Stensen duct demonstrates classic "sausage" pattern characteristic of chronic parotitis.

duct injection of methyl violet to cause inflammation and sclerosis with pan-ductal fibrosis and gland atrophy has been advocated as a treatment.[25] When the symptoms of CP are severe and therapy is unsuccessful, parotid lobectomy is indicated.

HUMAN IMMUNODEFICIENCY VIRUS PAROTID DISEASE (DIFFUSE INFILTRATIVE LYMPHOCYTOSIS SYNDROME)

The oral region often serves as a target for the human immunodeficiency virus (HIV), with approximately 5% of HIV patients developing parotid enlargements (**Fig. 6**A).[26] These parotid gland (PG) swellings are usually bilateral, cystic, and associated with a generalized lymphadenopathy. Simultaneously, there also exists a persistent circulating CD8 lymphocytosis and diffuse visceral CD8 infiltrations. This symptom complex has been defined as the diffuse infiltrative CD8 lymphocytosis syndrome (DILS), with an immunogenetically distinct group (HLA-DR5) being most susceptible.[27] With viral replication, a massive parotid lymphoproliferation can also develop and cause an enlarged PG. However, bilateral benign parotid lymphoepithelial cysts (LEC) are the more likely cause of the swellings (see **Fig. 6**B). The LEC may originate from abnormally included glandular epithelium within an intraparotid lymph node. It also has been suggested that the lymphoid proliferation leads to duct obstruction and dilatation that mimics a true cyst.[28]

Multiple cysts are usually seen in each gland (**Fig. 7**). Even when the problem is clinically unilateral, imaging studies often confirm the existence of bilateral involvement. The swellings are large and cosmetically deforming, and can be either firm from the lymphoid hyperplasia or soft reflecting the presence of the LEC. Eating causes no fluctuation in size, and palpation indicates that the swellings are painless. Cervical lymphadenopathy is common. The PG swellings do not indicate HIV progression because DILS patients manifest a relatively benign disease progression in comparison with patients who do not have DILS.

Serology will diagnose the presence of HIV disease. The diagnosis of DILS is made when the aforementioned clinical PG picture is integrated with the serologic demonstration of a significant elevation of CD8 levels. Early recognition of the voluminous reactive lymphoid hyperplasia is essential. Although the LEC has not demonstrated progression to malignancy, the glandular interstitial lymphoproliferation may be a precursor to a mucosa-associated lymphoid tissue (MALT) lymphoma.

Parotidectomy was initially considered the treatment of choice for LEC. No treatment became an option because of the surgical morbidity associated with what is

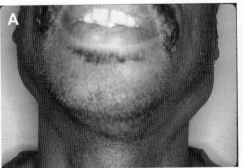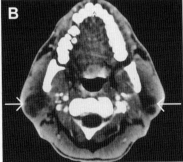

Fig. 6. (A) Human immunodeficiency virus (HIV) disease with bilateral parotid swelling. (B) CT scan (axial view) of HIV disease (same patient). Bilateral parotid cystic involvement is present (arrows).

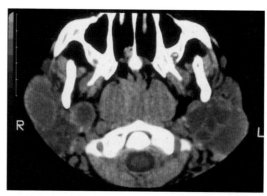

Fig. 7. CT scan (axial view) of HIV disease. Bilateral multicystic parotid enlargement.

essentially a cosmetic issue. Low-dose radiation therapy provides long-term cosmetic control of the LEC with few side effects and failures. Monitoring for the onset of a MALT lymphoma can be accomplished with periodic fine-needle aspiration biopsies. The introduction of highly active antiretroviral therapy (HAART) has resulted in effective reduction and control of the parotid swellings, and is sufficient to alleviate the cosmetic concerns of the patient.[29]

Unfortunately, collateral damage from HAART, in the form of metabolic disorders, is now recognized. A lipodystrophy syndrome from HAART therapy can develop, and is defined as a triad of significant body fat redistribution, dyslipidemia, and insulin resistance.[30,31] The fat redistribution can manifest itself in different regions as fatty hypertrophy or atrophy. A "buffalo hump," neck thickening, and breast and waist hypertrophy may develop. Wasting from fat atrophy may be noted with thinning of the extremities, the buttocks, and malar areas.[30] Patients can develop paraparotid fat depositions that simulate PG enlargement (**Fig. 8**). A definitive diagnosis is achieved when the CT scan demonstrates the increased presence of subcutaneous fat in the paraparotid region.[31]

EPIDEMIC PAROTITIS (MUMPS)

Epidemic parotitis (EP), or mumps, is a viral parotitis caused by a paramyxovirus.[32] An acute contagious disease primarily affecting children younger than 15 years, EP has a predilection for glandular and nervous tissue, and confers a lifelong immunity. After contact with airborne saliva droplets of an infected individual, viral entry into the nose or mouth is followed by viral proliferation in the salivary glands or in the surface epithelium of the respiratory tract. A generalized systemic infection results with detectable viral particles in saliva, serum, urine, and cerebrospinal fluid.[32]

The onset of clinical symptoms occurs 14 to 18 days after exposure, although there are patients who demonstrate no clinical signs of EP. Before the clinical symptoms of EP develop, a 2- to 3-day prodrome of fever, headache, myalgia, and malaise is present. Classically only parotid enlargement, unilateral or more often bilateral, is observed (**Fig. 9**).[33] Involvement of the PG is also signaled by glandular pain, trismus, and dysphagia. After the incubation period, the parotid swellings peak in 1 to 5 days. Initially one gland becomes swollen with contralateral involvement following within 5 days, but simultaneous involvement of both glands also occurs.[32] Palpation of the swollen parotids will reveal them to be very firm and tender. Viral edema causes the observed parotid swelling, but because the physical expansion of the gland is limited

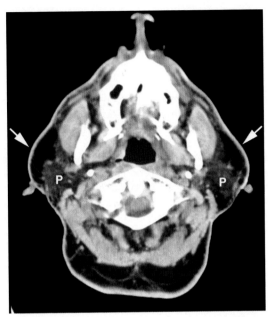

Fig. 8. CT scan (axial view) showing lipodystrophy syndrome with paraparotid fat deposition (*arrows*) around parotids (P) in an HIV patient.

by its tense fibrous capsule, mounting intraparotid pressure leads to the significant pain associated with EP. Examination of the salivary return at the Stensen orifice will reveal a clear but somewhat diminished salivary flow. The PG swellings last for 5 to 7 days, during which time the patient is contagious and should be isolated.

Submandibular or sublingual salivary gland symptoms may also develop with or without parotid signs. Additionally and particularly in adults, complications such as orchitis, meningitis, encephalitis, pancreatitis, and oophoritis may be observed. Because the disease confers immunity, support for a firm diagnosis of EP can be derived from a history of never having had mumps. A history of exposure to the virus 2 to 3 weeks before the onset of symptoms and a compatible clinical picture of parotitis facilitate diagnosis. Laboratory testing for diagnostic antibodies and the presence of viral particles in saliva, blood, urine, or cerebrospinal fluid confirm the diagnosis.

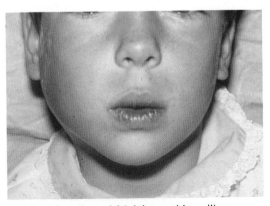

Fig. 9. Epidemic parotitis with unilateral (*right*) parotid swelling.

Vaccination with live attenuated virus contained in the measles-mumps-rubella (MMR) vaccine serves as the best preventive measure. Because EP is a self-limiting disease, treatment is symptomatic and supportive.

SIALOLITHIASIS

Sialolithiasis, or salivary stones, are calcium concretions within the salivary duct system that most frequently involve the submandibular salivary gland (SMSG) (**Fig. 10**). Approximately 83% of salivary stones are found in the SMSG while 10% involve the PG, and 7% are located in the sublingual and minor salivary glands.[34] These stones occur equally in both sexes and in any age category, and can be single or multiple, unilateral or bilateral, and in the intraglandular or extraglandular duct systems. The SMSG is more susceptible than the PG to stone formation, primarily because of its greater salivary concentration of calcium and phosphate salts, and because of the relative viscosity of its mucus secretions in comparison with the PG's aqueous serous secretions.[35] Although the exact evolution of sialolithiasis is unknown, 3 prerequisites seem to be causally implicated. Initially a nidus, a complex glycoprotein gel, develops. The nidus is probably caused by a subclinical retrograde duct infection that initiates a change in the saliva's mucoid molecule.[35,36] Salivary stasis, the second prerequisite, results from the nidal obstruction. The third element, a precipitation of salts into the glycoprotein matrix, ensues. With continued mineral deposition, a clinically apparent sialolith becomes evident.

Because most stones involve the SMSG, the following description of the diagnostic signs, symptoms, and therapy for sialolithiasis is mostly focused on the SMSG system. The SGC has noted 3 different clinical manifestations for the presence of salivary stones. First, there may be total absence of symptoms, with the sialolith identified only as an incidental finding during an imaging study. More often, a history of intermittent swellings of the involved gland, associated with eating, is elicited. During meals, the increased salivary production meeting the obstructive stone results in salivary retention and glandular swelling. Because the sialolith only partially blocks the duct lumen, saliva seeps past the stone and the glandular swelling subsides. This process may repeat itself with varying periods of remission. Eventually the third clinical manifestation, an acute suppurative process, will develop. Bacterial infection, secondary to the salivary stasis caused by the obstructing stone, is the culprit. An extraoral persistent, painful, indurated, and infected gland swelling becomes apparent (**Fig. 11A**). The swelling does not subside between meals, and eating exacerbates the symptoms.

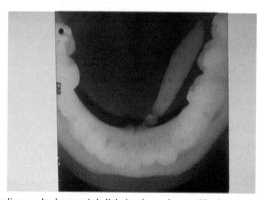

Fig. 10. Occlusal radiograph shows sialolith in the submandibular duct.

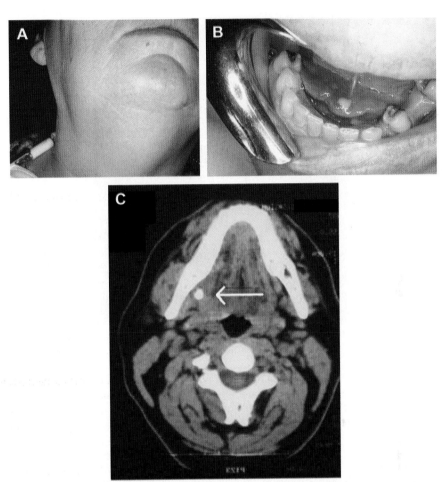

Fig. 11. (*A*) Extraoral view of acute submandibular salivary gland swelling. (*B*) Intraoral view (same patient). Inflamed mouth floor with pus exiting from submandibular duct orifice. (*C*) CT scan (axial view) with no contrast (same patient) shows sialolith posterior segment submandibular duct (*arrow*).

Intraorally the floor of the mouth along the course of the submandibular duct is swollen, erythematous, tender, and indurated. Pus can be observed exiting from the duct's orifice (see **Fig. 11**B). Systemic toxicity is not uncommon.

The history and clinical picture are essential features in the successful diagnosis of sialolithiasis. Palpation may also disclose the stone's position, but sialoliths in the more proximal segment of the submandibular duct cannot be readily palpated because the duct in this location courses through the tissues at a deep level. Imaging serves as the key diagnostic tool. A dental occlusal film of the mouth floor will often successfully reveal a sialolith in the anterior two-thirds of the submandibular duct. However, a CT scan is required for stones that are posteriorly positioned within the submandibular duct or hilus (see **Fig. 11**C). The CT scan also serves as the best means of diagnosing a stone in the PG system (**Fig. 12**). The value of CT is derived from the procedure being exquisitely sensitive to minute amounts of calcification. The scan will establish the precise position of the stone within the duct, and simultaneously assess

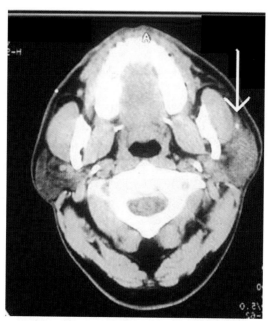

Fig. 12. CT scan (axial view, no contrast) shows a sialolith at junction of parotid duct with gland (*arrow*). Note increased parotid density caused by inflammatory infiltrate.

the status of the implicated gland. Contrast should be avoided because a contrast-enhanced blood vessel can mimic the appearance of a stone. Sialography is a venerable technique that can reveal the presence of a sialolith and its effect on the ductal system. Ultrasonography has limited diagnostic value because of its poor sensitivity in the imaging of small stones.

Until recently, an intraoral surgical approach has been widely used to remove stones in the submandibular duct anterior to the mandibular second molar or in the anterior 2 cm of the parotid duct. Stones in the hilar area of the submandibular duct or proximally placed in the Stensen duct may require an extraoral surgical approach that involves gland removal and sialolithectomy. Newer surgical approaches have now been described to surgically remove posteriorly placed submandibular stones via an intraoral approach.[37] Alternatively, lithotripsy or lasers have been used to fragment stones.[38] Failure occurs when the sialolith is larger than 7 mm or when the fragments fail to flush out, probably because of the lack of adequate salivary hydrostatic pressure.[39] Sialendoscopy has diagnostic value and has also become a popular means of noninvasive removal of duct stones.[40] Instrument miniaturization has made it possible to use a 1.1-mm diameter flexible endoscope that can enter the duct orifice. With visualization of the sialolith, an attached Dormia basket is used to grasp and remove the stone. The success of the sialendoscopic technique is limited by its failure to negotiate the anatomic bend in the most proximal segment of the submandibular duct and its inability to deal with larger sialoliths. To overcome the problem of a large stone, a combined lithotripsy and endoscopic procedure has been suggested.[41]

SJÖGREN SYNDROME

Sjögren syndrome (SS), a multisystem autoimmune disease mostly affecting women, causes hypofunction of the salivary and lacrimal glands. Only the lacrimal and salivary glands are involved in primary SS, the sicca syndrome. Secondary SS, the triad, is associated with a systemic autoimmune disease, usually rheumatoid arthritis, lupus erythematosus, or systemic sclerosis. Histologically a florid lymphoproliferation in the exocrine salivary (**Fig. 13**) and lacrimal glands leads to parenchymal replacement and the clinically observed hyposalivation and hypolacrimation. Systemic involvement can develop, including pulmonary disease, vasculitis, lymphadenopathy, Raynaud phenomenon, autoimmune thyroiditis, hepatosplenomegaly, achlorhydria, leukopenia, and thrombocytopenia.

The established criteria for the diagnosis of SS, endorsed by the American College of Rheumatology, are based on objective testing rather than subjective symptomatology.[42] The diagnosis of SS, which applies to individuals with the signs and symptoms suggestive of SS, is achieved in patients who have at least 2 of the following 3 objective features:

1. Positive serum anti-SSA and/or anti-SSB, or a positive rheumatoid factor and antinuclear antibody titer of 1:320 or higher
2. Labial salivary gland biopsy with a focal lymphocytic sialadenitis and a focus score of 1 or more foci per 4 mm^2
3. Keratoconjunctivitis sicca with an ocular staining score of 3 or higher

In patients with SS, marked salivary volume reductions become apparent. Burning sensation, difficulty with swallowing dry foods, loss of taste, and mucosal pain from the pressure created by removable dentures all cause patients concern. In addition, the tongue often takes on a cobblestone appearance, and candidiasis can become a problem. Rampant dental caries, resulting from the significant hyposalivation and loss of saliva's protective properties, are a marker of SS (**Fig. 14**).

PG swellings frequently develop in association with SS. Recurrent PG swellings, inflammatory and obstructive in nature, mimic the symptoms of CP. These swellings result from an ascending ductal infection that is assisted by the decreased salivary duct lavage. Occasionally a painless, persistent, neoplastic-like swelling will be observed. Such a condition may represent the onset of a MALT lymphoma, a B-cell lymphoma.

Imaging can be of value in the diagnosis of SS. Parotid sialography will usually demonstrate the sialectic pattern seen in the presence of dilated minor ducts (**Fig. 15**). Anechoic and hypoechoic areas, reflecting dilated ducts and

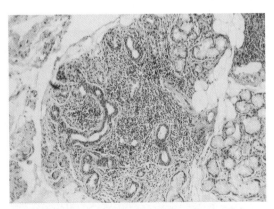

Fig. 13. Sjögren syndrome. Positive labial gland biopsy with glandular parenchyma replaced by a lymphoproliferation and duct ectasia (H&E stain, magnification ×100).

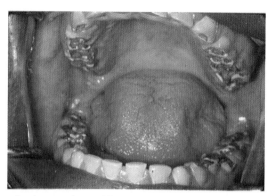

Fig. 14. Rampant caries in a patient with Sjögren syndrome.

lymphoproliferative masses, can be identified by ultrasonography. Close scrutiny of a parotid CT scan often will show multiple pinpoint lucencies reflecting duct dilations.

Prompt diagnosis is imperative because local and systemic symptomatology can be palliated. Continued observation is mandatory because of the propensity for lymphoma development. A primary oral concern is the extensive level of dental caries often observed in SS patients. Aggressive fluoride therapy in the form of topical applications, mouthwashes, and toothpaste should be encouraged. Some success in increasing salivary production has been attained with the use of pilocarpine or cevimeline. Salivary production can also be stimulated with sugarless sour candy or sugarless chewing gum. Oral moisturizers and artificial salivas are available commercially.

Traditional systemic therapy includes hydroxychloroquine (Plaquenil), but the results are questionable. Interferon, cyclosporine, methotrexate, azathioprine, and corticosteroids have been used with limited success. Rituximab has seen suggested for the severe inflammatory manifestations of SS.[43]

IMMUNOGLOBULIN G4–RELATED SIALADENITIS

Recently, immunoglobulin G4 (IgG4)-related sialadenitis has been identified and defined as a sclerosing SGD with a predilection to involve the SMSG, often bilaterally (**Fig. 16**). Mikulicz disease, a bilateral, painless, persistent symmetric swelling of the

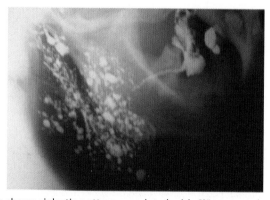

Fig. 15. Sialogram shows sialectic pattern associated with Sjögren syndrome.

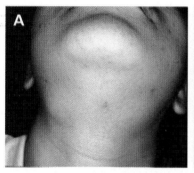
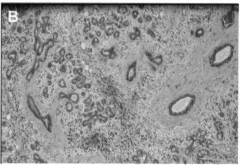

Fig. 16. (*A*) Bilateral submandibular salivary gland swellings in immunoglobulin G4 disease. (*B*) Microscopic view shows marked sclerosis and duct ectasia with absence of submandibular gland parenchyma (same patient) (H&E stain, magnification ×100).

parotid and SMSGs, previously thought to be a subtype of SS, is now considered a manifestation of IgG4-related sialadenitis.[44,45] Kuttner tumor, first described by Kuttner as a chronic sclerosing sialadenitis, is also now defined as an IgG4-related sclerosing disease.[44,45]

A diagnosis of IgG4 sialadenitis is based on its recognition as a systemic sclerosing disease with extensive infiltrations of IgG4-positive plasma cells and lymphocytes into various organs. Autoimmune pancreatitis, tubulointerstitial nephritis, and retroperitoneal fibrosis are the most frequently observed systemic extrasalivary gland lesions. Serum IgG4 levels are usually elevated. Patients respond to steroid therapy, and recovery of gland function can be expected.

SARCOIDOSIS

Sarcoidosis is a multisystem, noncaseating granulomatous disorder of unknown etiology with a possible genetic predisposition.[46] It commonly affects young adults, and has a predilection for the lungs and hilar lymph nodes. Respiratory symptoms, bilateral hilar lymphadenopathy and/or pulmonary infiltrates, and skin and ocular lesions are classic signs of sarcoidosis. Swelling of parotid glands has been reported to occur in 6% of patients with sarcoidosis (**Fig. 17**A).[47] SMSG involvement is not as common, but 58% of the labial salivary glands will show the pathognomonic granuloma (see **Fig. 17**B).[48] The major glandular swellings are usually bilateral, firm, persistent, and painless. Spontaneous regression of the swellings can occur. The gland swellings

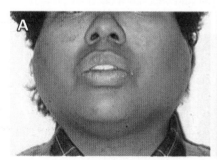
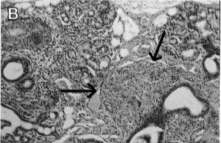

Fig. 17. (*A*) Sarcoidosis. Bilateral parotid swelling. (*B*) Sarcoidosis (same patient). Labial gland histology shows granuloma (*arrows*) (H&E stain, magnification ×150).

may develop simultaneously with systemic signs or after the onset of systemic sarcoidosis, or even herald the onset of systemic disease.[49] Hyposalivation results from replacement of parenchymal cells by the multiplying granulomas.

Uveoparotid fever, or Heerfordt syndrome, is a clinical triad of symptoms associated with sarcoidosis. Inflammation of the uveal tract of the eye, bilateral parotid swelling, and cranial nerve involvement, usually seventh nerve paralysis, characterize the syndrome.

Diagnosis is established when the clinical and radiographic findings are integrated with the histology while other granulomatous diseases are excluded. Microscopic evidence from the biopsy of a minor salivary gland (labial gland) can reveal the noncaseating cell granulomas. Alternatively, an incisional biopsy of a swollen major gland will provide similar evidence. Serology usually reveals an increase of the angiotensin-converting enzyme, a nonspecific sign, resulting from its production by the epithelioid cells in the granulomas. Gallium scintigraphy causes the radioisotope to accumulate in the nasopharynx and parotid and lacrimal glands, and mimic the dark facial markings seen in the giant panda.

Observation is a viable therapeutic option because of spontaneous remissions. However, the increased tendency of sarcoid patients to develop lymphomas demands close monitoring. Corticosteroids represent the primary therapeutic approach, but a variety of immunosuppressives has also been proved to be successful. Infliximab has been used effectively to treat refractory cases.[50]

RECURRENT PAROTITIS IN CHILDREN

Recurrent parotitis in children (RPC), or juvenile parotitis with sialectasis, is observed in children, with the highest incidence between 3 and 6 years of age (**Fig. 18**). The condition involves males slightly more than females, and has a marked tendency to regress with puberty. Both parotids are usually involved, but the swellings tend to be unilateral in presentation. Swellings are sudden in onset and may be accompanied by pain and fever. Recurrences are common and tend to occur 1 to 5 times each year. Each episode lasts 3 to 7 days and usually subsides without treatment.

The saliva in RPC often contains visible flocculations, of questionable origin, which may aggregate to form obstructive mucous plugs that may serve as the precipitator of the parotid swellings. It may be that as the pressure of the obstructed retained saliva increases, spontaneous plug extrusion occurs. Salivary flow resumes, and the parotid swelling subsides provided infection is not a factor.

The etiology of RPC has not been determined. Because no serologic test exists for RPC, diagnosis must be based on the clinical symptomatology and imaging via sialography or ultrasonography.[51,52] Sialography will demonstrate a sialectic pattern (see

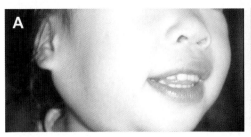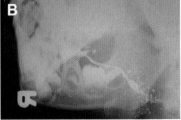

Fig. 18. (*A*) Recurrent parotitis in child. (*B*) Same patient. Sialogram shows pathognomonic sialectic pattern.

Fig. 18B) while ultrasonography will show multiple round hypoechoic areas. Each sonolucent area reflects the histologic presence of duct dilation and a surrounding periductal lymphocytic infiltration. The mechanism initiating this histologic process is not understood.

NEOPLASMS

Salivary gland tumors represent 3% to 6% of all adult head and neck tumors seen in the United States.[53] The mean age for a malignant tumor is between 55 and 65 years, and benign growths occur 10 years earlier.[53] Most neoplasms (70%–85%) occur in the PG while 8% to 15% develop in the SMSG and less than 1% involves the sublingual gland.[54] Minor salivary gland neoplasms are responsible for 5% to 8% of the total (**Fig. 19**).[54] In general, the smaller the salivary gland, the more likely it is to harbor a malignant growth. Parotid tumors are malignant in 15% to 25% of cases, while 37% to 43% of the tumors in the submandibular system and 80% of the tumors in the sublingual and minor salivary glands are malignant.[54]

Diagnosis of a salivary gland neoplasm depends on a detailed history and clinical examination. Obviously a definitive diagnosis is based on histologic examination of the lesion. Benign tumors tend to be slow-growing, localized, and subjectively painless masses (**Fig. 20**). Palpation indicates that they are circumscribed, movable, soft or firm, and painless. There are no facial nerve deficits or cervical lymphadenopathies. Malignant tumors tend to grow rapidly, can be painful, are not well circumscribed, and may demonstrate central necrosis (**Fig. 21**). These tumors are firm, infiltrate the surrounding tissues, and become fixed in position. Parotid malignancies often invade the facial nerve and cause facial motor loss. Because of the malignancy's ability to metastasize, cervical lymphadenopathy is a diagnostic sign.

Imaging studies (CT, MRI, ultrasonography) are key components in achieving a diagnosis. The imaged margins of the mass, the lesion's composition, and its location in the gland are helpful in differentiating a benign from a malignant growth and determining the surgical approach. A fine-needle aspiration biopsy often can demonstrate sufficient cytologic data for an exact histologic diagnosis. Nevertheless, a tissue specimen from an incisional biopsy represents the gold standard in diagnosis.

Histologically the pleomorphic adenoma is the most commonly occurring benign salivary gland tumor. It tends to be lobulated, and has a thin and often incomplete capsule with small tumor projections that extend into the surrounding normal glandular parenchyma. These histologic elements inhibit successful surgical removal via blunt dissection. The papillary cystadenoma lymphomatosum, or Warthin tumor is the second most common benign parotid growth. It is unique in that it can occur

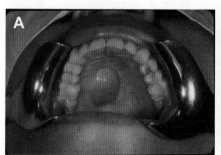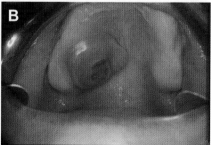

Fig. 19. (*A*) Benign salivary gland tumor (palate). (*B*) Malignant salivary gland tumor (palate). Note ulceration.

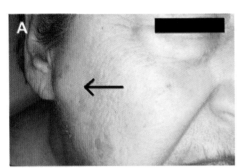
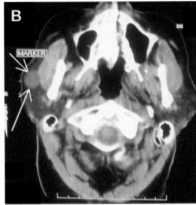

Fig. 20. (A) Benign parotid neoplasm (arrow). (B) Same patient. Benign parotid neoplasm (arrows) seen on CT scan, axial view.

bilaterally. A third parotid benign epithelial tumor, the oncocytoma, is usually seen in older patients.

The mucoepidermoid carcinoma is the most common malignant lesion of the PG, and presents itself in both low-grade and high-grade varieties. The adenoid cystic carcinoma is the most frequent salivary malignancy to involve the submandibular gland. This tumor has an indolent but relentless growth pattern as it extends along perineural lymphatics.

Surgery remains the treatment of choice for all salivary gland tumors. The usual benign parotid tumor is best removed via a superficial lobe parotidectomy. The SMSG, containing a benign tumor, lends itself to a total gland extirpation because of its anatomic configuration and its well-defined capsule. Malignant lesions demand extensive surgery whose success is defined by obtaining adequate margins. Cervical lymphadenopathy is performed as either a therapeutic or prophylactic procedure. Radiation and chemotherapy are used when necessary.

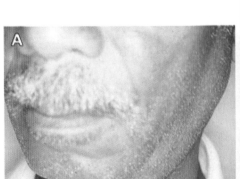
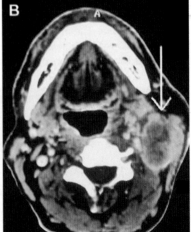

Fig. 21. (A) Malignant parotid neoplasm. (B) CT scan of the same patient. Malignant neoplasm (arrow) with central necrosis.

RADIATION SIALADENITIS
External Beam Radiation

More than 50,000 patients receive head and neck cancer treatments with external beam radiation (EBR) each year.[55] A major concern is the hyposalivation that develops when EBR involves the salivary glands and exceeds 15 to 20 Gy.[56] Salivary production by serous acini is readily affected within 1 week, whereas the mucous acini of the submandibular/sublingual salivary gland complex seem to be more resistant and are only damaged at higher dose levels. In addition, although the acini are primarily afflicted, the ducts usually remain intact. Some recovery of salivary secretion can be anticipated provided a dose of less than 26 Gy has been administered.[57] It has been reported that irreversible hyposalivation results from doses of greater than 40 Gy, with the surviving glandular tissue functioning only at levels of 5% to 15% of normal.[58] Cumulative doses of 60 Gy cause glandular atrophy and fibrosis with only minimal saliva production.[59]

The marked reduction in salivary secretion from EBR causes significant patient discomfort. Not only does salivary volume diminish but its consistency becomes extremely viscous, a result of saliva's serous element being more affected proportionately than the secretions from the more radiation-resistant mucous acini. With the loss of saliva's lubricating, buffering, and antimicroorganism powers, mucositis, rampant caries (**Fig. 22**), candidiasis, dysgeusia, dysphagia, and trismus may be encountered.

Combining the patient's medical history with the clinical examination facilitates a diagnosis of EBR hyposalivation. Treatment begins with preventive measures that include the use of 3-dimensional and intensity-modulated radiotherapeutic approaches. The aim is to limit salivary gland irradiation while targeting the neoplasm. Amifostine, a cytoprotectant, may also serve to limit injury to the salivary glands.

Treatment of the oral conditions resulting from EBR includes a variety of palliative techniques. Aggressive fluoride therapy is necessary to control the extensive dental caries that will develop with the significant salivary loss. The sialogogues pilocarpine or cevimeline can be prescribed, along with the adjunctive use of sugarless chewing gum or sour candy, to stimulate any residual surviving salivary parenchyma. Artificial salivas, moisturizers, and lubricant mouthwashes are available commercially to ameliorate the subjective discomfort originating from a dry mouth. Candidiasis can be treated with antifungals. Oral hygiene must be scrupulously maintained, and dehydration should be avoided.

Radioactive Iodine

Radioactive iodine (^{131}I) (**Box 1**) plays an effective role in the treatment of differentiated papillary and follicular thyroid carcinomas. This radioisotope targets these thyroid cancers, but simultaneously a significant proportion of the administered ^{131}I is concentrated

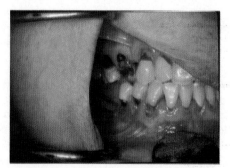

Fig. 22. Cancericidal radiation has caused hyposalivation and rampant cervical caries.

Box 1
Radiation sialadenitis

Radiation to the salivary glands, whether delivered by external beam radiation for head and cancer or in the form of ingested radioactive iodine (^{131}I) used for the treatment of thyroid cancer, will inevitably lead to radiation sialadenitis and its concomitant symptomatology.

---

and secreted into the saliva by the salivary glands. The sodium iodide symporter molecule, the transport mechanism, resides in duct epithelium. As the ^{131}I passes through the duct epithelium into the duct lumen, the lining cells become damaged. A thickening of the duct's epithelial lining, a metaplasia, and luminal obstruction by an inflammatory exudate develop. Dose-related and time-related damage to the salivary tissues becomes manifest, most often in the PG. Transient obstructive swellings and pain associated with eating occur. Almost immediately after ^{131}I therapy 39% of the patients develop these problems, whereas some patients develop symptoms months later.[60,61]

The effect of ^{131}I on the excretory ducts and gland parenchyma are independent of each other. The usual therapeutic ^{131}I dose varies between 50 and 130 mCi. At these levels, gland swelling from duct wall damage and obstruction becomes apparent. After 7 years symptom resolution occurs, with only 5% of patients reporting salivary gland problems.[60] Aggressive thyroid malignancies, with or without metastases, require higher doses of ^{131}I. The secreting parenchyma will then be affected and hyposalivation, with its collateral issues of mucositis, dysgeusia, oral dryness, oral burning, and dysphagia, becomes a frequent patient complaint.

Diagnosis of a ^{131}I gland injury is made by relating the medical history to the clinical findings. The extent of gland injury can be determined by a scintigraphic study (**Fig. 23**). Abnormalities in glandular uptake and secretory ability will be observed in asymmetric combinations of the major salivary glands.

Preventive treatment starts with the use of sialogogic agents, such as sour candy or pilocarpine, whose aim is to have the damaging radioisotope pass through the salivary glands as rapidly as possible. The cytoprotectant amifostine has also been used to protect the salivary glands. However, these preventive approaches have had questionable success. Obstructive symptoms can be treated by probing, sialendoscopic procedures, and sialogogues to increase secretion, followed by forceful gland massage to flush the duct. Dexamethasone duct irrigations have met with some success. Oral dryness can be treated in the same manner as for those patients who develop similar symptomatology from EBR.

IODIDE MUMPS

Iodide mumps, first described in a kidney-impaired patient after undergoing intravenous pyelography,[62] can develop after any imaging procedure that uses iodine-based contrast medium. Patients usually exhibit painless bilateral parotid or submandibular gland swellings that are rapid in onset, and gradually disappear over a 6-day period.[63] No long-term consequences occur.

The etiologic key for the salivary gland swellings is the plasma iodide level. Increased levels result from the intravenous introduction of large amounts of iodine-containing compounds, the contrast dyes, and may be facilitated by an inadequately functioning kidney. Extremely high levels of plasma iodide can damage the salivary duct epithelium whose sodium iodide symporter molecule transports the iodide into the duct lumen. Duct wall inflammation will lead to obstruction with salivary gland swelling.[64] Some immediate reactions are allergic and may be accompanied by urticaria, bronchospasms, and angioneurotic edema. Delayed swellings probably

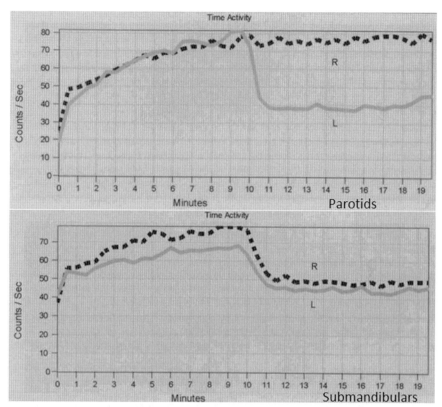

Fig. 23. Scintigram of salivary glands following administration of therapeutic radioactive iodine. Left (L) parotid and both submandibular glands show normal uptake and release of radioisotope. Right (R) parotid demonstrates normal uptake but failure to secrete isotope at 10-minute mark because of obstructed parotid duct.

represent toxic reactions. Steroids and antihistamines are used for prevention, while therapy includes anti-inflammatory medications or observation.

NEUROLOGIC IMPAIRMENT AND THE SALIVARY GLANDS

Some surgical procedures in the head and neck region can result in damage to a salivary gland's nerve supply. The resulting iatrogenic neurologic impairment manifests in several ways (**Box 2**).

SIALOCELE

A parotid sialocele, a subcutaneous accumulation of saliva, usually results from a traumatic event. Laceration of the parotid duct or one of its intraglandular tributaries causes salivary leakage. Most commonly the problem originates from external trauma (knife wound, automobile accident) that sections the duct. Mobilization of the superficial musculoaponeurotic sheath during a rhytidectomy, parotidectomy, temporomandibular surgery, or any surgical procedure performed in close proximity to the parotid that inadvertently traumatizes a duct may also initiate the onset of a sialocele.[65,66]

Clinically a soft, cyst-like swelling develops. The swelling involves the face's parotid/masseteric area, and tends to be painless unless it becomes secondarily infected. An

---

Box 2
Manifestations of iatrogenic neurologic impairment

1. Auriculotemporal syndrome (ATS), also known as Frey syndrome, is characterized by sweating, flushing, and warmth in the preauricular and temporal areas when saliva is stimulated (eating) **(Fig. 24)**. Besides supplying parasympathetic secretory fibers to the parotid, the auriculotemporal nerve (ATN) transmits sensory fibers to the preauricular region and sympathetic fibers to preauricular sweat glands. The ATN sympathetic fibers also serve as vasoconstrictors in the preauricular area. Parotidectomy can sever the ATN's sympathetic and parasympathetic innervation to these structures. Subsequently, regenerating parasympathetic nerve fibers enter the axon sheath of the severed postganglionic sympathetic fibers that formerly supplied sweat glands and blood vessels in the overlying skin. Masticatory stimulation of the ATN will result in facial sweating, with preauricular flushing and warmth from vasodilation, signifying the presence of the ATS.

2. The chorda tympani nerve (CTN) courses through the middle ear in intimate relation with the stapes. Not infrequently, stapes surgery for otosclerosis damages the CTN. Altered taste and hyposalivation can develop. The CTN is responsible, after synapsing in the submandibular ganglion, for secretory stimulation of the submandibular/sublingual salivary gland complex. A damaged CTN causes a decreased salivary production from this complex, which is responsible for producing approximately 68% of resting whole saliva. Therefore, these patients may describe clinical symptoms consistent with dryness only during oral rest. With salivary stimulation from food, a compensatory increase in parotid secretion occurs, producing sufficient saliva to overcome the subjective xerostomia.[126]

3. First-bite syndrome (FBS) is characterized by severe pain in the parotid area with the first bite of food.[127] Surgery performed in the area of the parapharyngeal space may traumatize the sympathetic chain's superior cervical ganglion (SCG) and its postganglionic fibers. These fibers run with the external carotid artery as a plexus to innervate the parotid gland and face. Injury to the SCG or plexus leads to loss of sympathetic innervation to the parotid. It is hypothesized that with salivary stimulation from food there is a release of parotid parasympathetic neurotransmitters that cross over to stimulate sympathetic receptors on the duct myoepithelial cells, which have developed denervation supersensitivity. The increased response of these cells is thought to cause the spasms of pain arising from stimulation by the first bite of food.

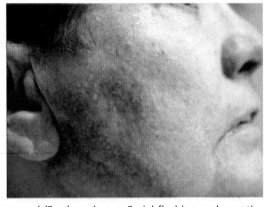

Fig. 24. Auriculotemporal (Frey) syndrome. Facial flushing and sweating are evident.

extraoral fistula can develop if the swelling is not treated. Fine-needle aspiration of salivary fluid and imaging, combined with a history of trauma and its associated clinical symptomatology, serve to establish the diagnosis.

Conservative treatment involves repeated aspirations followed by aggressive compression and the adjunctive use of antisialogogic medications. Botulinum toxin, sclerotherapy, and radiation have been used therapeutically. Surgical repair of the parotid duct is only feasible when performed shortly after the traumatic event. Parotidectomy is advocated when conservative approaches fail.

DILATATION OF STENSEN DUCT

Dilatation of the Stensen duct (DSD) may have a congenital background. These dilations are first noticed by patients as a unique and peculiar facial swelling, somewhat tubular in configuration, located along the course of the Stensen duct (**Fig. 25**). These horizontal distentions have a long-standing presence, with periods during which they become more prominent. The painless swellings of the cheek have no obvious cause, can occur at any age, are unrelated to eating, and are usually unilateral in presentation.[67,68] Palpation indicates that the swellings tend to be soft and defined. If secondary infection intervenes, the swellings become painful and indurated. Aggressive massage causes an emptying of collected saliva from the distended noninfected parotid duct. A decrease in the size of the deformity results, but total remission is not achieved.

Imaging, combined with the clinical picture, facilitates DSD diagnosis. A CT scan will clearly demonstrate the distended parotid duct as it courses along the lateral border of the masseter muscle (see **Fig. 25**B). If there is infection or history of infection, the changes associated with CP will be observed. Sialography can also serve to reveal the presence of the duct dilatation.

Conservative management by milking the swelling and evacuating the retained saliva into the oral cavity is an option. Duct orifice marsupialization with its suturing

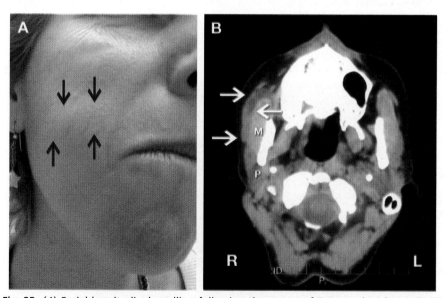

Fig. 25. (A) Facial longitudinal swelling following the course of Stensen duct (*arrows*). (B) Same patient (CT scan, axial view) with significant dilation of right Stensen duct (*arrows*). M, masseter muscle; P, parotid gland.

to the buccal mucosa has been suggested.[69] Surgical parotidectomy is advocated when there is a history of repeated infectious episodes.[68]

SUBMANDIBULAR DUCT ATRESIA

Submandibular salivary duct orifice atresia is a developmental anomaly observed in the newborn. The SMSG develops during the 10th to 12th weeks of embryonic life. At approximately 28 weeks of fetal life, a hollowing out of its duct lumen occurs.[70] Anterior duct atresia results when the hollowing process is incomplete and fails to incorporate the orifice area. Salivary retention, posterior to the imperforate orifice, develops. A cyst-like swelling in the mouth floor, mimicking a ranula, is the end result (**Fig. 26**A). MRI reveals an elongated, dilated, tubular, segmentally lobed structure in the mouth floor that is consistent with the anatomic course of the Wharton duct (see **Fig. 26**B).[71] Surgical success is achieved by filleting the distended duct and suturing its wings to the adjoining mouth floor mucosa.

SALIVARY GLAND APLASIA

Aplasia of the parotid or SMSGs is not always subjectively symptomatic. Any one or group of these salivary glands may be absent, and their absence can be seen in a variety of unilateral or bilateral combinations.[72] Furthermore, salivary gland aplasia may occur alone or in association with other anomalies, particularly defects in the lacrimal apparatus.[73] Intraorally there is an absence of the involved gland's orifice and papilla. Salivary production diminishes, but some mucosal moisture may be present, reflecting the continued presence and function of the minor salivary glands and any unaffected major gland.[74–79] The hyposalivation will inevitably lead to extensive dental breakdown (**Fig. 27**), oral burning, lip dryness, and dysphagia.

HYPERPLASIA OF SUBLINGUAL SALIVARY GLAND

Hyperplasia of sublingual salivary gland (SLSG) manifests itself as an observed enlargement of the intraoral sublingual fold beneath which the SLSG lies. Palpation indicates that the swelling is painless, normal in tone, and not circumscribed. For

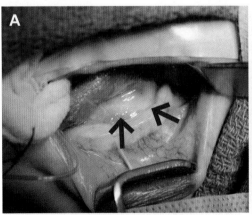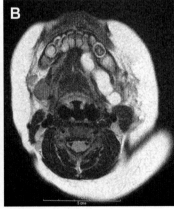

Fig. 26. (*A*) Submandibular duct atresia in an infant. Swelling of mouth floor (*arrows*) mimics a ranula. (*B*) Submandibular duct atresia (same patient). Magnetic resonance imaging reveals segmented duct.

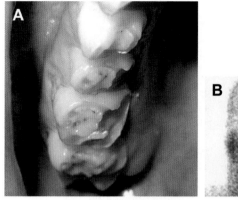
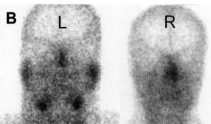

Fig. 27. (*A*) Salivary gland aplasia has caused unique dental chipping pattern. (*B*) Scintigraphy (L) demonstrates radioisotope pickup by salivary glands in normal patient. Right scintigram (R) demonstrates absence of parotid and submandibular gland radioisotope concentration because of gland aplasia in the same patient.

unknown reasons, the SLSG can become hyperplastic and balloon into an edentulous area (**Fig. 28**).[80–84] The swelling may be unilateral or bilateral, and may involve the entire length of the SLSG as the gland extends in the mouth floor from the region of the lingual frenum to the posterior molar area. The growth impetus seems to be initiated by an edentulous mandibular segment.[80,81] Histologically moderate inflammation may be present, but usually no abnormality is evident. An increased number of normal-appearing SLSG acini will be noted. Usually no treatment is indicated.

RANULA

A ranula represents a submucosal mucus extravasation phenomenon that develops as a result of leakage from an SLSG duct. The SLSG is an elongated gland that runs in an anterior-posterior direction in the mouth floor and lies on the oral aspect of the mylohyoid muscle. It consists of 10 to 15 individual lobes each with its own duct, the duct of Rivinus. Secretory leakage occurs when the duct wall is lacerated, probably from trauma. The rapid accumulation of fluid is cyst-like in appearance and presents itself as either an intraoral or extraoral swelling.

The intraoral ranula is recognized as a fluid-containing painless bluish swelling on the mouth floor (**Fig. 29**). As it increases in size and/or becomes subject to oral trauma,

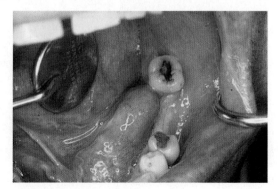

Fig. 28. Hyperplasia of sublingual salivary gland.

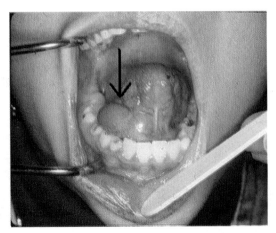

Fig. 29. Intraoral ranula (*arrow*).

it spontaneously breaks, and the swelling collapses. With healing, recurrences are to be anticipated.

The extraoral ranula, or deep-plunging ranula, occurs when an SLSG lobe and its duct extend through a naturally occurring dehiscence in the mylohyoid muscle, and secretions become manifest extraorally in the cervical area (**Fig. 30**A). Clinical diagnosis of the unilateral, painless, persistent, cervically plunging ranula can be substantiated with a CT scan (see **Fig. 30**B). The scan will reveal a unilateral lucency located in the submental/submandibular region that displaces or infiltrates around adjacent anatomic structures.

Successful treatment of the oral ranula is best accomplished by surgically removing the culpable SLSG lobe. The surgical void should be packed with an iodoform strip and maintained for 10 days so as to incite irritation. An inflammatory response with fibrosis usually seals off any leaking duct that was not removed surgically.[84] With

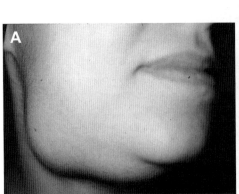
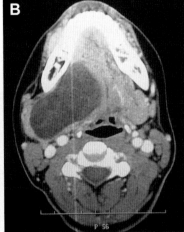

Fig. 30. (A) Plunging ranula, extraoral swelling. (B) Plunging ranula (same patient). CT scan reveals large-lucency posterior mouth floor with extension into the submandibular area.

removal of the packing, rapid healing by second intention occurs. Recurrences are a problem, but are minimalized with this procedure.

Treatment of the plunging ranula requires surgical removal of the entire SLSG. Recurrences after this procedure probably result from segments of the SLSG that have unknowingly been left intact during surgery.

MINOR SALIVARY GLANDS

Scattered throughout the oral cavity are lobules of minor salivary glands. These exocrine glands, approximately 1000 in number, measure 1 to 5 mm in size, lie just beneath the surface epithelium, and are located in the soft tissues of the lips, buccal mucosa, floor of mouth, hard and soft palates, tongue, and tonsillar pillars. These unencapsulated, mostly mucous, glands are generally absent in the anterior hard palate and gingiva. Minor glands can be subject to many of the conditions that involve the major salivary glands, but are also subject to several unique conditions not usually associated with the major glands.

Mucocele

In areas where the ducts of minor salivary glands are subject to trauma, lower lip, or inner cheek, duct laceration may occur. The resulting salivary leakage will pool into the submucosal connective tissue. This extravasation phenomenon, the mucocele, is clinically recognized as a visible cyst-like swelling superficially located, poorly circumscribed, bluish in color, painless, and having a diameter of at least 1 cm (**Fig. 31**). Because it is thin walled and subject to trauma, there is a tendency for it to rupture, collapse, and then recur. Successful therapy for these swellings is best attained via an excisional approach that encompasses the swelling and a peripheral margin of normal tissue, and includes the contiguous culpable minor salivary gland.

Superficial Mucocele

Superficial mucoceles (SMs) are rare superficially located variants of the more common mucocele. SMs usually occur in women, on noninflamed mucosa as single or multiple tense vesicles 1 to 4 mm in size, and most frequently involve the soft palate (**Fig. 32**). SMs are asymptomatic, tend to rupture within a few days, heal, and recur.

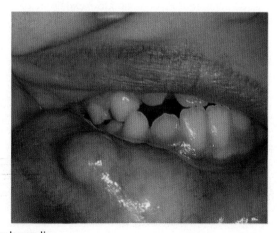

Fig. 31. Mucocele lower lip.

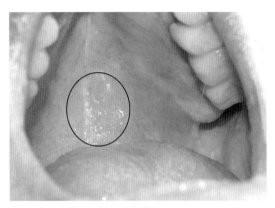

Fig. 32. Superficial mucoceles palate (*encircled*).

Histologically a superficial accumulation of extravasated sialomucin causes a cleavage at the epithelial-connective tissue interface, whereas the more common classic mucocele manifests itself in the submucosal connective tissue.[85,86] The etiology and a definitive therapeutic approach to SMs have not been determined.

Necrotizing Sialometaplasia

Necrotizing sialometaplasia (NS) is a benign, ulcerative, self-limiting inflammatory disease of the minor salivary glands (**Fig. 33**).[87] It probably results from a compromised vasculature supplying salivary gland tissue. The palatine salivary glands represent the most frequent group involved. Trauma, localized vasculitis, cocaine use, radiation, and sickle cell anemia represent factors that may interfere with the adequate blood flow of the greater palatine artery.[88,89] Ischemia with tissue infarction results. A deep crater-like ulcer with sharp margins appears. NS is self-limiting and will heal spontaneously by second intention within 6 to 12 weeks. The significance of NS rests in the fact that it may be misdiagnosed clinically and histologically as a squamous cell or mucoepidermoid carcinoma.

Cheilitis Glandularis

Cheilitis glandularis is an inflammatory condition that usually involves the vermilion of the lower lip and secondarily implicates the underlying minor salivary glands. Chronic

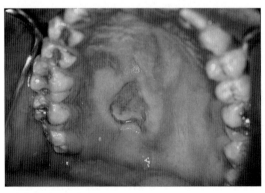

Fig. 33. Necrotizing sialometaplasia.

irritation from the sun, wind, smoking, alcohol, and so forth is thought to be the cause.[90,91] Enlargement and induration of the lower lip, with varying degrees of infection and mucopurulent discharge from visibly dilated duct openings, are observed. Treatment involves removal of all irritants, antibiotics, and steroids. Vermilionectomy becomes an option when the response to conservative therapy is poor.[91]

Stomatitis Nicotina

Heavy smoking can lead to oral mucosal changes referred to as stomatitis nicotina (SN) (**Fig. 34**). Keratosis, characterized by a white/gray appearance of the palate, develops in response to the heat and/or tobacco irritants. Eventually a raised papule, measuring up to 5 mm with a center depression containing a reddened palatine duct orifice, will be seen. The raised papules are thought to represent hyperplasia of the underlying palatine mucous glands.[92] Because SN is reversible, no treatment other than cessation of smoking is indicated.

DIAGNOSTIC ROLE OF THE LABIAL SALIVARY GLAND

The inner aspect of the lower lip harbors numerous superficially located labial salivary glands (LSG). Their surgical accessibility affords the practitioner the opportunity to harvest these glands as an aid in diagnosing a variety of systemic diseases (**Box 3**) (**Fig. 35**).

FALSE POSITIVES

The largest group of patients seen in the SGC comprises the false positives; that is, patients who present with a variety of subjective complaints or objective conditions that mimic a salivary problem. Because the false positives encompass multiple entities, only those that are most frequently observed in the SGC are reviewed here.

Somatoform Disease

Surprisingly, most false-positive patients who have salivary concerns fall into the somatoform disease (SD) category. These patients have psychological disorders that manifest themselves with a physical complaint that has no organic basis. Most complaints involve hyposalivation or sialorrhea, often limited to a precise oral area. Others are somewhat bizarre and include constant drooling, expectoration, or swallowing of what the patient believes is abnormal saliva. No such activity is usually observed during the clinical examination. Patients often state that the saliva has a

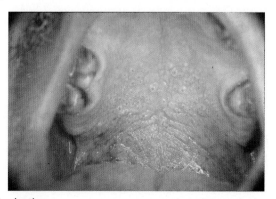

Fig. 34. Stomatitis nicotina.

Box 3
Diagnostic role of the labial salivary gland

Sjögren syndrome

The biopsy and microscopic examination of an LSG is, as previously stated, 1 of the 3 objective tests advised for the diagnosis of SS.[42] Serology and ocular staining are the other 2 clinical elements used for diagnosing SS. A histologic SS diagnosis is based on demonstrating 1 or more foci of lymphocytic cells, predominantly CD4 lymphocytes, in 4 mm^2 of LSG tissue (see **Fig. 13**).

Sarcoid

Sarcoid, a multisystem granulomatous disease, makes its presence known in 58% of biopsied LSGs.[50] Pathognomonic histologic features include the presence of a noncaseating granuloma, containing epithelioid and giant cells, surrounded by a periphery of lymphocytes and fibroblasts (see **Fig. 17**B).

Diffuse infiltrative CD8 lymphocytosis syndrome component of human immunodeficiency virus

DILS component of HIV disease can be subjected to an LSG biopsy for diagnostic purposes. Two or more lymphocytic foci within 4 mm^2 of tissue will be observed. A focus is 50 or more lymphocytes. The appearance is similar to that seen in SS, but differs in that the lymphocytic infiltration in DILS is dominated by CD8 cells, whereas CD4 cells are in the majority in SS.[93]

Amyloidosis

Amyloidosis represents a group of disorders whose common denominator is the extracellular deposition of amyloid protein into diverse tissues and organs. The LSG biopsy is a reliable test for diagnosis because a Congo red stain can demonstrate amyloid distributed periductally in an LSG.[94]

Chronic graft-versus-host disease

Chronic graft-versus-host disease (cGvHD) is the major cause of morbidity and mortality in patients undergoing bone marrow transplants. The histologic features in the LSG of patients with oral cGvHD include lymphocytic infiltration, acinar loss, fibrosis, and a predominance of CD8 cells.[95]

Sclerosing polycystic adenosis

Sclerosing polycystic adenosis (SPA) is a reactive sclerosing process that involves both major and minor salivary glands, and shares the features of the fibrocystic disease associated with the mammary gland. The entity has been identified in minor salivary glands.[96–109]

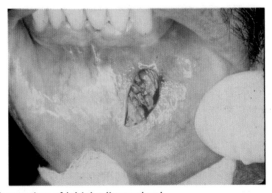

Fig. 35. Surgical harvesting of labial salivary gland.

bitter taste, frequently metallic, that it is granular, thick, or slimy, and coats specific oral areas, causing food to adhere to teeth, or may be frothy (a normal condition that results from aeration of accumulated saliva by the tongue's movement) (**Fig. 36**).

Common denominators in SD patients include a history of emotional disturbances, anxiety, or depression that requires the use of psychotherapeutic medications. Frequently the patient traces the start of the problem to some oral event such as a dental procedure, oral trauma, or a new oral hygiene product. The oral incident only serves to focus the patient's attention on the mouth. Stressful work conditions or difficult social or family situations often contribute to the SD. Patients may bring written detailed chronologic histories of their symptoms, medications, and medical visits. Questioning usually reveals that the salivary problem intensifies as the day progresses, and there is difficulty with sleep. The patient blames oral dryness for frequent night awakenings when, in reality, the mental state is the cause. Concurrently many patients will have other conditions, such as burning mouth syndrome, parafunctional habit (PFH), or atypical oral pain, all thought to have psychogenic aspects.

The triad of dysgeusia, burning sensations of the oral cavity, and a perceived abnormal saliva indicate a diagnosis of SD. Volume measurements in these patients with disturbed perceptions of hyposalivation or sialorrhea are normal. Many of these patients take multiple anticholinergic medications, and will develop clinical hyposalivation only when the mouth is at rest. Any oral stimulation (eg, eating) overrides the medication's anticholinergic effect on the resting gland.[35] Conversely, salivary volume of patients with salivary gland abnormality will be diminished both at rest and when stimulated.

Accurate early categorization negates invasive procedures. The absence of a demonstrable organic basis for the patient's complaint indicates the need for reassurance or psychiatric consultation.

Masseteric Hypertrophy

Masseteric hypertrophy (MH) is a common condition often mistaken for parotid enlargement because of the masseter muscle's proximity to the gland. MH is an asymptomatic persistent enlargement of one or both masseter muscles resulting from hypertrophy initiated by clenching, bruxing, or continuous gum chewing (**Fig. 37**). MH occurs primarily in younger individuals because generally, the elderly have deteriorated dentition that prevents masticatory activation of the masseters.

Anatomically, most of the masseteric thickness is along the inferior portion of the mandibular ramus where the facial contour normally tapers. In the presence of MH,

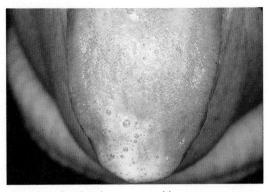

Fig. 36. Normal frothy saliva that has been aerated by tongue movement.

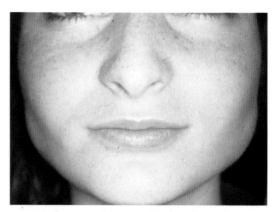

Fig. 37. Bilateral masseteric hypertrophy caused by bruxing.

the face takes on a rectangular configuration from increased muscle bulk in the region of facial narrowing. In contradistinction to MH, parotid swelling accentuates facial ovality because the major portion of the gland is situated at a higher facial level, adjacent to the ear. In addition, on activation a previously flaccid masseter becomes firm and displays a discrete and prominent facial outline. Tooth attrition attributed to bruxing/clenching may be present.

Other than increased masseter muscle fiber length and diameter, histology reveals no abnormalities. Therapy therefore often includes reassurance, muscle relaxation, dental bite plate construction, and behavioral modification. For cosmetic reasons, botulinum toxin injections have been advocated to inactivate the masseter and cause muscle atrophy.[110]

Lymphadenopathy

Diagnosis of cervicofacial lymphadenopathy and its differentiation from sialadenopathy are based on an understanding of lymph node anatomy, and knowledge of the systemic abnormalities that can lead to lymphadenopathy. It is the close proximity of these nodes to adjacent salivary glands that creates diagnostic dilemmas in differentiating an enlarged extranglandular node from a supposed salivary gland swelling.

The most common cause of an enlarged lymph node seen in the SGC is lymphadenitis initiated by bacterial infection (**Fig. 38**). Cervicofacial lymphadenopathies have also been observed in HIV disease, granulomatous disease, autoimmune disease, lymphomas, and metastatic malignancies. However, the sudden onset of pain and swelling in a movable and circumscribed node suggests the presence of a lymphadenitis.

A simple method to differentiate an inflamed node from sialadenitis is to observe whether expressed saliva exiting from the suspected salivary gland's duct is cloudy from the contained pus associated with sialadenitis. Neoplastic nodes tend to be painless, persistent, and fixed in position, and increase in size with time. Palpation and imaging are helpful in identifying the presence of a lymphadenopathy. Tissue biopsy or fine-needle aspiration biopsy facilitate diagnosis and guide the therapeutic approach.

Paraglandular Opacities

A variety of paraglandular opacities exists and can complicate the differential diagnosis of salivary stones. However, the pain and swelling initiated by eating and associated with sialolithiasis are absent.

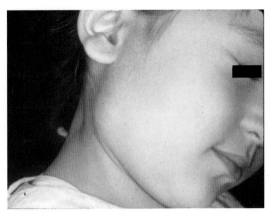

Fig. 38. Lymphadenitis secondary to ear infection.

Calcified lymph node
Healing of an inflamed lymph node can result in calcification of the node. Obviously such a node, if it is in close proximity to a salivary gland, can be confused with a sialolith. Metastatic disease from the thyroid or breast, lymphoma, and granulomatous diseases such as sarcoid, tuberculosis (**Fig. 39**), and/or histoplasmosis can cause nodal calcifications.

Tonsilloliths
Tonsilloliths develop in the tonsillar crypt where a precipitation of salts from stagnant crypt saliva takes place.[111] A mandibular radiograph can show these tonsillar spherical calcifications superimposed on the mandibular ramus (**Fig. 40**A). Their misinterpretation as parotid stones can be avoided by considering the absence of the signs and symptoms associated with salivary duct obstruction. Conclusive evidence for a tonsillolith is obtained when viewing an axial view of a CT scan, which reveals the opacities to be medial to the mandibular ramus and in close relation to the pharyngeal space (see **Fig. 40**B).

Phleboliths
Phleboliths, or calcified thrombi, are usually multiple in their presentation, and usually associated with intramuscular hemangiomas (IMH) or vascular malformations (VM).[112]

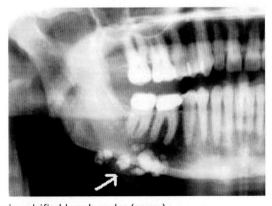

Fig. 39. Tuberculosis; calcified lymph nodes (*arrow*).

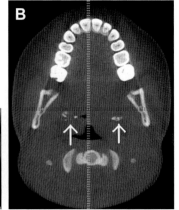

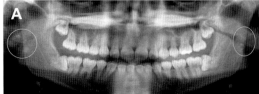

Fig. 40. (*A*) Panoramic radiograph. Tonsilloliths superimposed on ramus (*encircled*). (*B*) CT scan (axial view) with tonsilloliths present medial to ramus (*arrows*).

The stagnant blood flow in the IMH or VM favors thrombus formation, which can calcify to form a phlebolith. Clinically, patients with an IMH or VM frequently present the benign neoplastic picture of a chronic, slow-growing swelling that does not fluctuate in size. These vascular entities with their phleboliths are often seen in masseteric or submandibular locations, whereupon confusion with sialolithiasis results. Diagnostic differentiation is aided by the knowledge that phleboliths radiographically have a unique lamellated concentric-ring target pattern (**Fig. 41**).

Carotid artery calcifications

Carotid artery calcifications are often found at the bifurcation of the common carotid artery following atheroma formation and calcium deposition. This arterial wall opacity is classically located posterior and inferior to the mandibular angle at the level of the junction of the third and fourth cervical vertebrae (**Fig. 42**).[113] Radiographs, taken routinely in dental offices or when an oral problem requires a CT scan, afford the opportunity to diagnose the presence of a carotid artery calcification, often as an

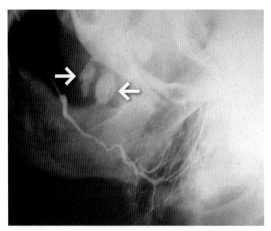

Fig. 41. Phleboliths (*arrows*) in association with masseteric intramuscular hemangioma (IMH). Normal parotid sialogram with some posterior displacement by the IMH.

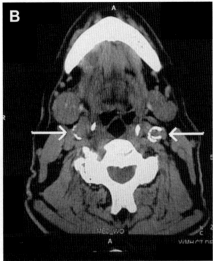

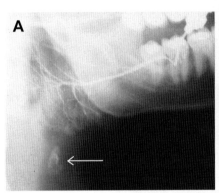

Fig. 42. (A) Calcification of carotid artery wall (*arrow*). Normal parotid sialogram. (B) CT scan, axial view. Bilateral carotid artery calcifications (*arrows*).

incidental finding.[114] The extent of the calcification and vascular lumen stenosis may indicate a need for medical referral.

Neuromuscular Dysfunction

Management of accumulated saliva requires an intact functioning neuromuscular swallowing system. The inability to swallow causes saliva to excessively pool in the floor of the mouth. Parkinson disease and amyotrophic lateral sclerosis (ALS) are examples of diseases that are associated with this condition. Because these patients accumulate saliva and because their head is usually in a forward-leaning position, they tend to visibly drool. In patients with ALS associated labial incompetence develops, which inhibits normal lip sealing and may be an additional cause of drooling.

Therapeutically, antisialogogic agents (anticholinergics, antihistamines, psychotherapeutics) can be used to reduce the normal but unmanageable salivary volume. Botulinum toxin injections into the salivary glands have met with some success.[115,116] Low-dose radiation and surgical repositioning of the salivary ducts are alternative therapies.

Dental Conditions

Saliva is recognized as the key component in preventing dental caries. Many patients with extensive dental damage are seen in the SGC based on the assumption that some salivary deficiency has caused the dental problem. Sufficient hyposalivation to initiate dental caries only exists in patients with SS, and those who have received radiation to head and neck areas that incorporates the salivary glands. Rampant caries in patients who have not been irradiated and do not have SS usually is dietary in origin.[117] Extremely high sucrose intake from large quantities of soft drinks, fruit juices, constant sucking on mints and candies, and continuous use of sugared gum is the usual offender (**Fig. 43**A).

Dental attrition represents wear of tooth enamel and/or dentin, and is most often seen in patients with a parafunctional habit (PFH) (see **Fig. 43**B). Abrasion is the wearing away of tooth structure by an extraoral foreign object such as a toothbrush. Dental

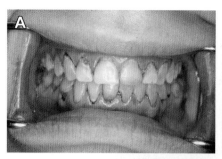
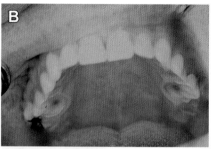
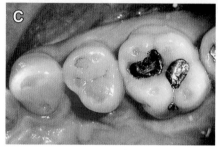

Fig. 43. (*A*) Extensive cervical decay from constant use of sugared mints. (*B*) Dental attrition caused by bruxing. (*C*) Constant wine sipping has caused loss of occlusal masticatory enamel with exposure of dentin (*yellow*). A peripheral enamel rim (*white*) is present. Enamel loss on molar has caused contact pitting.

corrosion develops from acidic effects on tooth structure. Dietary intakes of foods with high acidic content such as sipping of wine, whose pH approximates 2.9, can cause corrosive dental damage (see **Fig. 43**C).[118,119] Regurgitated gastric acids from reflux disease will also destroy tooth structure.

GASTROESOPHAGEAL REFLUX DISEASE

Gastroesophageal reflux (GER) is considered a normal retrograde flow of gastric contents, particularly acid, into the esophagus.[120] GER by itself is physiologic and does not produce esophageal mucosal damage because of its rapid removal by esophageal peristalsis. Unfortunately GER can intensify, become more frequent, and cause gastroesophageal reflux disease (GERD), whose clinical symptoms include heartburn and regurgitation. It has been estimated that 10% to 30%, of the adult population is affected by GERD.[121,122]

The lower esophageal sphincter (LES), which consists of smooth muscle, guards against the retrograde movement of gastric contents. An incompetent LES allows for the repeated incursions of refluxed acid, pepsin, and bile that lead to corrosive effects on the esophageal mucosa. Cellular damage with an epithelial metaplasia occurs, referred to as Barrett esophagus (BE), and places these patients at increased risk for the development of a malignancy.

Normal LES function can be inhibited mechanically in the presence of a hiatal hernia.[123] Inadequate function of the LES has also been reported in pregnant women. Their increased circulating hormones, particularly progesterone, interfere with the contractility of the smooth-muscled LES.[124]

Limitation of the effect of gastric acids on the esophageal wall is mediated through a protective esophageal salivary reflex (ESR).[125] With the onset of heartburn, the ESR

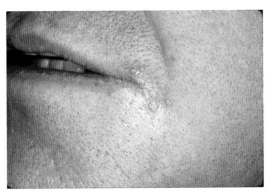

Fig. 44. Commissural cheilitis and dermatitis caused by chronic nocturnal drooling associated with gastroesophageal reflux disease.

causes hypersalivation, or water brash. On swallowing, salivary lavage of the esophageal wall occurs. In addition, the contained salivary bicarbonate acids act to buffer the effect of any residual gastric acid. Consequently, significant damage to the esophageal wall and the onset of BE are discouraged.

An oral history and examination is extremely helpful in uncovering the existence of GERD. Nocturnal drooling with pillow wetting results from the encouragement of GERD by the patient's supine position. The chronic water brash from the ESR, mixed with regurgitated gastric acids displaced into the mouth, will then lead to tissue excoriation and maceration in the lip commissure area from drooling (**Fig. 44**).[119] Studies of salivary flow during episodes of heartburn will substantiate the existence of significant volume increases. Additional evidence for GERD may be obtained through a dental examination. Tooth corrosions from GERD's acid effect will be apparent.

The oral effects of GERD can be ameliorated through prescribed acid-suppressing medications that include omeprazole, lansoprazole, and other antacids. Avoidance of spicy foods, alcohol, chocolate, and large meals are helpful in treating heartburn and the associated hypersalivation. Elevation of the head during sleep is advised.

REFERENCES

1. Mandel L, Vakkas J, Saqi A. Alcoholic (beer) sialosis. J Oral Maxillofac Surg 2005;63:402–5.
2. Chilla R. Sialadenosis of the salivary glands of the head: studies on the physiology and pathophysiology of parotid secretion. Adv Otorhinolaryngol 1981;26:1–38.
3. Scully C, Bagan JV, Eveson JW, et al. Sialosis: 35 cases of persistent parotid swelling from two countries. Br J Oral Maxillofac Surg 2008;46:468–72.
4. Donath K, Seifert G. Ultrastructural studies of the parotid gland in sialadenosis. Virchows Arch A Pathol Anat Histol 1975;365:119–35.
5. Donath K. Wangenschwellung bei sialadenose. HNO 1979;27:113–8.
6. Ihrler S, Rath C, Zengel P, et al. Pathogenesis of sialadenosis: possible role of functionally deficient myoepithelial cells. Oral Surg Oral Med Oral Pathol Oral Radiol Endod 2010;110:218–23.
7. Mandic R, Teymoortash A, Kann PH, et al. Sialadenosis of the major salivary glands in a patient with central diabetes insipidus-Implications of aquaporin water channels in the pathomechanism of sialadenosis. Exp Clin Endocrinol Diabetes 2005;113:205–7.

8. Teymoortash A, Wiegand S, Borkeloh M, et al. Variations in the expression and distribution pattern of AQP5 in acinar cells of patients with sialadenosis. In Vivo 2012;26:951–5.

9. Rabinov K, Kell T, Gordon PH. CT of the salivary glands. Radiol Clin North Am 1984;22:145–9.

10. Casper RC. The pathophysiology of anorexia nervosa and bulimia nervosa. Annu Rev Nutr 1986;6:299–316.

11. Mandel L, Abai S. Diagnosing bulimia nervosa with parotid gland swelling: case report. J Am Dent Assoc 2004;135:613–6.

12. Soloman LW, Merzianu M, Sullivan M, et al. Necrotizing sialometaplasia associated with bulimia: case report and literature review. Oral Surg Oral Med Oral Pathol Oral Radiol Endod 2007;103:e39–42.

13. Imai T, Michizawa M. Necrotizing sialometaplasia in a patient with an eating disorder: palatal ulcer accompanied by dental erosion due to binge-purging. J Oral Maxillofac Surg 2013;71:879–85.

14. Mandel L, Kaynar A, Wazen J. Pneumoparotid: a case report. Oral Surg Oral Med Oral Pathol 1991;72:22–4.

15. McGreevy AE, O'Kane AM, McCaul D, et al. Pneumoparotitis: a case report. Head Neck 2013;35:E55–9.

16. Potet J, Arnaud FX, Valbousquet L, et al. Pneumoparotid, a rare diagnosis to consider when faced with unexplained parotid swelling. Diagn Interv Imaging 2013;94:95–7.

17. Bonchek LI. Salivary gland enlargement during induction of anesthesia. JAMA 1969;209:1716–8.

18. Ismail EA, Seoudi TM, Al-Amir M, et al. Neonatal suppurative parotitis over the last 4 decades: report of three new cases and review. Pediatr Int 2013;55:60–4.

19. Mandel L. Differentiating acute suppurative parotitis from acute exacerbation of a chronic parotitis: case reports. J Oral Maxillofac Surg 2008;66:1964–8.

20. Brook I. Acute bacterial suppurative parotitis: microbiology and management. J Craniofac Surg 2003;14:37–40.

21. Bhatty MA, Piggot TA, Soames JV, et al. Chronic non-specific parotid sialadenitis. Br J Plast Surg 1998;51:517–21.

22. Mandel L, Witck EL. Chronic parotitis diagnosis and treatment: case report. J Am Dent Assoc 2001;132:1707–11.

23. Wang SL, Zou ZJ, Wu QC, et al. Sialographic changes related to clinical and pathologic findings in chronic obstructive parotitis. Int J Oral Maxillofac Surg 1992;21:364–8.

24. Nahlieli O, Bar T, Schacham R, et al. Management of chronic recurrent parotitis: current therapy. J Oral Maxillofac Surg 2004;62:1150–5.

25. Wang S, Li J, Zhu X, et al. Gland atrophy following retrograde injection of methyl violet as a treatment in chronic obstructive parotitis. Oral Surg Oral Med Oral Pathol Oral Radiol Endod 1998;85:276–81.

26. Soberman N, Leonidas JC, Berdon W, et al. Parotid enlargement in children seropositive for human immunodeficiency virus. AJR Am J Roentgenol 1991; 157:553–6.

27. Itescu S, Brancato LJ, Buxbaum J, et al. A diffuse infiltrative CD8 lymphocytosis syndrome in human immunodeficiency virus (HIV) infection: a host immune response associated with HLA-DR5. Ann Intern Med 1990;112:3–10.

28. Mourad WF, Hu KS, Shourbaji RA, et al. Radiation therapy for benign lymphoepithelial cysts of parotid glands in HIV patients. Laryngoscope 2013;123:1184–9.

29. Syebele K, Bütow KW. Comparative study of the effect of antiretroviral therapy on benign lymphoepithelial cyst of parotid glands and ranulas in HIV-positive patients. Oral Surg Oral Med Oral Pathol Oral Radiol Endod 2011;111:205–10.
30. Morse CG, Kovacs JA. Metabolic and skeletal complications of HIV infection: the price of success. JAMA 2006;296:844–54.
31. Mandel L, Alfi D. Drug-induced paraparotid fat deposition in patients with HIV: case reports. J Am Dent Assoc 2008;139:152–7.
32. Katz SL, Gershon AA, Hotez PJ. Infectious diseases of children. New York: Mosby Year Book Inc; 1998. p. 280–9.
33. McQuone SJ. Acute viral and bacterial infections of the salivary glands. Otolaryngol Clin North Am 1999;32:793–811.
34. Lustmann J, Regev E, Melemed Y. Sialolithiasis; a survey on 245 patients and a review of literature. Int J Oral Maxillofac Surg 1990;193:135–8.
35. Mandel ID. Sialochemistry in diseases and clinical situations affecting salivary glands. Crit Rev Clin Lab Sci 1980;12:321–66.
36. Harrison JD. Causes, natural history, and incidence of salivary stones and obstructions. Otolaryngol Clin North Am 2009;42:927–47.
37. Park HS, Pae Y, Kim KY, et al. Intraoral removal of stones in the proximal submandibular duct: usefulness of a surgical landmark for the hilum. Laryngoscope 2013;123:934–7.
38. Gundlach P, Scherer H, Hopf J, et al. Endoscopic-controlled laser lithotripsy of salivary calculi: in vitro studies and initial clinical use. HNO 1990;38:247–50.
39. Capaccio P, Toretta S, Ottaviani F, et al. Modern management of obstructive salivary disease. Acta Otorhinolaryngol Ital 2007;27:161–72.
40. Katz P. Endoscopy of the salivary glands. Ann Radiol (Paris) 1991;34:110–3.
41. Nahlieli O, Schacham R, Zaguri A. Combined external lithotripsy and endoscopic techniques for advanced sialolithiasis cases. J Oral Maxillofac Surg 2010;68:347–53.
42. Shiboski SC, Shiboski CH, Criswell SA, et al. American College of Rheumatology classification criteria for Sjögren's syndrome: a data-driven, expert consensus approach in the Sjögren's International Collaborative Clinical Alliance Cohort. Arthritis Care Res 2012;64:45–87.
43. Quartuccio L, Farbis M, Salvin S, et al. Controversies on rituximab therapy in Sjögren syndrome-associated lymphoproliferation. Int J Rheumatol 2009;2009: 424935.
44. Himi T, Takano K, Yamanoto M, et al. A novel concept of Mikulicz's disease as Ig G4-related disease. Auris Nasus Larynx 2012;39:9–17.
45. Harrison JD, Rodriquez-Justo M. Commentary on Ig G4-related sialadenitis: Mikulicz's disease, Küttner tumour, and eponymy. Histopathology 2011;58: 1164–6.
46. Vairaktaris E, Vassilliou S, Yapijakis C, et al. Salivary gland manifestations of sarcoidosis: report of three cases. J Oral Maxillofac Surg 2005;63:1016–21.
47. Greenberg G, Anderson R, Sharpstone P, et al. Enlargement of the parotid gland due to sarcoidosis. Br Med J 1964;2:861–2.
48. Nessan V, Jacoway J. Biopsy of minor salivary glands in the diagnosis of sarcoidosis. N Engl J Med 1979;301:922–4.
49. Mandel L, Kaynar A. Sialadenopathy: a clinical herald of sarcoidosis: report of two cases. J Oral Maxillofac Surg 1994;52:1208–10.
50. Mandel L, Wolinsky B, Chalom EC. Treatment of refractory sarcoidal parotid gland swelling in a previously reported unresponsive case: case report. J Am Dent Assoc 2005;136:1282–5.

51. Shimizu M, Usmuller J, Donath K, et al. Sonographic analysis of recurrent parotitis in children: a comparative study with sialographic findings. Oral Surg Oral Med Oral Pathol 1988;86:606–15.

52. Mandel L, Bijoor R. Imaging (computed tomography, magnetic resonance imaging; ultrasound, sialography) in a case of recurrent parotitis in children. J Oral Maxillofac Surg 2006;64:984–8.

53. Ward MJ, Levine PA. Salivary gland tumors. In: Close LG, Larson DL, Shah JP, editors. Essentials of head and neck oncology. 1st edition. New York: Thieme; 1998. p. 73–81.

54. Spiro RH. Salivary neoplasms: overview of a 35-year experience with 2807 patients. Head Neck Surg 1986;8:177–84.

55. Randall K, Stevens J, Yepes JF, et al. Analysis of factors influencing the development of xerostomia during intensity-modulated radiotherapy. Oral Surg Oral Med Oral Pathol Oral Radiol 2013;115:772–9.

56. Fall-Dickson JM, Berger AM. Oral manifestations and complications of cancer therapy. In: Berger AM, Shuster JL, Von Roenn JH, editors. Principles and practice of palliative care and supportive oncology. 3rd edition. Philadelphia: Lippincott Williams & Wilkins; 2007. p. 205–20.

57. Eisbruch A, Ten Haken RK, Kim HM, et al. Dose, volume and function relationships in parotid salivary glands following conformal and intensity modulated irradiation of head and neck cancer. Int J Radiat Oncol Biol Phys 1999;45: 577–87.

58. Grotz KA, Wustenberg P, Kohnen R, et al. Prophylaxis or radiogenic sialadenitis and mucositis by coumarin/troxerutine in patients with head and neck cancer–a prospective randomized placebo-controlled double-blind study. Br J Oral Maxillofac Surg 2001;39:34–9.

59. Ship JA, Eisbruch A, D' Hondt E, et al. Parotid sparing study in head and neck cancer patients receiving bilateral radiation therapy: 1 year results. J Dent Res 1997;76:807–13.

60. Grewal RK, Larson SM, Pentlow CE, et al. Salivary gland side effects commonly develop several weeks after initial radioactive iodine ablation. J Nucl Med 2009; 50:1605–10.

61. Mandel SJ, Mandel L. Radioactive iodine and the salivary glands. Thyroid 2003; 13:265–71.

62. Sussman RM, Miller J. Iodide 'mumps' after intravenous urography. N Engl J Med 1956;255:433–4.

63. Christensen J. Iodide mumps after intravascular administration of nonionic contrast medium. Acta Radiol 1995;36:82–4.

64. Bohora S, Harikrishnan S, Tharakan J. Iodide mumps. Int J Cardiol 2008;130: 82–3.

65. Araujo M, Centurion BS, Albuquerque DF, et al. Management of a parotid sialocele in a young patient: case report and literature review. J Appl Oral Sci 2010; 18:432–6.

66. Mandel L. Bilateral parotid duct obstruction after rhytidectomies: case report. J Oral Maxillofac Surg 2012;70:449–52.

67. Mandel L. The grossly dilated Stensen's duct: case reports. J Oral Maxillofac Surg 2007;65:2089–94.

68. Wang Y, Yu GY, Huang MX, et al. Diagnosis and treatment of congenital dilatation of Stensen's duct. Laryngoscope 2011;121:1682–6.

69. Baurmash H. Sialectasis of Stensen's duct with an extraoral swelling: a case report with surgical management. J Oral Maxillofac Surg 2007;65:1170–2.

70. Kawahara K, Hotta F, Myachi H, et al. Congenital dilation of the submandibular duct: report of a case. J Oral Maxillofac Surg 2000;58:1170–2.
71. Mandel L, Alfi D. Diagnostic imaging for submandibular duct atresia: literature review and case report. J Oral Maxillofac Surg 2012;70:2819–22.
72. McDonald FG, Mantas J, Mc Ewen CG, et al. Salivary gland aplasia: an ectodermal disorder? J Oral Pathol 1986;15:115–7.
73. Fracaro MS, Linnett VM, Hallett KB, et al. Submandibular gland aplasia and progressive dental caries: a case report. Aust Dent J 2002;47:347–50.
74. Mandel L. An unusual pattern of dental damage with salivary gland aplasia. J Am Dent Assoc 2006;137:984–9.
75. Smyth AG, Ward-Booth RP, High AS. Polycystic disease of the parotid glands: two familial cases. Br J Oral Maxillofac Surg 1993;31:38–40.
76. Brown E, August M, Pilch BZ, et al. Polycystic disease of the parotid glands. AJNR Am J Neuroradiol 1995;16:1128–31.
77. Ficarra G, Sapp JP, Christensen RE, et al. Dysgenetic polycystic disease of the parotid gland: report of a case. J Oral Maxillofac Surg 1996;54:1246–9.
78. Mathison CC, Hudgins PA. Bilateral submandibular gland aplasia with hypertrophy of sublingual glands. Otolaryngol Head Neck Surg 2008;138:119–20.
79. Haktanir A. CT and MR findings of bilateral submandibular gland aplasia associated with hypertrophied symmetrical sublingual glands herniated through mylohyoid defects. Dentomaxillofac Radiol 2012;41:79–83.
80. Mandel L, Romao M. Sublingual salivary gland enlargement. N Y State Dent J 2004;70:24–7.
81. Domaneschi C, Mauricio AR, Modolo F, et al. Idiopathic hyperplasia of the sublingual glands in totally or partially edentulous individuals. Oral Surg Oral Med Oral Pathol Oral Radiol Endod 2007;103:374–7.
82. Sober AJ, Gorden P, Roth J, et al. Visceromegaly in acromegaly: evidence that clinical hepatomegaly or splenomegaly (but not sialomegaly) are manifestations of a second disease. Arch Intern Med 1974;134:415–7.
83. Manetti L, Bogazzi F, Brogioni S, et al. Submandibular salivary gland volume is increased in patients with acromegaly. Clin Endocrinol 2002;57:97–100.
84. Baurmash H. A case against sublingual gland removal as primary treatment of ranulas. J Oral Maxillofac Surg 2007;65:117–24.
85. Everson JW. Superficial mucoceles: pitfall in clinical and microscopic diagnosis. Oral Surg Oral Med Oral Pathol 1988;66:318–22.
86. Jensen JL. Superficial mucoceles of the oral mucosa. Am J Dermatopathol 1990;12:88–92.
87. Abrams A, Melrose R, Howell F. Necrotizing sialometaplasia. Cancer 1973;32:130–5.
88. Anneroth G, Hansen L. Necrotizing sialometaplasia. Int J Oral Surg 1982;11:283–91.
89. Mandel L, Kaynar A, DeChiara S. Necrotizing sialometaplasia in a patient with sickle cell anemia. J Oral Maxillofac Surg 1991;49:757–9.
90. Stoopler ET, Carrasco L, Stanton DC, et al. Cheilitis glandularis: an unusual histopathologic presentation. Oral Surg Oral Med Oral Pathol Oral Radiol Endod 2003;95:312–7.
91. Nico MM, deMelo JN, Lourenco SV. Cheilitis glandularis: a clinicopathological study in 22 patients. J Am Acad Dermatol 2010;62:233–8.
92. Reddy C, Kameswari V, Ramulu C, et al. Histopathological study of stomatitis nicotina. Br J Cancer 1971;25:403–10.
93. Basu D, Williams FM, Ahn CW, et al. Changing spectrum of the diffuse infiltrative lymphocytosis syndrome. Arthritis Rheum 2006;55:466–72.

94. Caporali R, Bonacci E, Epis O, et al. Safety and usefulness of minor salivary gland biopsy: retrospective analysis of 502 procedures performed at a single center. Arthritis Rheum 2008;59:714–20.

95. Soares AB, Faria PR, Magna LA, et al. Chronic GVHD in minor salivary glands and oral mucosa: histopathological and immunohistochemical evaluation of 25 patients. J Oral Pathol 2005;34:368–73.

96. Noonan VL, Kalmar JR, Allen CM, et al. Sclerosing polycystic adenosis of minor salivary glands: report of three cases and review of the literature. Oral Surg Oral Med Oral Pathol Oral Radiol Endod 2007;104:516–20.

97. Meer S, Altini M. Sclerosing polycystic adenosis of the buccal mucosa. Head Neck Pathol 2008;2:31–5.

98. Ah-See KW, McLaren K, Maran AG. Wegener's granulomatosis presenting as major salivary gland involvement. J Laryngol Otol 1996;110:691–3.

99. Almouhawis HA, Leao JC, Fedele S, et al. Wegener's granulomatosis: a review of clinical features and an update in diagnosis and treatment. J Oral Pathol Med 2013;42:507–16.

100. Zhang JZ, Zhang CG, Chen JM. Thirty-five cases of Kimura's disease (eosinophilic lymphogranuloma). Br J Dermatol 1998;139:542–3.

101. Boccato P, Mannara GM, Rinaldo A, et al. Kimura's disease of the intraparotid lymph nodes fine needle aspiration biopsy findings. ORL J Otorhinolaryngol Relat Spec 1999;61:227–31.

102. Som PM, Biller HF. Kimura disease involving parotid gland and cervical nodes: CT and MR findings. J Comput Assist Tomogr 1992;16:320–3.

103. Irish JC, Kain K, Keystone JS, et al. Kimura's disease: an unusual cause of head and neck masses. J Otolaryngol 1994;23:88–91.

104. Kilty SJ, Yammine NV, Corsten MJ, et al. Castleman's disease of the parotid. J Otolaryngol 2004;13:396–400.

105. Yi AY, DeTar M, Becker TS, et al. Giant lymph node hyperplasia of the head and neck (Castleman's disease): a report of five cases. Otolaryngol Head Neck Surg 1995;113:462–6.

106. Lei J, Zhao LY, Liu Y, et al. Castleman's disease of the neck: report of 4 cases with unusual presentations. J Oral Maxillofac Surg 2011;69:1094–9.

107. Smith BC, Ellis GL, Slater LJ, et al. Sclerosing polycystic adenosis of major salivary glands: a clinicopathologic analysis of nine cases. Am J Surg Pathol 1996; 20:161–70.

108. Skalova AG, Gnepp DR, Simpson RH, et al. Clonal nature of sclerosing polycystic adenosis of salivary glands demonstrated by using the polymorphism of the human androgen receptor (HUMARA) locus as a marker. Am J Surg Pathol 2006;30:939–44.

109. Shields DW, Snead OC. Benign epilepsy with centrotemporal spikes. Epilepsia 2009;50(Suppl 8):10–5.

110. Mandel L, Tharakan M. Treatment of unilateral masseteric hypertrophy with botulinum toxin: case report. J Oral Maxillofac Surg 1999;57:1017–9.

111. el-Sharif I, Shembesh FM. A tonsillolith seen on MRI. Comput Med Imaging Graph 1997;21:205–8.

112. Baker LL, Dillon WP, Hieshima GB, et al. Hemangiomas and vascular malformations of the head and neck: MR characterization. AJNR Am J Neuroradiol 1993;14:307–14.

113. Friedlander AH, Baker JD. Panoramic radiography: an aid in detecting patients at risk of cerebrovascular accident. J Am Dent Assoc 1994;125:1598–603.

114. Levy C, Mandel L. Calcified carotid artery imaged by computed tomography. J Oral Maxillofac Surg 2010;68:218–20.

115. Lagalla G, Millevolte M, Capecci M, et al. Botulinum toxin type A for drooling in Parkinson's disease: a double blind, randomized, placebo-controlled study. Mov Disord 2006;21:704–7.
116. Giess R, Naumann W, Werner E, et al. Injections of botulinum toxin type A into the salivary glands improve sialorrhea in amyotrophic lateral sclerosis. J Neurol Neurosurg Psychiatry 2000;69:121–3.
117. Burt BA, Pai S. Sugar consumption and caries risk: a systematic review. J Dent Educ 2001;65:1017–23.
118. Mandel L. Dental erosion due to wine consumption. J Am Dent Assoc 2005;136: 171–5.
119. Mandel L, Tamari K. Sialorrhea and gastroesophageal reflux. J Am Dent Assoc 1995;126:1537–41.
120. Ranjitkar S, Kaidonis JA, Smales RJ. Gastroesophageal reflux disease and tooth erosion. Int J Dent 2012;2012:479850.
121. Kim TH, Kwang JL, Yeo M, et al. Pepsin detection in the sputum/saliva for the diagnosis of gastroesophageal reflux disease in patients with clinically suspected atypical gastroesophageal reflux disease symptoms. Digestion 2008; 77:201–6.
122. Yuksel ES, Hong SK, Strugala V, et al. Rapid salivary pepsin test; Blinded assessment of test performance in gastroesophageal reflux disease. Laryngoscope 2012;122:1312–6.
123. Mittal RK, Lange RC, Mc Callum RW. Identification and mechanism of delayed esophageal acid clearance in subjects with hiatus hernia. Gastroenterology 1987;92:130–5.
124. Olans LB, Wolf JL. Gastroesophageal reflux in pregnancy. Gastrointest Endosc Clin N Am 1994;4:699–712.
125. Shafik A, El-Sibai O, Shafik AA, et al. Effect of topical esophageal acidification on salivary secretions: identification of the mechanism of action. J Gastroenterol Hepatol 2005;20:1935–9.
126. Mandel L. Hyposalivation after undergoing stapedectomy. J Am Dent Assoc 2012;143:39–42.
127. Mandel L, Syrop SB. First-bite syndrome after parapharyngeal surgery for cervical schwannoma. J Am Dent Assoc 2008;139:1480–3.

Index

Note: Page numbers of article titles are in **boldface** type.

A

Abrasions, 1262
Abscess
 dental (apical), 1244–1246
 periodontal, 1254–1257
Acetaminophen, for migraine, 1394
Actinic cheilosis, 1301, 1304
Acupuncture, for TMDs, 1375
Acyclovir
 for herpes simplex virus infections, 1329–1331
 for postherpetic neuralgia, 1390
Advanced Trauma Life Support, 1261
Alcohol use, as cancer risk factor, 1303–1304, 1307
Allelic imbalance, cancer and, 1305
Alveola, injuries of, 1265–1269
Alveolar mucosa, clinical examination of, 1237
Alveolar process, tori of, 1293–1294
Amalgam tattoo, 1291–1293
American Academy of Orofacial Pain classification, of TMDs, 1355–1356
American Association of Dental Research, TMD treatment recommendations of, 1368
Amitriptyline, for migraine, 1394
Amlexanox, for recurrent aphthous stomatitis, 1335
Amoxicillin, for periodontal disease, 1247
Amyloidosis, 1436
Anesthesia dolorosa (peripheral painful trigeminal traumatic neuropathy), 1388
Anesthesia mumps, 1410
Anesthetic injection
 for glossopharyngeal neuralgia, 1388
 for occipital neuralgia, 1388
 for TMD diagnosis, 1364
Aneuploidy, cancer and, 1305
Angular cheilitis, 1326
Ankyloglossia, 1285
Anorexia, salivary gland disorders in, 1409
Antibiotics
 for displaced teeth, 1269
 for periodontal disease, 1247, 1249
Anticonvulsants
 for migraine, 1394
 for peripheral painful trigeminal traumatic neuropathy, 1388
 for trigeminal neuralgia, 1386

Med Clin N Am 98 (2014) 1451–1465
http://dx.doi.org/10.1016/S0025-7125(14)00160-6
0025-7125/14/$ – see front matter © 2014 Elsevier Inc. All rights reserved.

medical.theclinics.com

C

United States Postal Service

Statement of Ownership, Management, and Circulation
(All Periodicals Publications Except Requestor Publications)

1. Publication Title Medical Clinics of North America	**2. Publication Number** 3 3 7 – 3 4 0	**3. Filing Date** 9/14/14
4. Issue Frequency Jan, Mar, May, Jul, Sep, Nov	**5. Number of Issues Published Annually** 4	**6. Annual Subscription Price** $255.00

7. Complete Mailing Address of Known Office of Publication (*Not printer*) (*Street, city, county, state, and ZIP+4®*)

Elsevier Inc.
360 Park Avenue South
New York, NY 10010-1710

Contact Person
Stephen R. Bushing

Telephone (*Include area code*)
215-239-3688

8. Complete Mailing Address of Headquarters or General Business Office of Publisher (*Not printer*)

Elsevier Inc., 360 Park Avenue South, New York, NY 10010-1710

9. Full Names and Complete Mailing Addresses of Publisher, Editor, and Managing Editor (*Do not leave blank*)

Publisher (*Name and complete mailing address*)

Linda Belfus, Elsevier Inc., 1600 John F. Kennedy Blvd., Suite 1800, Philadelphia, PA 19103-2899

Editor (*Name and complete mailing address*)

Jessica McCool, Elsevier Inc., 1600 John F. Kennedy Blvd., Suite 1800, Philadelphia, PA 19103-2899

Managing Editor (*Name and complete mailing address*)

Adrianne Brigido, Elsevier Inc., 1600 John F. Kennedy Blvd., Suite 1800, Philadelphia, PA 19103-2899

10. Owner (*Do not leave blank. If the publication is owned by a corporation, give the name and address of the corporation immediately followed by the names and addresses of all stockholders owning or holding 1 percent or more of the total amount of stock. If not owned by a corporation, give the names and addresses of the individual owners. If owned by a partnership or other unincorporated firm, give its name and address as well as those of each individual owner. If the publication is published by a nonprofit organization, give its name and address.*)

Full Name	Complete Mailing Address
Wholly owned subsidiary of	1600 John F. Kennedy Blvd, Ste. 1800
Reed/Elsevier, US holdings	Philadelphia, PA 19103-2899

11. Known Bondholders, Mortgagees, and Other Security Holders Owning or Holding 1 Percent or More of Total Amount of Bonds, Mortgages, or Other Securities. If none, check box → None

Full Name	Complete Mailing Address
N/A	

12. Tax Status (*For completion by nonprofit organizations authorized to mail at nonprofit rates*) (*Check one*)
The purpose, function, and nonprofit status of this organization and the exempt status for federal income tax purposes:
☐ Has Not Changed During Preceding 12 Months
☐ Has Changed During Preceding 12 Months (*Publisher must submit explanation of change with this statement*)

PS Form 3526, August 2012 (Page 1 of 3 (Instructions Page 3)) PSN 7530-01-000-9931 **PRIVACY NOTICE:** See our Privacy policy in www.usps.com

---

13. Publication Title Medical Clinics of North America		**14. Issue Date for Circulation Data Below** September 2014

15. Extent and Nature of Circulation		**Average No. Copies Each Issue During Preceding 12 Months**	**No. Copies of Single Issue Published Nearest to Filing Date**
a. Total Number of Copies (*Net press run*)		1,868	1,901
b. Paid Circulation (By Mail and Outside the Mail)	(1) Mailed Outside-County Paid Subscriptions Stated on PS Form 3541. (*Include paid distribution above nominal rate, advertiser's proof copies, and exchange copies*)	956	954
	(2) Mailed In-County Paid Subscriptions Stated on PS Form 3541 (*Include paid distribution above nominal rate, advertiser's proof copies, and exchange copies*)		
	(3) Paid Distribution Outside the Mails Including Sales Through Dealers and Carriers, Street Vendors, Counter Sales, and Other Paid Distribution Outside USPS®	363	454
	(4) Paid Distribution by Other Classes Mailed Through the USPS (e.g. First-Class Mail®)		
c. Total Paid Distribution (*Sum of 15b (1), (2), (3), and (4)*)	▶	1,319	1,408
d. Free or Nominal Rate Distribution (By Mail and Outside the Mail)	(1) Free or Nominal Rate Outside-County Copies Included on PS Form 3541	141	148
	(2) Free or Nominal Rate In-County Copies Included on PS Form 3541		
	(3) Free or Nominal Rate Copies Mailed at Other Classes Through the USPS (e.g. First-Class Mail)		
	(4) Free or Nominal Rate Distribution Outside the Mail (Carriers or other means)		
e. Total Free or Nominal Rate Distribution (Sum of 15d (1), (2), (3) and (4))	▶	141	148
f. Total Distribution (Sum of 15c and 15e)	▶	1,460	1,556
g. Copies not Distributed (See instructions to publishers #4 (page #3))	▶	408	345
h. Total (Sum of 15f and g)	▶	1,868	1,901
i. Percent Paid (15c divided by 15f times 100)	▶	90.34%	90.49%

16. Total circulation includes electronic copies. Report circulation on PS Form 3526-X worksheet.

17. Publication of Statement of Ownership
If the publication is a general publication, publication of this statement is required. Will be printed in the November 2014 issue of this publication.

18. Signature and Title of Editor, Publisher, Business Manager, or Owner

Stephen R. Bushing — Inventory Distribution Coordinator

Date: September 14, 2014

I certify that all information furnished on this form is true and complete. I understand that anyone who furnishes false or misleading information on this form or who omits material or information requested on the form may be subject to criminal sanctions (including fines and imprisonment) and/or civil sanctions (including civil penalties).

PS Form 3526, August 2012 (Page 2 of 3)